Anti-Obesity Drug Discovery and Development

(Volume 3)

Edited By

Atta-ur-Rahman, *FRS*
Honorary Life Fellow, Kings College, University of Cambridge,
Cambridge, UK

&

M. Iqbal Choudhary
H.E.J. Research Institute of Chemistry, International Center for Chemical
and Biological Sciences, University of Karachi, Karachi, Pakistan

Anti-Obesity Drug Discovery and Development

Volume # 3

Editors: Prof. Atta-ur-Rahman and Dr. M. Iqbal Choudhary

eISSN (Online): 2210-2698

ISSN (Print): 2467-9615

eISBN (Online): 978-1-68108-187-8

ISBN (Print): 978-1-68108-188-5

©2017, Bentham eBooks imprint.

Published by Bentham Science Publishers – Sharjah, UAE. All Rights Reserved.

First published in 2017.

BENTHAM SCIENCE PUBLISHERS LTD.
End User License Agreement (for non-institutional, personal use)

This is an agreement between you and Bentham Science Publishers Ltd. Please read this License Agreement carefully before using the ebook/echapter/ejournal (**"Work"**). Your use of the Work constitutes your agreement to the terms and conditions set forth in this License Agreement. If you do not agree to these terms and conditions then you should not use the Work.

Bentham Science Publishers agrees to grant you a non-exclusive, non-transferable limited license to use the Work subject to and in accordance with the following terms and conditions. This License Agreement is for non-library, personal use only. For a library / institutional / multi user license in respect of the Work, please contact: permission@benthamscience.org.

Usage Rules:

1. All rights reserved: The Work is the subject of copyright and Bentham Science Publishers either owns the Work (and the copyright in it) or is licensed to distribute the Work. You shall not copy, reproduce, modify, remove, delete, augment, add to, publish, transmit, sell, resell, create derivative works from, or in any way exploit the Work or make the Work available for others to do any of the same, in any form or by any means, in whole or in part, in each case without the prior written permission of Bentham Science Publishers, unless stated otherwise in this License Agreement.
2. You may download a copy of the Work on one occasion to one personal computer (including tablet, laptop, desktop, or other such devices). You may make one back-up copy of the Work to avoid losing it. The following DRM (Digital Rights Management) policy may also be applicable to the Work at Bentham Science Publishers' election, acting in its sole discretion:

- 25 'copy' commands can be executed every 7 days in respect of the Work. The text selected for copying cannot extend to more than a single page. Each time a text 'copy' command is executed, irrespective of whether the text selection is made from within one page or from separate pages, it will be considered as a separate / individual 'copy' command.
- 25 pages only from the Work can be printed every 7 days.

3. The unauthorised use or distribution of copyrighted or other proprietary content is illegal and could subject you to liability for substantial money damages. You will be liable for any damage resulting from your misuse of the Work or any violation of this License Agreement, including any infringement by you of copyrights or proprietary rights.

Disclaimer:

Bentham Science Publishers does not guarantee that the information in the Work is error-free, or warrant that it will meet your requirements or that access to the Work will be uninterrupted or error-free. The Work is provided "as is" without warranty of any kind, either express or implied or statutory, including, without limitation, implied warranties of merchantability and fitness for a particular purpose. The entire risk as to the results and performance of the Work is assumed by you. No responsibility is assumed by Bentham Science Publishers, its staff, editors and/or authors for any injury and/or damage to persons or property as a matter of products liability, negligence or otherwise, or from any use or operation of any methods, products instruction, advertisements or ideas contained in the Work.

Limitation of Liability:

In no event will Bentham Science Publishers, its staff, editors and/or authors, be liable for any damages, including, without limitation, special, incidental and/or consequential damages and/or damages for lost data and/or profits arising out of (whether directly or indirectly) the use or inability to use the Work. The entire liability of Bentham Science Publishers shall be limited to the amount actually paid by you for the Work.

General:

1. Any dispute or claim arising out of or in connection with this License Agreement or the Work (including non-contractual disputes or claims) will be governed by and construed in accordance with the laws of the U.A.E. as applied in the Emirate of Dubai. Each party agrees that the courts of the Emirate of Dubai shall have exclusive jurisdiction to settle any dispute or claim arising out of or in connection with this License Agreement or the Work (including non-contractual disputes or claims).
2. Your rights under this License Agreement will automatically terminate without notice and without the need for a court order if at any point you breach any terms of this License Agreement. In no event will any delay or failure by Bentham Science Publishers in enforcing your compliance with this License Agreement constitute a waiver of any of its rights.
3. You acknowledge that you have read this License Agreement, and agree to be bound by its terms and conditions. To the extent that any other terms and conditions presented on any website of Bentham Science Publishers conflict with, or are inconsistent with, the terms and conditions set out in this License Agreement, you acknowledge that the terms and conditions set out in this License Agreement shall prevail.

Bentham Science Publishers Ltd.
Executive Suite Y - 2
PO Box 7917, Saif Zone
Sharjah, U.A.E.
Email: subscriptions@benthamscience.org

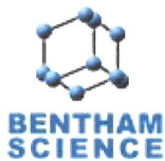

CONTENTS

PREFACE	i
LIST OF CONTRIBUTORS	iii
CHAPTER 1 CURRENT STATUS OF MEDICAL THERAPY AND NEW TARGETS FOR ANTI-OBESITY DRUG DEVELOPMENT	3
Chihiro Okuma, Yukihito Ishii and *Takeshi Ohta*	
INTRODUCTION	3
Approved Drugs	4
Phentermine	5
Mazindol	7
Fenfluramine/Dexfenfluramine	9
Orlistat	10
Shibutramine	12
Rimonabant	14
Qsymia	16
BELVIQ (Lorcaserin)	17
Contrave	19
New Drug Targets (Table 3)	20
Late Phase Clinical Development	21
Early Phase Clinical Stage Development or Pre-Clinical Development Stage Late Phase Clinical Development	27
Future Prospects	39
Obesity Animal Models	40
ob/ob Mouse	41
db/db Mouse	41
KK-Ay Mouse	41
TSOD Mouse	42
SDT fatty Rat	42
ZF Rat	42
ZDF Rat	43
cp/cp Rat	43
WBN/Kob fatty Rat	43
DIO Models	44
CONFLICT OF INTEREST	46
ACKNOWLEDGEMENTS	46
REFERENCES	46
CHAPTER 2 UNRAVELLING POTENTIAL ANOREXIGEN EFFECTS OF NESFATIN-1: HOW HOMEOSTATIC MECHANISMS HELP BALANCE EXCESS CALORIES	65
Carmine Finelli	
INTRODUCTION	65
Nesfatin-1/NUCB-2 and Anorexigenic Effect	67
The Oxytocin Pathway in Nesfatin-1's Inhibitory Effect on Food Intake	67
Nesfatin-1 and CRF	68
Nesfatin-1 and Anti-Obesity Treatment	69
Nesfatin-1 and Food Behaviour Control	70
Nesfatin-1 and Signaling Pathway	71
Nesfatin-1 and Eating Disorders	72
CONCLUSIVE REMARKS	73
CONFLICT OF INTEREST	74
ACKNOWLEDGEMENTS	74
ABBREVIATIONS	74
REFERENCES	75
CHAPTER 3 PROTEOMICS IN THE CHARACTERIZATION OF NEW TARGET THERAPIES IN PEDIATRIC OBESITY TREATMENT	80
Gillian E. Walker, Marilisa De Feudis, Marta Roccio, Gianni Bona and *Flavia Prodam*	
INTRODUCTION	80

	CHILDHOOD OBESITY: PATHOLOGICAL BASIS	83
	Genetic Considerations for Childhood Obesity	84
	Energy Homeostasis Dysregulation	85
	Pathophysiology of Adipose Tissue	87
	PROTEOMICS	89
	Gel Based Methods	90
	Non Gel Based Methods: Mass Spectrometry (MS)	92
	Chips	94
	Challenges	95
	PROTEOMIC STUDIES OF ADIPOSE TISSUE	96
	WAT Depots	96
	WAT Secretome	101
	BAT	103
	Stromal-Vascular Fraction (SVF)	106
	PROTEOMIC STUDIES IN ADIPOCYTES: STEM CELLS AND CELL LINES	107
	Adipogenesis: Adipo-proteomics	108
	Murine 3T3-L1 Preadipocytes	108
	Adipocyte-Derived Stem Cells (ASCs)	111
	Adipocyte Secretome	111
	Post-Translational Modifications (PTMs)	113
	PROTEOMIC PROFILING: TISSUES AND CIRCULATION	114
	Fetal Programming: Tissue-Specific Biomarkers	115
	Circulating Biomarkers	116
	Urine Biomarkers	119
	OUTLOOKS	119
	CONFLICT OF INTEREST	121
	ACKNOWLEDGEMENTS	121
	ABBREVIATIONS	121
	REFERENCES	122

CHAPTER 4 RELATIONSHIP BETWEEN HORMONAL MILIEU AND OXIDATIVE STRESS IN CHILDHOOD OBESITY: A PHYSIOPATHOLOGICAL BASIS FOR ANTIOXIDANT TREATMENT AND PREVENTION OF CARDIOVASCULAR RISK 149

Antonio Mancini, Francesco Leo, Chantal Di Segni, Sebastiano Raimondo and *Aurora Natalia Rossodivita*

	INTRODUCTION	150
	OBESITY AND OXIDATIVE STRESS	152
	Hormones and Inflammatory Molecules Produced by or Related to Adipose Tissue	154
	Oxidative Stress in Childhood Obesity	160
	HORMONAL REGULATION OF ANTIOXIDANT SYSTEMS AND THEIR DERANGEMENT IN CHILDHOOD OBESITY	162
	Growth Hormone (GH)	162
	Thyroid	165
	Adrenal Glands	168
	Gonads	174
	Adipose tissue (Leptin and Kisspeptin)	179
	ANTIOXIDANT-ENRICHED DIET AS A TREATMENT FOR OBESITY	180
	CONCLUSION	183
	CONFLICT OF INTEREST	184
	ACKNOWLEDGEMENTS	184
	REFERENCES	184

CHAPTER 5 THE ROLE OF GUT MICROFLORA IN OBESITY - DOES THE DATA PROVIDE AN OPTION FOR INTERVENTION? 204

Parth J. Parekh, Edward C. Oldfield, IV, Amrit Lamba and *David A. Johnson*

	INTRODUCTION	204
	OBESITY AND THE MICROFLORA: A BRIEF OVERVIEW	205
	DATA AND OPTIONS FOR INTERVENTION	209
	Antibiotics	210
	Probiotics	213

  Prebiotics 216
  Synbiotics 218
  The Role of Fecal Transplant 218
CONCLUSION 219
CONFLICT OF INTEREST 219
ACKNOWLEDGEMENTS 220
REFERENCES 220

SUBJECT INDEX 228

PREFACE

An epidemic of obesity is among the most important global healthcare challenges of the 21st century, causing considerable morbidity and mortality in a large segment of human population. Obesity has been identified as the largest preventable cause of numerous diseases. Obese and overweight population are at risk for a number of conditions, including high cholesterol levels, high blood pressure, heart diseases, diabetes, bone problems, skin diseases, neurological and psychological disorders, and increased chances of various malignancies. At individual level, obesity adversely effects the state of health and the quality of life, whereas at national level, it is a significant burden on the current healthcare systems. Unfortunately existing anti-obesity drugs are associated with numerous side effects, and are only prescribed when the benefits of treatment outweigh their risks.

The regulation of body weight is a complex process which involves cascades of mechanisms, including a variety of neuropeptides and transmitters in the brain, and endocrine and metabolic signalling molecules. Many of these processes are only superficially understood and extensive research is being conducted to decipher the complex biomolecular pathways behind the obesity syndrome. Understanding these inherent pathways, as well as the role of other factors, such as dietary habits, physical activities, gut microflora, *etc.* is critically important in devising successful strategies to combat obesity epidemics, including the discovery and development of improved treatments.

The 3rd volume of the book series entitled "*Anti-Obesity Drug Discovery and Development*" presents the most exciting recent developments in the field of obesity and its treatment. This book comprises five authoritative reviews ranging from identification of new drug targets to novel pharmacological and non-pharmacological interventions.

The first chapter by Ohta *et al.* presents a comprehensive account of recent literature on various treatment options available for obesity. Primary treatment of obesity disorder involves dietary restrictions, and exercise. However, in many cases, pharmacotherapy is imperative. The authors have categorised anti-obesity drugs into three classes, *i.e.* appetite suppressors, agents which inhibit nutritional absorptions, and drugs which accelerate energy expenditures. Various molecular targets in all three categories have been described, with merits and demerits of drugs developed against them.

Nesfatin-1 is a peptide which has attracted considerable attention as a possible antibody treatment of obesity. Nesfatin-1 is secreted by peripheral tissues, central and peripheral nervous system and it can pass the blood-brain barrier. It is involved in the regulation of energy homeostasis related with food regulation and water intake. It suppresses the urge for food independently from the leptin pathway and increases insulin secretion of the pancreatic beta islet cells. The use of Nesfatin-1 for the treatment of obesity has been widely investigated. Finelli has contributed a comprehensive review in chapter 2 on the potential of Nesfatin-1 as a new treatment for obesity and related disorders, its effects on other physiological parameters and the proposed mechanisms of action.

In chapter 3, Walker *et al.* focus on obesity in children, and identification of appropriate drug targets. Paediatric obesity is a growing menace with increasing prevalence globally. Overweight and obese children are at high risk of becoming overweight adolescents and adults, developing chronic diseases, such as heart disease and diabetes later in life. They are also more prone to develop stress, sadness, and low self-esteem. Adipose tissues (AT) play an important role in obesity. AT dysfunction leads to chronic inflammation, weight homeostasis, and insulin resistance. Understanding AT dysfunction at receptors and secondary messenger pathways is critically important in understanding the unique features of paediatric obesity at molecular levels. The authors have reviewed recent advances in the field of proteomics technologies with reference to their use in identifying key components of adipose proteome. This helps in understanding the pathogenesis of adipose tissue dysfunction in obesity

Mancini *et al*. have contributed a chapter on vascular, histopathological and metabolic changes that occur in obese children, which in many cases lead to metabolic syndrome, such as insulin resistance, type 2 diabetes, dyslipidemia, endothelial dysfunctions and cardiovascular disorders. The authors have focussed on the role of neuroendocrine peptides and cytokines in chronic inflammation and oxidative stress (OS). These mediators of chronic inflammation and OS are produced in adipose tissues, and are thus, directly responsible for endothelial dysfunction and insulin resistance. An extensive commentary on the role of oxidative stress in the onset of various obesity related diseases, such as atherogenesis and diabetes, is presented. Based on this, the authors have moved on to discuss the strategies to lower the chronic inflammation and oxidative stress in childhood obesity in order to prevent metabolic syndrome.

Gut microflora are perceived to play an important role in the prevention of various diseases, including obesity. Comparative studies have been conducted on bacterial flora of obese and lean individuals, and substantial differences were recorded. The disequilibrium in the composition of microorganisms that inhabit the human body can cause various diseases. High-throughput sequencing techniques and new tools used in bioinformatics have indicated strong relationships between the gut microbiota, and host's physiology. Disruption of the ecological equilibrium in the gut is called dysbiosis. Diet is a strong determinant of gut microbial balance. In chapter 5, Johnson *et al*. present a comprehensive discussion on state-of-the-art understanding of the role of intestinal dysbiosis in the on-set of obesity disorder. They reviewed the most recent literature on the restoration of microflora in gut as a novel therapeutic option against the obesity epidemics. Strategies for the manipulation of intestinal microflora, such as antibiotic therapy against xenobiotic flora, supplementation of normal flora through probiotics and prebiotics and symbiotics (combination of probiotics and prebiotics), fecal microbiota transplant, *etc*. have been discussed. The role of intestinal microflora in metabolic programming is also extensively discussed.

In brief, the above cited reviews contributed by leading researchers in the field make this volume an interesting and useful reading for scientists and graduate students. We wish to express our felicitation and gratitude to all the authors for their excellent and scholarly contributions for the 3rd volume of this reputed series. We also greatly appreciate the efforts of the entire team of Bentham Science Publishers for efficient processing and timely management of the publication. The efforts of Ms. Faryal Sami (Assistant Manager Publications), Mr. Shehzad Naqvi (Senior Manager Publications) and the leadership of Mr. Mahmood Alam (Director Publications) are specially praiseworthy. We hope that like the previous volumes of this internationally recognized book series, the current compilation will also receive a wide readership and appreciation.

Prof. Dr. Atta-ur-Rahman *FRS*
Honorary Life Fellow
Kings College
University of Cambridge
Cambridge
UK

Prof. Dr. M. Iqbal Choudhary
H.E.J. Research Institute of Chemistry
International Center for Chemical
and Biological Sciences, University of Karachi
Karachi
Pakistan

List of Contributors

Antonio Mancini	Departments of Medical Sciences and Pediatrics, Catholic University of the Sacred Heart, Rome, Italy
Aurora Natalia Rossodivita	Departments of Medical Sciences and Pediatrics, Catholic University of the Sacred Heart, Rome, Italy
Amrit Lamba	Department of Internal Medicine, Tulane University, New Orleans, USA
Chantal Di Segni	Departments of Medical Sciences and Pediatrics, Catholic University of the Sacred Heart, Rome, Italy
Carmine Finelli	Department of Emergency and Internal Medicine, S. Maria della Pietà Nola's Hospital, *Via* della Repubblica 1, 80035 Nola (Na), Italy
Chihiro Okuma	Central Pharmaceutical Research Institute, Japan Tobacco Inc., Takatsuki, Japan
David A. Johnson	Department of Internal Medicine, Division of Gastroenterology and Hepatology, Eastern Virginia Medical School, Norfolk, USA
Edward C. Oldfield	Department of Internal Medicine, Eastern Virginia Medical School, Norfolk, USA
Francesco Leo	Departments of Medical Sciences and Pediatrics, Catholic University of the Sacred Heart, Rome, Italy
Flavia Prodam	Division of Pediatrics, Department of Health Sciences, Università Del Piemonte Orientale, Novara, Italy
Gianni Bona	Division of Pediatrics, Department of Health Sciences, Università Del Piemonte Orientale, Novara, Italy
Gillian E. Walker	Laboratory of Clinical Pediatrics, Department of Health Sciences, Università del Piemonte Orientale, *Via* Solaroli, Italy
Marilisa De Feudis	Laboratory of Clinical Pediatrics, Department of Health Sciences, Università del Piemonte Orientale, *Via* Solaroli, Italy
Marta Roccio	Laboratory of Clinical Pediatrics, Department of Health Sciences, Università del Piemonte Orientale, *Via* Solaroli, Italy
Parth J. Parekh	Department of Internal Medicine, Division of Gastroenterology and Hepatology, Tulane University, New Orleans, USA
Sebastiano Raimondo	Departments of Medical Sciences and Pediatrics, Catholic University of the Sacred Heart, Rome, Italy
Takeshi Ohta	Central Pharmaceutical Research Institute, Japan Tobacco Inc., Takatsuki, Japan
Yukihito Ishii	Central Pharmaceutical Research Institute, Japan Tobacco Inc., Takatsuki, Japan

Anti-Obesity Drug Discovery and Development

CHAPTER 1

Current Status of Medical Therapy and New Targets for Anti-Obesity Drug Development

Chihiro Okuma, Yukihito Ishii and Takeshi Ohta[*]

Central Pharmaceutical Research Institute, Japan Tobacco Inc., Takatsuki, 569-1125 Osaka, Japan

Abstract: Obesity is considered to be caused by an imbalance in individual energy. The basic therapies for obesity are appropriate dietary restriction for the purpose of decreasing energy intake and effective exercise for the purpose of promoting energy expenditure. At present, drug therapies for obesity are secondary treatments. Therapeutic strategies using pharmacotherapy are divided into the following three types: 1) suppressing appetite, 2) inhibiting nutritional absorption, and 3) accelerating energy expenditure. Mazindol and Phentermine have long been recognized as drugs for increasing satiety, and Orlistat and Cetilistat have been developed as drugs that inhibit lipid absorption from the intestine. Moreover, ß3 agonists have been developed to accelerate energy combustion. In this chapter, we first introduce drugs that are on the market, after which drugs that are in clinical or preclinical stages of development will be introduced. Furthermore, obese animal models that are now available will be introduced in the last section.

Keywords: Animal model, Anti-obesity drug, DGAT inhibitor, MGAT inhibitor, MTP inhibitor, Obesity.

INTRODUCTION

The number of obese patients is rapidly increasing all over the world due to changes in lifestyle, such as habits of consuming high calorie diets and sedentary lifestyles. Obesity and obesity-related diseases, such as diabetes mellitus, dyslipidemia, and hypertension, deteriorate the quality of life (QOL) of patients and result in high medical expenses [1 - 3].

Energy homeostasis in the body is maintained by a balance between energy intake and energy expenditure. When the former exceeds the latter, overt energy is accumulated in adipose tissues, resulting in obesity. Regulating food intake and

---

[*] **Corresponding author Takeshi Ohta:** Central Pharmaceutical Research Institute, Japan Tobacco Inc., Takatsuki, 569-1125 Osaka, Japan; Tel: +81-72-681-9700; Fax: +81-72-681-9722; takeshi.ota@jt.com

energy expenditure and integrating this balance is important in preventing obesity [4, 5]. Lifestyle modifications, such as diet therapy and exercise, as well as medications, chiefly occupy the treatments for obesity and related diseases; however, bariatric surgery is sometimes performed on patients with overt obesity (ex. Body mass index (BMI) over 35) [6 - 8].

Basically, medical therapy is a pivotal step in reducing excess fat accumulation. To reduce excess fat accumulation and excess body weight, several anti-obesity drugs that reduce appetite or lipid absorption in the intestine have been developed. Mazindol is now available only in Japan [9]. In the 1990s, another type of anti-obesity drug, Orlistat, was approved in the U.S. and Europe. Orlistat inhibits lipid absorption in the intestine and is now also available [10, 11]. Thereafter, Sibutramine and Rimonabant were developed; however, both drugs were withdrawn because of adverse effects [12]. Drug combinations, including Qsymia and Contrave, have been developed [13] and serotonin (5HT2c)-R agonist Lorcaserin was approved by the FDA in 2012 [14].

In addition, a variety of drugs with various mechanisms, such as microsomal triglyceride transfer protein (MTP) inhibitors, diacylglycerol acyltransferase 1 (DGAT1) inhibitors, monoacylglycerol acyltransferase (MGAT) inhibitors, and protein tyrosine phosphatase 1B (PTP1B) inhibitors, have been investigated in clinical and basic research stages of development [15 - 20]. Several anti-obesity drugs were withdrawn because of adverse effects; however, a tremendous amount of research to develop novel anti-obesity drugs is still ongoing all over the world. In this chapter, we focus on the effects of these drugs and will introduce preclinical and clinical data.

Approved Drugs

Anti-obesity drugs launched in the past years are shown in Table **1**. Ten drugs have been launched to date, but the six drugs were withdrawn because of the severe side effects. The drug properties, including efficacy and adverse events, are shown in Table **2**. Efficacy indexed by body weight change was approximately 5-10 kg decrease in body weight. Mazindol showed pronounced clinical efficacy, -14.2 kg, whereas the decrease in BELVIQ, - 5.8 kg, was mild as compared with the other drugs. Adverse events related to the central nervous system, such as nervousness, anxiety, and dizziness, were observed as responses to TAAR1 agonists, monoamine-reuptake inhibitors, and serotonin receptor agonists. Moreover, digestive symptom, such as, oily stool, faecal urgency, and oily spotting was observed in orlistat. Detailed features of each anti-obesity drug are included in Table **2**.

Table 1. Anti-obesity drugs launched in the past years.

Drug	Mechanism of action	History in USA	History in EU
Phentermine	Trace amine-associated receptor 1 (TAAR1) agonist	1959:Approval	1999:Withdrawn
Mazindol	Monoamine-reuptake inhibitor	1973:Approval Withdrawn	Withdrawn
Fenfluramine	Serotonin receptor (5-HT$_{2B}$) agonist	1973:Approval 1997:Withdrawn	1997:Withdrawn
Dexfenfluramine	Serotonin receptor (5-HT$_{2B}$) agonist	1996:Approval 1997:Withdrawn	1997:Withdrawn
Orlistat	Lipase inhibitor	1999:Approval	1998:Approval
Sibutramine	Monoamine-reuptake inhibitor	1997:Approval	2001:Approval 2010:Withdrawn
Rimonabant	Cannabinoid receptor antagonist	Disapproval	2006:Approval 2008:Withdrawn
Qsymia (Qnexa)	Phentermine/topiramate	2012:Approval	Disapproval
BELVIQ (lorcaserin)	Serotonin receptor (5-HT$_{2C}$) agonist	2012:Approval	Disapproval
Contrave	Bupropion/naltrexone	2014:Approval	2015:Approval

Phentermine

Phentermine is a sympathomimetic amine (Fig. **1A**) and anorectic agent that is used for short-term therapy of obesity (less than 12 weeks) in combination with behavioral modification, caloric restriction and exercise. In 1959, phentermine received approval from the FDA as an appetite-suppressing drug, after which a hydrochloride form of the drug became available in the early 1970s. In 1999, phentermine was removed from the market in the EU; however, the drug is also currently sold as a generic in the U.S., and is still available in most countries, including the U.S [21, 22].

Table 2. Clinical efficacy and adverse events in anti-obesity drugs.

Drug	Body weight change (Administration period)	Adverse events
Phentermine	- 11.7 kg (24 weeks)	Insomia, Irritability, Agitation, Nervousness, Anxiety
Mazindol	- 14.2 kg (64 weeks)	Dry mouth, Constipation, Stomach discomfort, Nausea, Sleep disturbance, Dizziness

(Table 2) contd.....

Drug	Body weight change (Administration period)	Adverse events
Fenfluramine	- 8.7 kg (52 weeks)	Asthenia, Euphonia, Edema
Dexfenfluramine	- 9.8 kg (52 weeks)	Asthenia, Drowsiness, Polyuria, Nocturia, Dry mouth, Thirst
Orlistat	- 10.3 kg (52 weeks)	Oily stool, Faecal urgency, Oily spotting
Sibutramine	- 8.0 kg (52 weeks)	Insomnia, Nausea, Dry mouth, Constipation.
Rimonabant	- 12.2 kg (52 weeks)	Depression, Nausea, Dizziness, Influenza, Anxiety, Diarrhea, Insomnia
Qsymia (Qnexa)	-10.2 kg (56 weeks)	Dry mouth, Paraesthesia, Constipation, Dizziness
BELVIQ (lorcaserin)	- 5.8 kg (56 weeks)	Headache, Dizziness, Nausea
Contrave	- 8.0 kg (56 weeks)	Nausea, Headache, Constipation, Dizziness, Dry mouth

Phentermine, which is a trace amine-associated receptor 1 (TAAR1) agonist, is a structural analogue of amphetamine (Fig. **1B**), and demonstrates some similarities in terms of mechanisms of action, such as suppressing appetite, but also demonstrates several of the central nervous system effects of amphetamine [23]. Amphetamine stimulates neurons to release and sustain the levels of neurotransmitters known as catecholamines, such as norepinephrine, serotonin, and dopamine. The elevation of catecholamines inhibits hunger signals and appetite. The pharmacological effects of phentermine in increasing weight loss are mediated by anorectic activity that is the result of catecholamine release from the appetite center of the brain. Phentermine is also considered to inhibit the reuptake of catecholamines through the inhibition or reversal of reuptake transporters [24, 25]. Phentermine may inhibit monoamine oxidase (MAO) enzymes, leaving more neurotransmitters available at the synapse. Phentermine works on the hypothalamus portion of the brain to stimulate adrenal glands to release norepinephrine. Moreover, phentermine works outside the brain to release epinephrine (adrenaline), causing fat cells to promote lipolysis. However, the principal basis of efficacy is hunger reduction. Phentermine is considered to indirectly increase the levels of leptin that signal satiety in the brain through catecholamine elevation. The elevation of catecholamine levels is also considered partially responsible for halting another chemical messenger, neuropeptide Y, which initiates eating, decreases energy expenditure and increases fat storage.

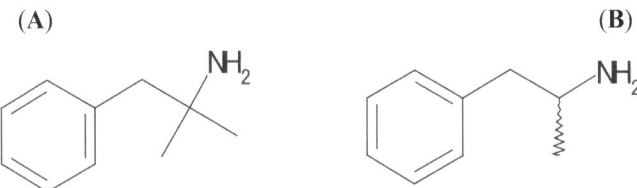

Fig. (1). Chemical structures of phentermine, 2-metyl-1-phenylpropan-2-amine (**A**) and amphetamine, (±)-1-phenylpropan-2-amine (**B**).

A double-blind clinical study, wherein 36 weeks of continuous and intermittent treatment with phentermine and placebo were evaluated, was reportedly conducted in 108 obese patients [26]. In this study, the weight loss effect reached a plateau after about 24 weeks of treatment. In patients who completed the study, weight loss in the intermittent phentermine group was as effective as that in the continuous group and was more effective than that in the placebo group. Phentermine treatment resulted in the reduction of appetite; however, the effectiveness in individual patients varied and was not clearly related to the degree of obesity, age, or dietary habits, thereby making a determination on the duration of appetite-reducing effects of phentermine difficult. In patients treated intermittently or continuously with the drug, a 56% decrease in weight during the last 16 weeks of treatment compared with 28% in the placebo group was observed. In all groups, weight loss diminished with duration of treatment. Adverse events related to central nervous system-stimulating effects, such as insomnia, irritability, agitation, nervousness, and anxiety, were observed.

Mazindol

Mazindol is also a sympathomimetic amine (Fig. **2**), which is similar to an amphetamine, and is used in short-term treatment (a few weeks) of overt obesity in combination with behavioral modification, caloric restriction and exercise in patients with a body mass index (BMI) that is 30 kg/m^2 or higher, or BMI that is 27 kg/m^2 or higher in the presence of risk factors, such as diabetes, hyperlipidemia and hypertension [27]. Mazindol reportedly suppresses food intake by stimulating beta-adrenergic receptors, inhibiting the feeding center and stimulating the satiety center in the hypothalamus. The drug is not currently available for the treatment of obesity in the EU and U.S., and only the use in treatment of Duchenne muscular dystrophy is approved in the U.S. This drug is also now available in Japan [25, 28].

In basic research studies, mazindol suppressed the firing rate of glucose-sensitive neurons in the lateral hypothalamus, suggesting that the drug directly suppresses a feeding center in the hypothalamus [29]. The direct inhibitory activity of hypothalamic leads to the inhibition of gastric acid release, which may contribute to the suppression of appetite [30]. Moreover, the drug treatment reportedly increased locomotor activity, which may contribute to an increase in energy expenditure [31]. Furthermore, the treatment attenuated hypersecretion of insulin in ventromedial-hypothalamic-lesioned (VMH) obese rats, suggesting that this phenomenon was induced by decreases in body weight due to anorectic effects and/or inhibition of vagal hyperactivity [32, 33]. Mazindol treatment also reduced glucose absorption in the small intestine of rats, and anti-obesity effects were expected based on the regulation of calorie intake (food intake) [34, 35]. The weight loss effects of mazindol were investigated in two types of obesity: VMH and diet-induced obesity (DIO) in rats [36]. Results demonstrated that weight loss was significantly higher in VMH obesity than in DIO obesity. This result suggests that mazindol is more effective in central nervous system-induced obesity than other types of obesity.

Fig. (2). Chemical structure of mazindol, (±)-5-(4-chlorophenyl)-3,5-dihydro-2H-imidazo[2.1-a]isoindol-5-ol

As mentioned above, mazindol is now only available in Japan, and data from clinical studies conducted in Japan was described as follows. In an open-label clinical study, mazindol was administered according to the flexible schedule (0.5–3 mg/day, every 2 or 4 weeks) for 14 weeks in simple or symptomatic obese patients [36]. Results demonstrated that patients treated with mazindol lost 4.6 kg of body weight and 9.2% of relative excess weight in 14 weeks. In female patients, mazindol treatment resulted in decreases of skinfold thickness. Appetite was suppressed by mazindol in 71.3% of the patients and this rate was similar to the percent that showed body weight loss (79.8%). Appetite suppression continued until the end of the study; however, the suppression rate decreased in the follow-up period for 4 weeks. In the double-blind study, in which mazindol was given for 12 weeks, treatment with the drug resulted in significant reductions in body weight and relative body weight, and skinfold thickness reductions. Side effects, such as dry mouth, constipation, stomach discomfort, nausea, sleep disturbance and dizziness, were observed; however, most were transient or mild.

Fenfluramine/Dexfenfluramine

Fenfluramine, similar to phentermine or mazindol, is a structural analogue of amphetamine (Fig. **3**) and was approved in the U.S. in 1973. Fenfluramine is a serotonergic anorectic drug, and reduces appetite by increasing serotonin levels in the brain. This compound is the racemic mixture of two enantiomers, dextrofenfluramine (D-fenfluramine) and levofenfluramine (L-fenfluramine). Since D-fenfluramine showed more potential for efficacy than that of L-fenfluramine, D-fenfluramine was approved as dexfenfluramine in 1996 [37, 38]. However, the drugs were withdrawn from the market in the U.S. in 1997 after reports of heart valve disease, and pulmonary hypertension, including a condition known as cardiac fibrosis [39, 40]. After the withdrawal of the drugs in the U.S., the drugs were also withdrawn from other countries around the world.

Fig. (3). Chemical structure of fenfluramine, (±)-N-ethyl-1-[3-(trifluoromethyl)phenyl]propan-2-amine.

Fenfluramine binds to the serotonin reuptake pump, and inhibits serotonin uptake and increases in serotonin levels. The elevation of serotonin leads to greater serotonin receptor activation, which in turn leads to the enhancement of serotonergic transmission in the center of feeding behavior located in the hypothalamus [41, 42]. The reason for the adverse effect of heart disease was also considered. The valvular abnormality seen with fenfluramine was the thickening of leaflet and chordae tendineae. The pathological findings in the heart are considered to involve heart valve serotonin receptors that regulate growth. Since fenfluramine stimulates serotonin receptors, this may lead to valvular abnormalities in patients using fenfluramine [43, 44].

In preclinical studies, the chronic administration of fenfluramine induced sustained body weight loss with normal food intake [45]. Unlike other appetite inhibitory drugs, fenfluramine suppresses rather than increases locomotor activity in animals. Another possible explanation for the sustained weight loss could be the disruption in intestinal absorption of nutrients. The chronic administration of dexfenfluramine, however, has no effect on the digestibility of a high-carbohydrate diet or a high-fat diet [45]. Therefore, the sustained weight loss observed in animals with chronic treatment of fenfluramine is neither caused by alterations in behavioral activity nor by nutrient absorption. These phenomena indicate that fenfluramine increases metabolic rate. The effects of fenfluramine in animals along with meal administration were investigated [46]. Fenfluramine at a dose of 20 mg/kg administered with a meal induced 10-20% increases in postprandial metabolic rate as indicated by an increase in oxygen uptake. Furthermore, the ability of fenfluramine to potentiate the thermic effects of food (TEF) for nutrients was evaluated. Results demonstrate that the drug potentiated TEF for carbohydrates, but had little effect on fat diets. Fenfluramine clearly increased energy expenditure. This result is considered to be one energic explanation for the sustained weight loss in the presence of normal food intake. Fenfluramine can potentiate TEF without having a calorigenic effect when administered alone; however, the details of the mechanism have not been fully elucidated. In a chronic treatment study for 6 weeks, fenfluramine treatment resulted in decreases in weights that were ~15% lower than results observed in control animals.

Numerous clinical studies, including open or double-blind studies, were conducted for fenfluramine and dexfenfluramine. Hudson reported results from an open-label study for 52 weeks comparing the effects of fenfluramine plus diet with diet alone [47]. The patients were given a low-carbohydrate diet. Mean weight loss was highest in patients treated with fenfluramine plus diet (80-120 mg Fenfluramine, -7.6%; Fenfluramine + diet, -8.7%; Control, -4.5%). The rate of weight loss was higher during the first 3 months of treatment than at subsequent intervals, and the weight loss effect reached a plateau after 6 months of therapy. In other open-label clinical studies, fenfluramine treatment resulted in 10-15% decreases in baseline weights [48 - 50]. Douglas *et al.* reported that there were no statistically significant weight differences in endpoints in a double-blind clinical study conducted for 52 weeks [51]. In clinical studies assessing dexfenfluramine treatment, the drug administered at a dose of 15 mg, twice a day, resulted in approximately 3-10% decreases in baseline weights [52 - 54]. In double-blind dexfenfluramine studies, the difference between active therapy and placebo for patients who completed the study assessments was approximately 3 kg. Several reports indicated that some patients might regain weight despite continued treatment [26, 49, 51].

Orlistat

Orlistat is a gastric and pancreatic lipase inhibitor, and is the first non-centrally acting anti-obesity agent that acts on the gastrointestinal tract. The main effect of the drug is suppression of fat absorption, thereby reducing caloric intake. Orlistat was approved for use in Europe in 1998, in the U.S. in 1999, and has been sold all over the world, including Asian countries. The drug is currently available as an over-the-counter drug in the UK and .U.S. Because of reports of an increased risk of serious liver injury with the use of orlistat, The FDA approved a revised label that includes added safety information regarding cases of liver injuries in 2010.

Orlistat is a hydrogenated derivative of lipstatin (Fig. **4**), which is produced by *Streptomyces toxytricini* [55]. Orlistat potently inhibits various lipases, such as pancreatic lipases, and carboxylester lipase, but minimally inhibits digestive enzymes such as amylase, trypsin and phospholipase. Because of its minimal absorption, the bioavailability of orlistat is less than 1%. In fact, the plasma concentration of orlistat was <5 ng/mL after a single dose of 800 mg [56]. Therefore, orlistat is considered to show effects in the digestive tract only. Inactivation of pancreatic lipase by orlistat suppresses the hydrolysis of dietary fat, *i.e.*, decomposition from triglycerides to absorbable fatty acids and monoacylglycerol. As undigested triglycerides are excreted in feces, the reduction of energy intake into the body has a favorable effect on body weight.

Fig. (4). Chemical structure of orlistat, (S)-((S)-1-((2S,3S)-3-Hexyl-4-oxooxetan-2-yl)tridecan-2-yl) 2-formamido-4-methylpentanoate.

In preclinical studies, the effects of orlistat on fat absorption were investigated through the measurement of plasma TG after olive oil loading in mice fed Western diets. Increases in triglyceride levels after oral fat loading were significantly reduced in orlistat-treated mice [57, 58]. Anti-obesity effects were investigated in a high-fat diet-induced obese model. Body weight and adipose tissue decreased in the orlistat administration group [57, 59]. Moreover, orlistat reduced the progression of atherosclerosis through a triglyceride-lowering effect based on the inhibition of fat absorption in ApoE knockout mice fed Western diets [58].

Sjöström *et al.* reported results from a double-blind study in which the effect of orlistat on weight loss and preventing weight regain in obese patients were evaluated [56]. Obese patients received orlistat 120 mg three times daily before meals over 2 years with a hypocaloric diet. In the first year of the clinical study, mean weight loss was highest in patients treated with orlistat compared with placebo (120 mg orlistat, -10.3kg; placebo, -6.3 kg from baseline). The percentage of patients with decreases in body weight that were >20% of initial body weight was 2.1% in the placebo group and 9.3% in the orlistat group. At the end of the second year, a recurrence of weight gain was prevented compared with placebo (differences in weight loss between orlistat and placebo were 3.6 kg) in patients who continued treatment with orlistat. Significant reductions in LDL cholesterol, and total cholesterol, and glucose and insulin level were also observed with orlistat treatment. In meta-analyses of 22 studies, the average weight reduction at 12 months was higher in patients in the orlistat group than those in the placebo group (-8.1kg *vs.* -5.2kg, respectively) [60]. A large 4-year prospective study (XENDOS study) was performed to evaluate the effect of orlistat on preventing the onset of type 2 diabetes in obese patients [61]. The cumulative incidence of diabetes was 9% in the placebo group, and 6.2% in the orlistat group. Orlistat reduced the progression to type 2 diabetes by 37%. In addition, orlistat improved other cardiovascular risks, such as blood pressure, waist circumference and dyslipidemia. The most common adverse effects with orlistat were gastrointestinal disorders, such as diarrhea, fecal incontinence, oily spotting, flatulence and dyspepsia [42, 62]. These adverse effects were observed in 15-30% of patients receiving orlistat treatment. Since orlistat partially suppresses the absorption of fat-soluble vitamins, co-prescriptions of daily vitamin supplements are recommended. Systemic side effects are rarely observed because of minimal systemic absorption.

Shibutramine

Sibutramine selectively inhibits noradrenaline/serotonin reuptake (Fig. **5**). The main effect of sibutramine is the suppression of energy intake by appetite suppression, and the drug also has an effect on increasing energy consumption [63, 64]. Initially, sibutramine was developed as an antidepressant agent; however, antidepressant effects were not confirmed in clinical studies. Nevertheless, sibutramine treatment resulted in significant weight reductions in phase 2 studies in patients with depression, and the drug was therefore developed as a treatment for obesity. Sibutramine was approved in the U.S. in 1997 and Europe in 1999 [65]. The drug was withdrawn from markets in 2010 due to increased risks of heart attack and stroke in patients with a history of cardiovascular disease [66, 67].

Sibutramine is a selective inhibitor of presynaptic reuptake of monoaminergic neurotransmitters serotonin (5-HT), noradrenaline (NA), and dopamine in the central nervous system. The increase in levels of these neurotransmitters enhances the suppressive effect on appetite [67]. Unlike the early structural analogues of amphetamine, such as phentermine and fenfluramine, sibutramine does not stimulate the secretion of catecholamines. Therefore, sibutramine does not cause neurotoxicity [68]. In addition to appetite suppression, sibutramine increases energy expenditure based on two different effects. One effect is that sibutramine prevents decreases in basal energy consumption following weight loss *via* melanocortin receptor 4 (MCR-4) activation [69, 70]. The other effect is the increase in thermogenesis through the activation of ß 3 adrenergic receptors [71].

Fig. (5). Chemical structure of sibutramine, (±)-Dimethyl-1-[1-(4-chlorophenyl)cyclobutyl]- N,N,3-trimethylbutan-1-amine.

In basic research studies, a single administration of sibutramine reduced cumulative food intake at 2, 4, and 8 hr after administration [72]. Chronic sibutramine treatment resulted in suppression of food intake and reduction of body weight gain in dietary-induced obese Wistar rats. Sibutramine also remarkably reduced fat weight compared to muscle in diet-induced obesity rats. Furthermore, sibutramine treatment also ameliorates insulin resistance, which is a characteristic parameter in this model of obesity. Unlike serotonin-releasing agents, sibutramine acts independently of the hypothalamic NPY signaling system, which controls appetite [73]. In a genetic obesity model, sibutramine treatment ameliorated impaired obesity, reduced food consumption and increased energy expenditure in ZF rats without changes in hypothalamic NPY and orexins [74].

Smith *et al.* reported results from a double-blind study for 12 months in which the effects of sibutramine on weight loss in obese patients given dietary advice were evaluated. Mean weight loss was highest in patients treated with 10 mg and 15 mg of sibutramine (10 mg sibutramine, -4.4 kg; 15 mg sibutramine, -6.4 kg; placebo, -1.6 kg from baseline). The percentage of patients with decreases in body weight

>5 kg was 20% in the placebo, 39% in the sibutramine 10 mg, and 57% in the sibutramine 15 mg groups. A significantly higher proportion of patients taking sibutramine lost >10 kg from baseline (10 mg sibutramine, 19% 15 mg sibutramine, 34%) compared with patients taking placebo (7%) [75]. Furthermore, sibutramine showed potential benefits by improving cardiometabolic risk factors, such as high glucose, insulin or lipid levels [76]. The Sibutramine Cardiovascular Outcomes (SCOUT) study was conducted to evaluate the long-term effects of sibutramine treatment on the rates of cardiovascular events and cardiovascular deaths among patients with high cardiovascular risk. The results from SCOUT showed that long-term sibutramine treatment increased the risk of nonfatal myocardial infarction and stroke, but not cardiovascular deaths [77]. From this study, the EMA and FDA recommended the suspension of use of sibutramine. The drug was withdrawn from the market in 2010.

Rimonabant

Rimonabant is a cannabinoid-1 (CB1) receptor antagonist (Fig. **6**), which controls the uptake of cannabinoid and is the first agent that targets the endocannabinoid system. The main effect is suppression of appetite. Rimonabant was approved for use in Europe in 2006, but was not approved in the United States. Due to the risk of serious psychiatric problems, including suicide, the drug was withdrawn from the market in 2009 [78].

The CB1 receptor is a member of the 7-transmembrane G protein-coupled receptor family [79]. This receptor is expressed mainly in the brain, in particular in the basal ganglia, hippocampus, cerebral cortex and hypothalamus. These receptors are also present in the testes, adrenal gland, ovaries and adipose tissues [79 - 81]. The CB1 receptor is coupled to Gi/o proteins, but the details of the second messenger transduction of CB1 receptor signaling are complex [80]. The two main endogenous cannabinoid agonists are anandamide and 2-arachidonoyl glycerol, which act as neurotransmitters or neuromodulators [82 - 84]. These endocannabinoids play important roles in energy homeostasis and regulation of appetite [85]. Peripheral sites of activity may also be regulated by endocannabinoids *via* CB1 receptors that are present in peripheral tissues, such as the liver, skeletal muscles and pancreas [86]. Delta(9)-tetrahydrocannabinol (THC), which binds equally to CB1 and CB2 receptors, was identified from the cannabis plant in 1974. Synthetic THC, like dronabinol, is used for the treatment of emesis or nausea after chemotherapy [87]. The structure of THC has been modified to develop selective CB1 receptor antagonists since the late 1980s. After lengthy research, Rinaldi-Carmona *et al.* ultimately designed the compound, rimonabant, which is a selective CB1 receptor antagonist that has 1000-fold CB1 selectivity over CB2 [88].

Fig. (6). Chemical structure of rimonabant, 5-(4-Chlorophenyl)-1-(2,4-dichloro-phenyl)-4-methyl- N-(piperidin-1-yl)-1H-pyrazole-3-carboxamide.

In preclinical studies, rimonabant transiently reduced food intake in ob/ob mice, db/db mice and Zucker fatty rats, which are genetically obese animal models. However, the effects of rimonabant on body weight were sustained when compared with inhibitory effects on food intake in those rodents [89]. Rimonabant also remarkably reduced fat weight compared to muscle in diet-induced obesity mice. Furthermore, continuous inhibition of the CB1 receptor resulted in improvements in hyperlipidemia and dyslipidemia, which are characteristic metabolic parameters in obese models [90]. Similar to rimonabant, CB1 receptor knockout mice were hypophagic, and resistant to the development of obesity induced by high-fat diets, and had improved insulin and leptin resistance in comparison with wild-type mice [91]. From these results, the anti-obesity effects of CB1 receptor antagonists were considered to be attributed not only to suppression of food consumption, but also to decreases in fat weight, TG accumulation and accelerated energy consumption. In fact, rimonabant treatment increased O2 consumption and soleus muscle glucose uptake in ob/ob mice [92].

Després *et al.* reported results from a phase 3 study; Rimonabant in Obesity (RIO)-Lipids, in which the effect of rimonabant on weight loss in overweight patients with dyslipidemia was evaluated [93]. The study compared treatment with 5 mg and 20 mg of rimonabant to placebo in a group of obese patients with untreated dyslipidemia for twelve months under dietary restrictions. The percentage of patients with decreases in body weight >5 kg was 28% in the placebo, 42% in the rimonabant 5 mg, and 75% in the rimonabant 20 mg groups. Improvement in cardiovascular risk factors was observed with 20 mg of rimonabant treatment. The changes observed included 16% reductions in triglycerides, 23% increases in HDL cholesterol and glucose tolerance improvement, as well as blood pressure reduction. Other key RIO studies, RIO-North America, RIO-Europe, and RIO-diabetes reported similar results, and the differences were only in the number and type of patients, and location [94 - 96]. In patients in RIO-North America from the U.S. and Canada with dyslipidemia and obesity, similar to RIO-Lipids, rimonabant decreased body weight and abdominal circumference, and improved hypertriglyceridemia, hypoHDLemia and insulin resistance [95]. RIO-Europe was conducted to study overweight patients with dyslipidemia and hypertension, not diabetes. In addition to weight loss, significant improvements in lipid and glycemic variables were observed with rimonabant treatment [94]. RIO-diabetes evaluated the effects on patients with type II diabetes for one year. Increases in the percentage of patients with hemoglobin A1C <7% and decreases in body weight were observed with rimonabant therapy [96]. In safety data obtained from these studies, the major side effects were nausea, diarrhea, depressive moods, depression and anxiety [83].

Qsymia

Qsymia is a combination oral product composed of phentermine hydrochloride and topiramate (Fig. 7), and the drug was approved by the FDA in 2012. Both Qsymia and BELVIQ (Term 2.8.) were approved in 2012, and these new drug approvals for anti-obesity therapy were the first in 13 years [3, 13, 97]. Phentermine is a sympathomimetic amine anorectic agent for short-term therapy mentioned previously in Section 2.1., and topiramate is an oral drug that is used to prevent seizures or epilepsy, and is an anti-seizure or anti-epileptic drug [98 - 100], that was approved by the FDA in 1997.

Fig. (7). Chemical structure of Qsymia, a combination of phentermine/topiramate. Topiramate, 2,3:4,5-Bis-o-(1-methylethylidene)-beta-D-fructopyranose sulfamate.

Epilepsy and seizures occur due to abnormal activity of nerves in the brain, and the abnormalities spread to smaller or larger portions of the brain. Although the exact mechanism of action for topiramate is unknown, the drug reportedly alters neurotransmitters, including Gamma-amino butyric acids (GABAs) in the brain [101, 102]. By altering the production or activity of neurotransmitters, topiramate is considered to inhibit the abnormal activity of nerves in the brain. Other studies also indicate that topiramate may directly suppress the nerves and lessen the likelihood of these nerves firing. Topiramate is considered to bind to certain membrane ion channel proteins at phosphorylation sites, thereby allosterically modulating channel conductance and inhibiting secondary protein phosphorylation [103]. Moreover, York *et al*. reported that topiramate reduced food intake acutely and increased the metabolic rate in rats fed a high-fat diet [104]. In the hypothalamus, the drug increased mRNA levels for neuropeptide-Y and reduced mRNA levels for neuropeptide-Y1 and Y5 receptors, corticotropin-releasing hormone and type II glucocorticoid receptors, but had no effect on mRNA levels of the leptin receptor. In peripheral tissues, topiramate reduced leptin mRNA levels in adipose tissue, and had no effect on uncoupling protein 1 mRNA levels in brown tissue, but had tissue-selective effects on uncoupling proteins 2 and 3 mRNA levels in fat and muscle.

In clinical studies, in particular in a phase 3 study, treatment with Qsymia resulted in significant weight loss compared with the placebo group [105, 106]. After 56 weeks of treatment, the percent of weight loss achieved with Qsymia was 10.6%, 8.4% and 5.1% with 15/92 mg of phentermine/topiramate, 7.5/46 mg, and 3.75/23 mg, respectively. The 52-week extension study (SEQUE study) showed sustained weight loss over 2 years, with 9.3% and 10.5% weight loss from baseline weights with 7.5/46 mg and 15/92 mg of phentermine/topiramate. Significant reductions in waist circumference, fasting triglyceride levels, and fasting glucose levels, were also observed with Qsymia treatment. Adverse effects, such as paresthesia, dizziness, dysgeusia, insomnia, constipation, and dry mouth, were observed in 5% or higher of patients in the study. In previous studies, phentermine monotherapy at a dose of 30 mg resulted in significant body weight loss [26]. In this clinical study, phentermine at a dose of 15 mg or lower resulted in significant sustained body weight loss, and a decrease in the dose of the drug with combination therapy is expected to lead to attenuation of adverse effects. Qsymia is a new, once-daily, controlled-release, combination weight-loss product approved as an adjunct to diet and exercise for chronic weight management of obese patients. Qsymia is modestly effective and a viable option for patients intending to losing weight.

BELVIQ (Lorcaserin)

BELVIQ has serotonergic properties and acts as an anorectic (Fig. **8**). In 2012, FDA approved the drug for use in the treatment of obese patients with a BMI of 30 or higher, or patients with a BMI of 27 or higher who have at least one weight-related health condition, such as hypertension, type 2 diabetes, or dyslipidemia [3, 97, 107]. Qsymia and BELVIQ were approved by the FDA; however, both drugs have been withdrawn in the EU.

Lorcaserin is a selective $5\text{-}HT_{2C}$ receptor agonist, and showed reasonable selectivity for $5\text{-}HT_{2C}$ receptor over other related targets [107 - 109]. Lorcaserin showed a 100-fold selectivity for $5\text{-}HT_{2C}$ *versus* the closely related $5\text{-}HT_{2B}$

receptor, and a 17-fold selectivity over the 5-HT$_{2A}$ receptor [108, 110, 111]. 5-HT$_{2C}$ receptors are located almost exclusively in the brain, such as the choroid plexus, cortex, hippocampus, cerebellum, amygdala, thalamus, and hypothalamus. Activation of 5-HT$_{2C}$ receptors in the hypothalamus is considered to activate proopiomelanocortin (POMC) production and consequently promote weight loss through satiety [112].

Fig. (8). Chemical structure of lorcaserin, (1R)-8-chloro-1-methyl-2,3,4,5-tetrahydro-1H-3-benzazepine.

In pharmacological studies using rats, lorcaserin treatment resulted in an acute reduction in food intake, and chronic treatment with lorcaserin for 4 weeks maintained on a high-fat diet resulted in dose-dependent reductions in food intake and body weight gain [108, 111]. A single oral administration of lorcaserin (at a dose of 3, 6. 12, or 24 mg/kg) resulted in reductions in cumulative food intake at 2, 4, 6, and 22 h, with significant decreases continuing throughout the 22 h duration of the study only at the highest dose (24 mg/kg). With chronic lorcaserin administration to male DIO rats, drug treatment (4.5, 9, and 18 mg/kg p.o., b.i.d.) significantly reduced food intake over the first 13 days of dosing, after which tolerance to the food intake suppressing effects of lorcaserin developed dose-dependently.

In Phase 2 studies, lorcaserin treatment resulted in significantly higher weight loss when compared with placebo groups [113 - 115]. At the end of 12 weeks, body weights in lorcaserin treatment groups decreased by 4.0 pounds (10 mg/day), 5.7 pounds (15 mg/day), and 7.9 pounds (20 mg/day). The weight loss in placebo groups was 0.7 pounds. Patients in the Phase 2 study were tracked for 2 weeks post-study completion and all groups regained weight more rapidly than the pace at which the weight had originally decreased. In Phase 3 studies of lorcaserin, the cumulative proportion of patients who achieved a weight loss of 5% or higher over 12 months was about 47% with lorcaserin treatment *versus* 20-25% in the placebo group [116, 117]. Adverse effects, such as nausea, vomiting, headache, and dizziness were reported. In two of the three Phase 3 studies, lorcaserin treatment did not result in an observed increase in the risk of cardiac valvulopathy; however, in the other Phase 3 study that focused on patients with diabetes, drug treatment was associated with an increased rate of new valvulopathy.

Contrave

Contrave is a combination drug of two approved drugs, bupropion and naltrexone (Fig. **9**) for the treatment of obesity [118 - 122]. The drug was marketed in the U.S. in 2014 and in the EU in 2015. Both bupropion and naltrexone have individually shown some evidence of efficacy in weight loss, and the combination therapy is expected to have a synergistic effect. A New Drug Application (NDA) for contrave was submitted to the FDA in 2010; however, the FDA decided that an extremely large-scale study of long-term cardiovascular effects of the drug would be needed, and the application was rejected.

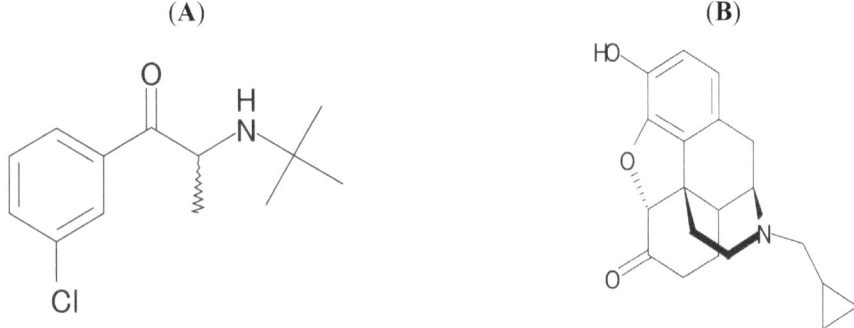

Fig. (9). Chemical structures of bupropion,(±)-2-(tert-Butylamino)-1-(3-chlorophenyl)propan-1-one (**A**) and naltrexone, 17-(cyclopropylmethyl)-4,5α-epoxy-3,14-dihydroxymorphinan-6-one (**B**).

Bupropion reportedly has several different biological targets and is widely known as a norepinephrine-dopamine reuptake inhibitor and neuronal nicotinic acetylcholine receptor-antagonist [123, 124]. Bupropion was approved by the FDA as an antidepressant in 1985, but a significant incidence of epileptic seizures at the recommended dose (400-600 mg) caused the withdrawal of the drug in 1986. Afterwards, bupropion was reapproved in 1989 at a lower maximum recommended dose [125, 126]. Bupropion was also approved by the FDA in 1997 for use as a smoking cessation aid. In basic research studies, bupropion was demonstrated as inhibiting norepinephrine-dopamine uptake and also inducing the release of dopamine and norepinephrine [127]. Moreover, pharmacological studies in rats undergoing nicotine withdrawal demonstrate that bupropion can dose-dependently lower changes in the brain-reward threshold and somatic signs of nicotine withdrawal [128]. Bupropion is one of the most widely prescribed antidepressants, and available evidence indicates that it is effective in clinical depression [129]. Bupropion has some features that distinguish it from other antidepressants, for instance, the drug does not cause sexual dysfunction [130, 131]. Furthermore, bupropion is reported to show anti-obesity effects. The drug, when used over a period of 6 to 12 months, causes weight loss of 2.7 kg over placebo, and the efficacy is not much different from that of several other medications, such as sibutramine, orlistat, and anferamone [60, 132].

Naltrexone is an opioid receptor antagonist used primarily for the management of alcohol dependence and opioid dependence. The main use of the drug is for the treatment of alcohol dependence, and was approved by the FDA in 1994 [133]. Naltrexone has generally been better studied for alcohol dependence than for treating opioid dependence; however, the use of the drug as a treatment for opioid addiction has already been approved in 1984 [134, 135]. Naltrexone is sometimes used as a treatment for other diseases, such as depersonalization disorder, tobacco dependence, self-injurious behaviors, and some behavioral addictions [136 - 138]. The most common adverse effects reported with naltrexone are non-specific gastrointestinal complaints, such as diarrhea and abdominal cramping.

Contrave, a bupropion and naltrexone combination therapy is reportedly useful for the potential treatment of obesity [119, 122, 139]. Greenway *et al.* reported results from a phase 3 study, in which the effect of naltrexone plus bupropion on weight loss in overweight and obese adults was evaluated [140]. In the phase 3 study conducted for 56 weeks, participants were randomly assigned to 3 groups, naltrexone 32 mg/day plus bupropion 360 mg/day, 16 mg/day plus bupropion 360 mg/day, or placebo. Results demonstrated that the mean change in body weight was -1.3% in the placebo group, -6.1% in the naltrexone 32 mg/day plus bupropion 360 mg/day group, and -5.0% in the naltrexone 16 mg/day plus bupropion 360 mg/day group. Adverse effects, such as headache, constipation, dizziness, vomiting, and dry mouth, were also more frequent in the naltrexone plus bupropion groups than in the placebo group. The combination of naltrexone plus bupropion is expected to be a useful therapeutic option for the treatment of obesity.

New Drug Targets (Table 3)

Table 3. Anti-obesity drugs under development.

Drug	Mechanism of action	Notes
Cetillistat	Gastrointestinal and pancreatic lipase inhibitor	Phase III 2014:Approval (in Japan)
Empatic	Bupropion/Zonisamide	Phase III
Liraglitide	GLP-1 agonist	Phase III 2014: Approval (in U.S.)
Tesofensine	Triple-monoamine inhibitor	Phase III
Beloranib	methionine aminopeptidase 2 inhibitor	Phase III
	MTP inhibitor	Inhibition of lipid absorption

(Table 3) contd.....

Drug	Mechanism of action	Notes
	DGAT1 inhibitor	Inhibition of lipid absorption
	MGAT2 inhibitor	Inhibition of lipid absorption
	SGLT2 inhibitor	Inhibition of glucose reabsorption
	PTP1B inhibitor	Activation of leptin signal

Late Phase Clinical Development

Cetilistat

Cetilistat is an inhibitor of gastric and pancreatic lipases that breaks down triglycerides in the intestine (Fig. **10**). This drug has the same mechanism of action as orlistat previously described above. The main effect is suppression of fat absorption from the intestine. Cetilistat was approved for use in Japan; however, Cetilistat has not been sold in the market [141]. The structure of cetilistat has highly lipophilic benzoxazinone, which raises the possibility of fewer side effects compared with orlistat. Cetilistat forms a covalent bond with the 152 serine residue in the active center of pancreatic lipase, and reversibly inhibits the activity of lipase. Inhibition of pancreatic lipase decreases TG absorption from the small intestine, and unabsorbed fat is excreted in the feces. The suppression of approximately 30% of triglyceride absorption reduces the energy intake into the body, and is expected to reduce body weight.

Fig. (10). Chemical structures of cetilistat, 2-(Hexadecyloxy)-6-methyl-4H-3,1-benzoxazin-4-one.

In preclinical *in vitro* studies, cetilistat inhibited pancreatic lipase activity in humans and rats with an IC_{50} of 5.95 nmol/L, and 54.8 nmol/L, respectively [142]. The inhibitory effects of cetilistat were more potent in human pancreatic lipase than in rats. The effects on fat absorption were investigated in *in vivo* measurements of plasma TG after fat loading in Sprague-Dawley rats. Plasma TG in the cetilistat administration group decreased in a dose-dependent manner. Anti-obesity effects were investigated in F344 rats fed a high-fat diet. Body weight and adipose tissues in the cetilistat administration group decreased dose-dependently; however, liver weight was not affected. Fecal TG and free fatty acid content increased dose-dependently with cetilistat treatment. The suppression of food intake was not observed in rats fed a high-fat diet after cetilistat treatment. The anti-obesity effect of cetilistat was suggested as being attributed to the suppression of fat absorption. Analysis of blood biochemistry values showed that cetilistat had lowering effects on plasma TG and leptin levels, but not glucose [142].

In clinical studies, Kopelman *et al.* reported results from a phase 2 study in which the effects of cetilistat on weight loss in overweight patients were evaluated [143]. Obese patients received cetilistat at a dose of 60 mg, 120 mg, or 240 mg for 12weeks with a hypocaloric diet. Body weights in cetilistat treatment groups significantly decreased by 3.3 kg (60 mg/day), 3.5 kg (120 mg/day), and 4.2 kg (240 mg/day), respectively. The proportion of patients who achieved a weight loss of 5% or higher were higher in all three doses compared with placebo. Significant reductions in waist circumference, LDL cholesterol, and total cholesterol level were also observed in all three doses of cetilistat treatment. Gastrointestinal adverse effects, such as flatulence, oily spotting and soft stools, were observed in cetilistat treatment groups. However these adverse effects were observed in only 1.8-2.8% of patients in cetilistat treatment groups. Kopelman *et al.* also reported the effects of cetilistat on obese patients with type II diabetes [144]. Diabetic obese patients on metformin received cetilistat at a dose of 40 mg, 80 mg, or 120 mg for 12 weeks with a reduced calorie diet. Mean weight loss was significant in patients treated with 80 mg and 120 mg of cetilistat (80 mg cetilistat, -3.9 kg; 120 mg cetilistat, -4.3 kg; placebo, -2.9 kg from baseline). Significant reductions relative to placebo were shown for HbA1c in 80 mg and 120 mg cetilistat treatment groups (80 mg cetilistat, -0.54%; 120 mg cetilistat, -0.51%; placebo, -0.37% from baseline). In cetilistat treatment groups, the incidence of gastrointestinal adverse effects was higher than placebo. However, the incidence of non-gastrointestinal adverse effects was similar in all patients including placebo.

Empatic

Empatic is a combination drug of two approved drugs, bupropion and zonisamide, for the treatment of obesity, and the drug is currently being tested in a phase 3 study. The drug is being developed by Orexigen Therapeutics, and the company published positive results from a phase 2b study in 2009 [145, 146]. According to the key top-line data report, patients completing 24 weeks of Empatic 360 (bupropion 360 mg/zonisamide 360 mg) therapy lost 9.9% of baseline body weight, or 22 pounds, compared to 1.7% for the placebo group. Empatic patients experienced significant weight loss as early as their first post-baseline visit at four weeks and, more importantly, patients continued to lose weight through the end of the study period, with no evidence of a plateau in weight loss. The sustained effectiveness for weight loss in the long-term is an advantage with empatic treatment. With many previous compounds, the duration was not sustained and the time to plateau of weight loss was earlier. Moreover, with emphatic treatment, improvements were observed in markers of cardiometabolic risk, such as waist circumference, triglycerides, fasting insulin, and blood pressure. The most commonly reported adverse effects were headache, insomnia, and nausea.

The combination consists of two prescription medications, bupropion and zonisamide, which were approved by the FDA for other diseases. Bupropion, as mentioned above, is a norepinephrine-dopamine reuptake inhibitor and neuronal nicotinic acetylcholine receptor-antagonist, and reportedly shows anti-obesity effects in clinical studies. Zonisamide is an anti-seizure drug chemically classified as a sulfonamide and is unrelated to other anti-seizure agents (Fig. **11**). The drug was discovered by Uno *et al*. in 1972 and was marketed by Dainippon Sumitomo Pharma in 1989 in Japan. In the U.S., drug development was delayed due to an adverse effect, urinary stone, and the drug was marketed in 2000. The drug is also marketed in Asia and Europe. The precise mechanisms of zonisamide treatment are unknown; however, the drug is considered to block sodium and T-type calcium channels, which leads to the suppression of neuronal hyper-synchronization. Moreover, other mechanisms of action, such as the inhibition of carbonic anhydrase and modulation of GABAergic and glutamatergic neurotransmission have been reported [147 - 150]. Zonisamide has also been investigated as a treatment for obesity and significant positive effects on body weight have been shown [151]. There are some clinical studies in this indication [152 - 155]. Shin *et al*. reported weight changes in obese patients 6 months after completing participation in a 12-month study, in which zonisamide at a dose of 200 or 400 mg was administered with lifestyle counseling. Results demonstrated weight changes from 12 to 18 months that were 0.5 kg in the placebo, 1.5 kg in the zonisamide 200 mg, and 2.4 kg in the zonisamide 400 mg groups. In a 1-year double-blind study, Gadde *et al*. also reported that the changes in body weight were -4.0 kg in the placebo, -4.4 kg in the zonisamide 200 mg, and -7.3 kg in the zonisamide 400 mg groups. In both clinical studies, treatment with zonisamide at a daily dose of 400 mg resulted in significant weight loss achieved with diet and lifestyle counseling; however, the incidence of adverse effects was also high.

Fig. (11). Chemical structure of zonisamide, benzo[d]isoxazol-3-ylmethanesulfonamide.

Tesofensine

Tesofensine (NS2330) is a novel triple monoamine, (serotonin, noradrenaline, and dopamine) reuptake inhibitor from the phenyltropane family of drugs that are used for the treatment of obesity (Fig. **12**) [156, 157]. Tesofensine was originally developed for the treatment of Alzheimer's disease and Parkinson's disease, but development for these applications was halted because of the limited efficacy in the treatment of these diseases in clinical studies [158 - 160]. However, in clinical studies, weight loss is reportedly observed with tesofensine in patients with Parkinson's or Alzheimer's disease [161]. Therefore, a decision was made to pursue the development of tesofensine for the treatment of obesity, and phase 2 studies have been successfully completed.

Tesofensine is a neurotransmitter-reuptake inhibitor that acts to increase noradrenaline, serotonin, and dopamine neurotransmission, and this main mechanism of action in basic research studies has also been reported. Larsen *et al.* showed that the drug enhanced hippocampal gene expression and new cell formation indicative of an antidepressant potential for this novel drug substance [162]. Tesofensine also indirectly potentiates cholinergic neurotransmission proven to have beneficial effects on cognition, including learning and memory. Chronic treatment with tesofensine increased brain-derived neurotrophic factor (BDNF) levels in the brain, and may have antidepressant effects [162].

Fig. (12). Chemical structure of tesofensine, (1R, 2R, 3S)-3-(3, 4-dichlorophenyl)-2-(ethoxymethyl)-8-methyl-8-.azabicyclo [3.2.1] octane.

In basic research studies, the mechanisms of action underlying the suppression of food intake and the effect on weight loss were investigated in DIO obese rat. Alex *et al.* reported that the mechanism of appetite inhibition is dependent on the drug's ability to indirectly stimulate the function of α-adrenoceptors and dopamine receptors [163]. Moreover, Hansen *et al.* reported that long-term treatment with tesofensine (28 days, 1.0 or 2.5 mg/kg p.o.) resulted in significant, dose-dependent and sustained weight loss of 5.7 and 9.9%, respectively [164]. In this study, sibutramine (7.5 mg/kg p.o.) or rimonabant (10 mg/kg p.o.) treatment also showed weight loss; however, the hypophagic effect of tesofensine was sustained for longer periods of time than sibutramine and rimonabant.

Furthermore, tesofensine stimulated energy expenditure.

Astrup *et al.* reported results from a phase 2 clinical study for obesity treatment [165]. Obese patients (BMI, 30-40) were prescribed an energy restricted diet and assigned to receive tesofensine at doses of 0.25 mg, 0.5 mg, or 1.0 mg or placebo (n=49-52) once daily for 24 weeks. After 24 weeks of treatment, the mean weight loss observed with placebo with the diet was 2.0%. Tesofensine administered at doses of 0.25 mg, 0.5 mg, and 1.0 mg with the diet restriction-induced mean weight losses that were 4.5%, 9.2%, and 10.6% greater than placebo, respectively, with the diet restriction. The most common adverse effects with tesofensine treatment were dry mouth, nausea, constipation, hard stools, diarrhea, and insomnia. Moreover, tesofensine treatment did not result in increases in blood pressure, whereas heart rate increased in the tesofensine 0.5 mg group. In a 48-week open-label study, tesofensine administered at a dose of 0.5 mg resulted in a total weight loss of 13-14 kg. Tesofensine at a dose of 0.5 mg might have potential to result in weight loss that is higher than that of currently approved drugs. These efficacy and safety findings are expected to be confirmed in phase 2 studies.

Liraglutide

Liraglutide is a glucagon-like peptide-1 (GLP-1) receptor agonist that enhances the glucose-dependent insulin secretion of pancreatic beta-cells (Fig. **13**) [166, 167], suppresses glucagon secretion [168, 169], reduces food intake [170, 171] and slows gastric emptying [172, 173]. Liraglutide was approved for use as a treatment for type 2 diabetes in Europe in 2009, and in the U.S. in 2010. Recently, Liraglutide was approved by the FDA as a treatment for obesity with some related comorbidities in late 2014.

Fig. (13). Chemical structure of liraglutide.

GLP-1 is an incretin peptide that is released from the intestinal L cell, which is primarily found in the ileum and the colon in response to the ingestion of nutrients

[174]. GLP-1 is processed from proglucagon and is rapidly broken down by the enzyme dipeptide peptidase 4 (DPP-4) to inactive metabolites [175]. Therefore, the half-life of GLP-1 is less than 2 minutes [176]. Because of this short duration, native GLP-1 is inappropriate for clinical treatment. These receptors are expressed in the pancreas, gut, and brain. These receptors are also present in the arcuate nucleus and the other hypothalamus, which are related to the regulation of appetite and food intake [177]. GLP-1 is known to have various physiological effects, including increasing insulin secretion, decreasing glucagon secretion, delaying gastric empting and suppressing appetite [178]. In order to be used for clinical therapy, the DPP-4 resistant GLP-1 agonist, liraglutide, was developed to overcome the short half-life of native GLP-1. Liraglutide has 97% homology with human GLP-1 and retains the activity of the GLP-1 receptor for 13 hr [179]. Liraglutide was shown to ameliorate glycemic control in patients with type 2 diabetes. In a phase 3 randomized controlled study, LEAD-3, Garber *et al.* reported that HbA1c reductions from baseline were -0.84% with liraglutide treatment at 1.2 mg and -1.14% with liraglutide treatment at 1.8 mg [180]. In addition to anti-diabetic effects, the body weight reductions from baseline were -2.05 kg and -2.45 kg with liraglutide administered at doses of 1.2 mg and 1.8 mg respectively in this study [180].

In basic research studies, the effects of liraglutide on obesity were investigated in DIO obese rats. After repeated dosing, liraglutide reduced body weight, fat weight and food consumption in gubra diet (high-fat and high-sugar diet) fed rats. Furthermore, liraglutide improved glucose tolerance in DIO obese rats [181]. In a genetic obesity model, liraglutide treatment ameliorated impaired obesity, glucose and lipid metabolism and reduced food consumption in ZDF rats [182].

Satiety and Clinical Adiposity – Liraglutide Evidence in Nondiabetic and Diabetic Subjects (SCALE) was designed to evaluate the safety and efficacy of liraglutide administered at a dose of 3 mg on body weight. In the SCALE Obesity and Prediabetes phase 3 study for 54 weeks, the average weight reduction was higher in patients in the liraglutide 3 mg group than those in the placebo group (-8% *vs.* -2.8%, respectively). The body weight of patients decreased by >5%, wherein the decrease was 63.5% in the liraglutide 3 mg group, and 26.6% in the placebo group [183]. The SCALE-Diabetes study evaluated obese or overweight patients with type 2 diabetes. At 56 weeks, weight losses of 6% and 5% were observed in the liraglutide 3 mg group and 1.8 mg group, respectively, compared with a loss of 2% in the placebo group. Greater than 5% weight reductions were observed in 50% of patients in the liraglutide 3 mg group and 35% of patients in the liraglutide 1.8 mg group. Furthermore, approximately 70% of patients receiving 3 mg liraglutide achieved <7% HbA1c [183]. The FDA approved liraglutide as a treatment option for obesity in December 2014.

Early Phase Clinical Stage Development or Pre-Clinical Development Stage
Late Phase Clinical Development

Beloranib

Beloranib is an inhibitor of methionine aminopeptidase 2 (MetAP2) that removes of methionine from newly synthesized proteins (Fig. **14**) [184, 185]. Suppression of MetAP2 has been shown to inhibit angiogenesis *via* a reduction in cell proliferation [186]. Therefore, beloranib was initially developed as an anticancer agent; however, MetAP2 treatment resulted in significant weight reductions in animal models of obesity and in human, and the drug was therefore developed as a treatment for obesity.

In basic research studies, the effects of beloranib on obesity were investigated in various obese animal models, which are C57Bl/6J mice, SD rats, Long-Evans Tokushima Otuska (LETO) rats and Long-Evans Tokushima Otuska fatty (OLETF) rats. After repeated dosing, beloranib reduced body weight and food consumption in all rat described in the above, especially obese models. Furthermore, beloranib treatment increased body temperature corresponding to an increase in energy expenditure [187]. Intracerebroventricular (ICV) injection of beloranib decreased food intake and body weight in ARJ lesion mice, but not normal mice. Anorexia effect of belranib might relate to central nervous system function [187].

Fig. (14). Chemical structure of beloranib. [(3R, 6R, 7S,8S)-7-methoxy-8-[(2R,3R)-2-methyl-3-(3-methylbut-2-enyl)oxiran-2-yl]-2-oxaspiro[2.5]octan-6-yl] (E)-3-[4-[2-(dimethylamino)ethoxy] phenyl]prop-2-enoate.

In clinical studies, Kim *et al*. reported results from a phase 2 study in which the effects of beloranib on weight loss in overweight patients were evaluated [188]. Obese patients (BMI, 30-50) were prescribed subcutaneously beloranib at doses of 0.6 mg, 1.2 mg, or 2.4 mg or placebo (n=38-35) twice weekly for 12 weeks. After 12 weeks of treatment, body weights in belranib treatment groups significantly decreased by 5.5 kg (0.6 mg), 6.9 kg (1.2 mg), and 10.9 kg (2.4 mg), respectively. Significant reductions in waist circumference, LDL cholesterol, and blood pressure were also observed with 2.4mg of beloranib treatment. Adverse effects, such as sleep disturbance, dry mouth and nausea, were observed in beloranib treatment groups. However these adverse effects were generally mild to modrate and transient. Phase 3 Trial of beloranib currently is being conducted in obese subjects with Prader-Willi Syndrome.

MTP Inhibitor

Microsomal triglyceride transfer protein (MTP) is localized in the endoplasmic reticulum in hepatocytes and enterocytes, and MTP leads the transfer of triglycerides (TG) and cholesteryl ester between membranes [189 - 191]. The protein participates in the assembly of TG-rich lipoproteins, such as chylomicron particles in the small intestine and very low-density lipoprotein (VLDL) particles in the liver, thereby also participating in the mobilization and secretion of TG-rich lipoproteins from enterocytes and hepatocytes [192]. Since enteric MTP has been shown to play a critical role in the absorption of fat or cholesterol, the inhibition of MTP in the small intestine is expected to induce the potential of weight loss as an anti-obesity drug.

Since the *in vivo* effects of MTP inhibitors were reported [190], it has also been pointed out that the inhibition of hepatic MTP could lead to the potent blockade of VLDL release, resulting in reduced plasma lipids but inducing fatty livers and hepatic dysfunction [193, 194]. In fact, while the potential benefits of MTP inhibition, such as lowering chylomicron-TG and VLDL-TG levels, were demonstrated in animal experiments and in clinical studies, several major toxicity issues have affected the clinical development of MTP inhibitors [193, 194]. In clinical studies of BAY 13-9952 and BMS-201038, for example, hepatotoxicity indicated by the elevation of levels of transaminases halted the development of these drugs. Therefore, compounds designed to show high selective inhibition for intestine-MTP have been developed and lipid-absorption inhibitors are expected to show pharmacological effects, including weight loss, without any hepatotoxicity.

Mera *et al.* designed a compound, JTT-130, that would be rapidly metabolized during the absorption process to avoid inhibition of hepatic MTP after oral administration (Fig. **15**) [195, 196]. Anti-obesity effects were investigated in Sprague-Dawley rats fed a 35% fat diet [18]. JTT-130 treatment decreased body weights and suppressed food intake (Fig. **16A, B**). Interestingly, the pharmacological effects were not observed in rats fed a 3.1% fat diet (Fig. **16C, D**), and JTT-130 showed anti-obesity effects in a dietary fat-dependent manner. The elevation of plasma levels of gut hormones, such as glucagon-like peptide-1 (GLP-1) and peptide YY (PYY), was observed in rats fed a 35% fat diet, and the elevation of gut peptides may be related with body weight loss with JTT-130 treatment.

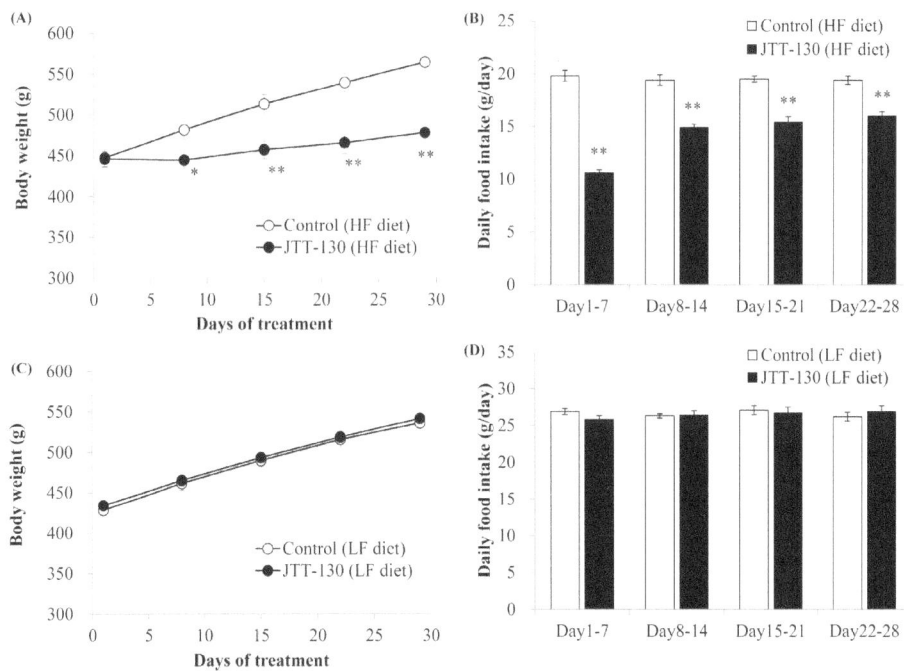

Fig. (15). Chemical structure of intestine-specific MTP inhibitor, JTT-130, and its metabolite.

Fig. (16). Effects of JTT-130 on body weight and food intake in Sprague-Dawley rats on a 35% fat diet (**A, B**) and a 3.1% fat diet (**C, D**). Rats in JTT-130 treatment groups were fed the drug as a 0.029% food admixture (approximately 10 mg/kg/day), beginning at 10 weeks of age.

Moreover, JTT-130 treatment resulted in increased O_2 consumption and CO_2 production on a 35% fat diet, suggesting the enhancement of energy expenditure (Fig. **17**). Considering that JTT-130 has no effects on lean mass, whereas there is a significant reduction of fat mass, the relative abundance of lean mass may lead to the elevation of O_2 consumption and CO_2 production. The elevation of plasma PYY and GLP-1 levels also seems to be associated with the elevation of O_2 consumption and CO_2 production.

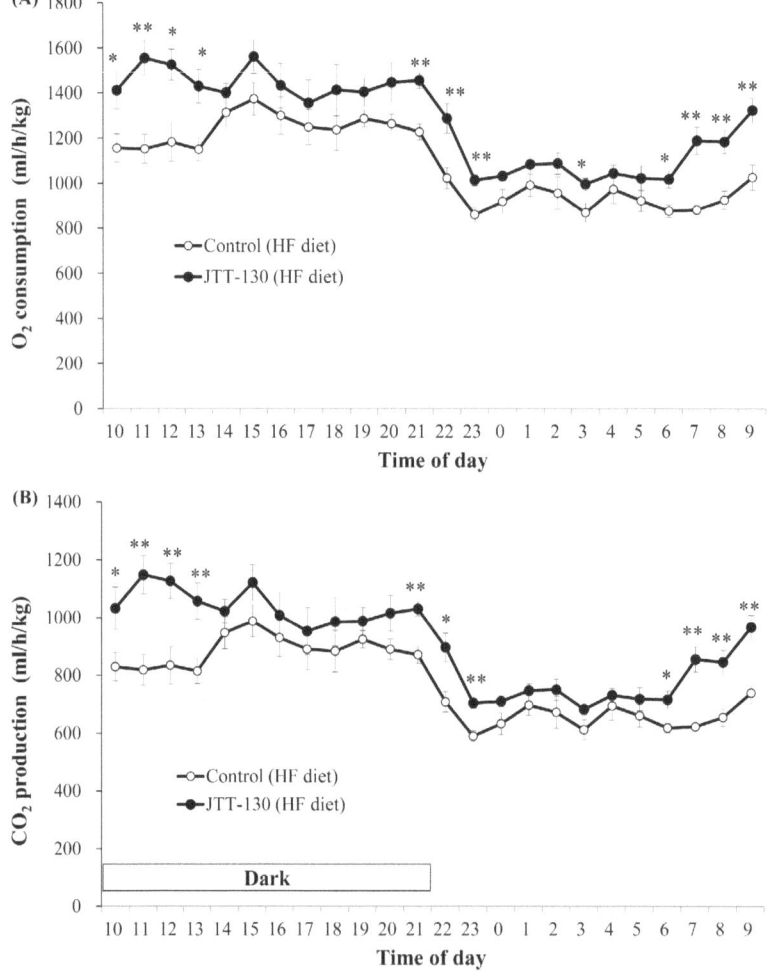

Fig. (17). Effects of JTT-130 on energy expenditure in Sprague-Dawley rats on a 35% fat diet were evaluated using indirect calorimetry after 4 weeks of treatment.

Furthermore, JTT-130 treatment has been reported as ameliorating impaired glucose and lipid metabolism in ZDF rats [197], and attenuating dyslipidemia in hyperlipidemic hamsters and rabbits. Intestine-specific MTP inhibitors are expected to be useful for the treatment of diabetes or atherosclerosis as well as obesity.

DGAT1 Inhibitor

Acyl CoA: diacylglycerol acyltransferase 1 (DGAT1) is an enzyme that catalyzes the final step of TG synthesis, *i.e.*, synthesis of triglycerides from diacylglycerol and fatty acyl-CoA. DGAT1 is expressed in various organs, and is especially highly expressed in the small intestine, fat tissue and testes [198]. The enzyme is involved in TG absorption from the small intestine and fat accumulation in adipose tissues [199, 200]. Indeed, DGAT1-knockout (-/-) mice showed resistance to the anti-obesity effects of a high-fat diet; wherein body weight gain suppressed, fat weight and hepatic TG contents decreased, and energy consumption in the liver and skeletal muscles accelerated, improvements in insulin and leptin resistance, in comparison with wild-type mice were observed [201]. Since the inhibition of DGAT1 is expected to result in two kinds of pharmacological effects; (1) inhibition of fat absorption in the intestine, (2) inhibition of fat synthesis in adipose tissues, DGAT1 inhibitors are likely to become a good therapeutic option for obesity. Tomimoto *et al.* reported anti-obesity effects with JTT-553, which was discovered as a novel DGAT1 inhibitor (Fig. **18**) [202]. First, the effects of JTT-553 on fat absorption were investigated through the measurement of plasma TG after olive oil loading in Sprague-Dawley rats.

Fig. (18). Chemical structure of DGAT1 inhibitor, JTT-553.

Plasma TG in the JTT-553 administration group decreased in a dose-dependent manner (Fig. **19**). In adipose tissues, JTT-553 also suppressed TG synthesis from radiolabeled free fatty acid in a dose-dependent manner (Fig. **20**). Anti-obesity effects were investigated in Sprague-Dawley rats fed a 35% fat diet. Body weight and visceral fat in the JTT-553 administration group decreased dose-dependently; however, the suppressive effects of JTT-553 on body weight were not observed with the 3.1% fat diet. Interestingly, the anti-feeding effects of JTT-553 were observed in rats fed a 35% fat diet, which was not observed in DGAT1-knockout (-/-) mice. A single administration of JTT-553 decreased food consumption depending on dietary fat content. The difference in appetite between DGAT1 inhibitor-treated and knockout mice remains unknown. The DGAT1 inhibitor was considered to suppress food consumption *via* the elevation of levels of gut hormones, such as glucagon-like peptide-1 (GLP-1), in plasma [203]. Furthermore, JTT-553 was administrated to B6D2F1 mice fed a 35% fat diet and anti-diabetic effects and anti-obesity effects were investigated at the same time. JTT-553 decreased body weight and food consumption, and treatment resulted in improvements in hyperinsulinemia and hyperlipidemia. In the glucose tolerance test, JTT-553 treatment resulted in ameliorations of insulin resistance. In addition, JTT-553 treatment resulted in significant reductions in fat mass, and increased glucose utilization of epididymal adipose tissues in the presence of insulin.

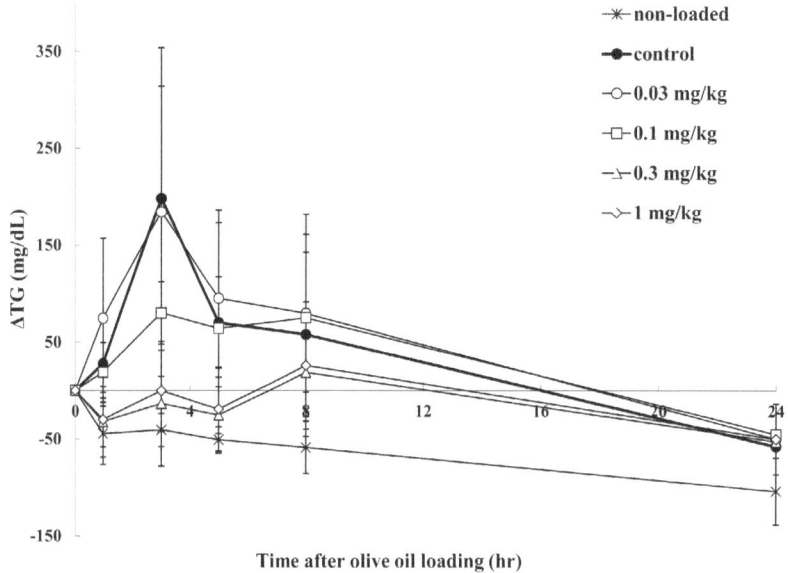

Fig. (19). Effects of JTT-553 on fat absorption in the small intestine.

There are some clinical reports of DGAT1 inhibitors, such as PF-04620110, AZD7687 and LCQ908 [17, 204, 205]. Denison *et al.* reported results from a clinical study in which healthy subjects received several doses (1-60 mg) of AZD7687 with 30, 45 and 60% fat energy content diet [206]. AZD7687 single-agent treatment reduced postprandial plasma TG levels dose-dependently in subjects given a 60% fat energy content diet. This effect on postprandial plasma

TG levels was not observed in subjects given a 30 and 45% fat energy content diet. There were no serious adverse events observed up to the highest dose. However, gastrointestinal adverse events, such as nausea, vomiting, and diarrhea, increased with the dose of AZD7687 administered with a 60% fat energy content diet. Because of this gastrointestinal intolerability, the dose escalation of AZD7687 was limited in subjects. The incidence of gastrointestinal adverse events was related to both the dose of the DGAT1 inhibitor and dietary fat content. The inhibition of fat absorption with DGAT inhibitors is considered to increase fatty acid and glycerides in the small intestine. The presence of fatty acid and glycerides in the gastrointestinal tract may be hypothesized as causing gastrointestinal adverse events. Similar adverse events were also observed in clinical studies of LCQ908. Therefore, DGAT1 inhibitors are expected to be used as an anti-obesity drug, if the hurdle with gastrointestinal adverse events can be overcome.

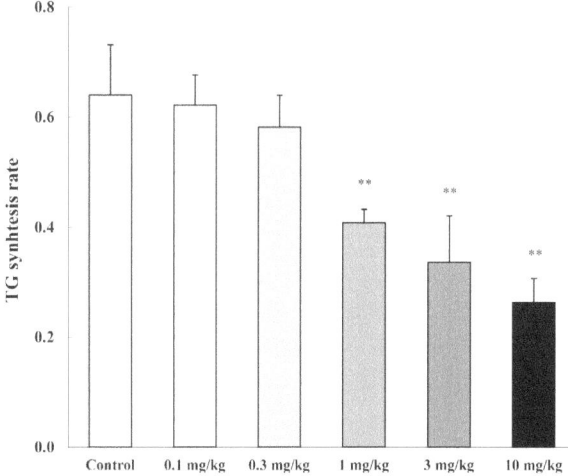

Fig. (20). Effect of JTT-553 on TG synthesis in mouse epididymal adipose tissue.

MGAT2 Inhibitor

Acyl CoA: monoacylglycerol acyltransferase (MGAT) 2 is an enzyme that catalyzes the esterification of monoacylglycerol, *i.e.*, synthesis of diglycerides from monoacylglycerol and fatty acyl-CoA [207, 208]. The genes encoding three MGATs, MGAT1, MGAT2, and MGAT3 have been identified [207, 209, 210]. MGAT1 is mainly expressed in the heart, lung, skeletal muscle and pancreas, but not in the small intestine. Both MGAT2 and MGAT3 are mainly expressed in human small intestine, whereas only MGAT2 is expressed in mouse small intestine [207].

MGAT2 is involved in the resynthesis of TG in the intestine, and plays an important role in the assembly and secretion of chylomicrons. In fact, MGAT2 KO mice demonstrated reduced fat uptake in the small intestine and delays in the absorption of fat into circulation [211]. In addition, the elevation of postprandial GLP-1 and not PYY levels were observed in MGAT2 KO mice fed a high-fat diet [212]. The chronic function of MGAT2 on metabolic disorders was investigated using MGAT2 KO mice. MGAT2 deficient mice were protected from high-fat diet-induced obesity and glucose intolerance [213]. Moreover, MGAT2 deficiency resulted in increased metabolic rates, decreased food consumption, and protection from obesity in genetically obese Agouti mice, suggesting that MGAT2 regulates energy balance [213 - 215]. The intestinal function of MGAT2 and the effect of this function on obesity were also investigated using intestine-specific MGAT2 KO mice [216]. Intestinal-specific deletion of MGAT2 altered TG metabolism in the small intestine and delayed fat absorption. These mice were protected from obesity and impaired glucose metabolism when fed a high-fat diet. Thus, there is considerable interest that inhibition of MGAT2 is a feasible target for obesity and other metabolic disorders caused by excess dietary calories. Although the physiological role of MGAT2 has been mainly investigated using genetically modified mice, the detailed pharmacological characteristics of MGAT2 inhibitors have not been reported. Recently, Okuma *et al.* reported the pharmacological profile of JTP-103237 (Fig. **21**), which was discovered as a novel MGAT2 inhibitor [217]. A single administration of JTT-103237 reduced plasma TG after lipid loading. In addition, JTT-103237 increased monoacylglycerol and fatty acid content, which are MGAT2 substrates, in the small intestine (Fig. **22**). A single administration of JTT-103237 tended to elevate plasma levels of glucagon-like peptide-1 (GLP-1) and peptide YY (PYY) after olive oil loading, and the anti-feeding effect of JTT-103237 was observed dependent of dietary fat content. After repeated dosing, JTT-103237 reduced body weight, fat weight and food consumption, and increased energy expenditure in high-fat diet fed mice. Furthermore, JTT-103237 improved glucose tolerance in diet-induced obese mice. Using JTT-103237, the role of hepatic MGAT2 activity was investigated in high sucrose very low fat diet (HSVLF) fed mice. The fat content of this diet is only 2.6% cal. The influence on reducing fat absorption with MGAT2 inhibitors was considered to be trivial. JTT-103237 reduced hepatic steatosis in HSVLF fed mice, through the suppression of TG synthesis related genes, such as SREBP-1c, fatty acid synthesis, and SCD-1 (Fig. **23**). The inhibition of hepatic MGAT2 activity is considered to directly reduce hepatic TG synthesis. From these findings, MGAT2 inhibition may prove to be a useful strategy target for treating obesity and related metabolic disorders.

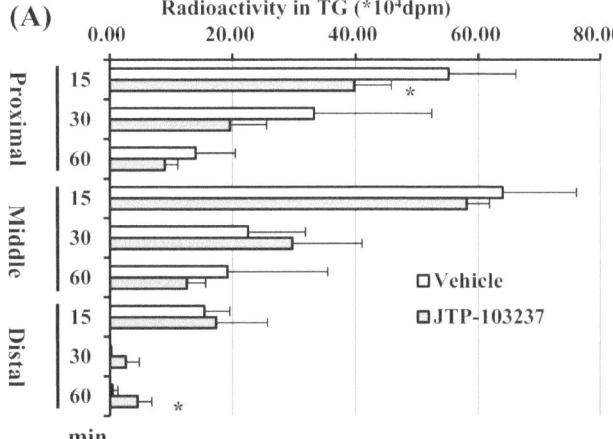

Fig. (21). Chemical structure of MGAT2 inhibitor, JTT-103237.

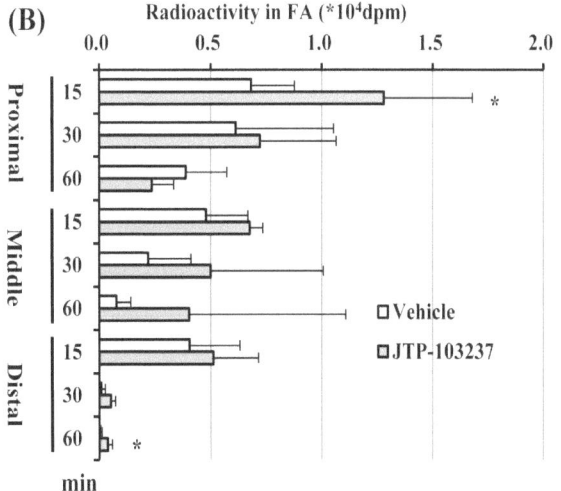

Fig. (22). Distribution of lipids in each segment of the small intestine after administration of lipid emulsions containing ^{14}C triolein in JTP-103237 treated mice. **A**: triglyceride content, **B**: fatty acid content.

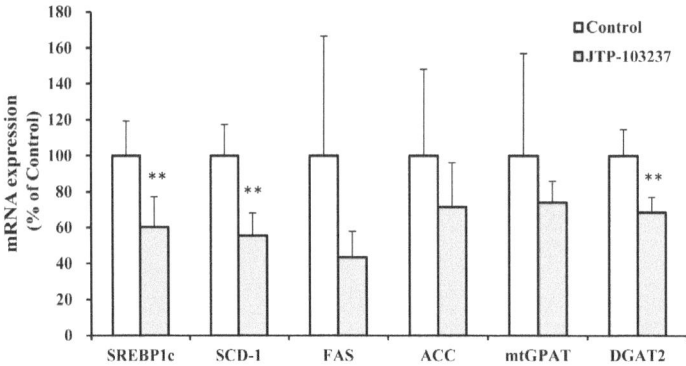

Fig. (23). Lipogenic gene expressions of liver in JTP-103237 treated mice.

Anti-Diabetic Drugs

There have been numerous reports in which anti-diabetic drugs showed effective potential for weight loss. Anti-obesity effects with protein tyrosine phosphatase 1B (PTP1B) inhibitors or sodium glucose cotransporter 2 (SGLT2) inhibitors are described below.

PTP1B Inhibitor

PTP1B is a 50-KD cytosolic tyrosine dephosphorylase consisting of 435 amino acids that are ubiquitously expressed in organs throughout the body. Originally, PTP1B was known to dephosphorylate phosphorylated insulin receptor (IR) β subunit and IR substrate in order to negatively regulate insulin signal transmission [218, 219]. PTP1B is also reportedly related to the negative regulation of leptin signal transmission and to the dephosphorylation of phosphorylated signal transducers and activators of transcription 3 (STAT3) [220, 221]. PTP1B KO mice were protected from diet-induced obesity, and neuronal PTP1B KO mice also showed increased leptin signaling in the hypothalamus, reductions in feeding, body weight and adiposity, and increases in energy expenditure [222, 223]. Ito *et al.* reported the anti-obesity effects of JTT-551, which was developed as a novel PTP1B inhibitor [20, 224].

First, a single administration of JTT-551 at a dose of 100 mg/kg was administered to DIO mice with or without leptin. Food intake in the JTT-551 administration group without leptin treatment did not result in the reduction; however, food intake in the JTT-551 group with leptin treatment resulted in significant reductions compared with that in the control group with leptin (Fig. **24**). STAT3 phosphorylation in the hypothalamus after administration of leptin and JTT-551 also increased.

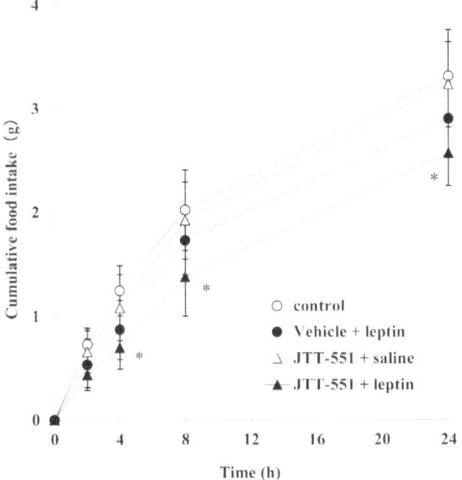

Fig. (24). Acute effects of JTT-551 on food intake in C57BL/6J mice on a 35% fat diet.

Moreover, eight-week-old DIO mice were given 10 or 100 mg/kg of JTT-551 contained in food for 6 weeks and chronic effects were investigated. In the JTT-551 100 m/kg group, cumulative calorie intake tended to decrease from 2 weeks after treatment and significantly decreased from 6 weeks after treatment (Fig. **25A**). Body weight with JTT-551 treatment tended to decrease dose-dependently and the decreases in the JTT-551 100 mg/kg group were significant from 5 to 6 weeks after treatment (Fig. **25B**).

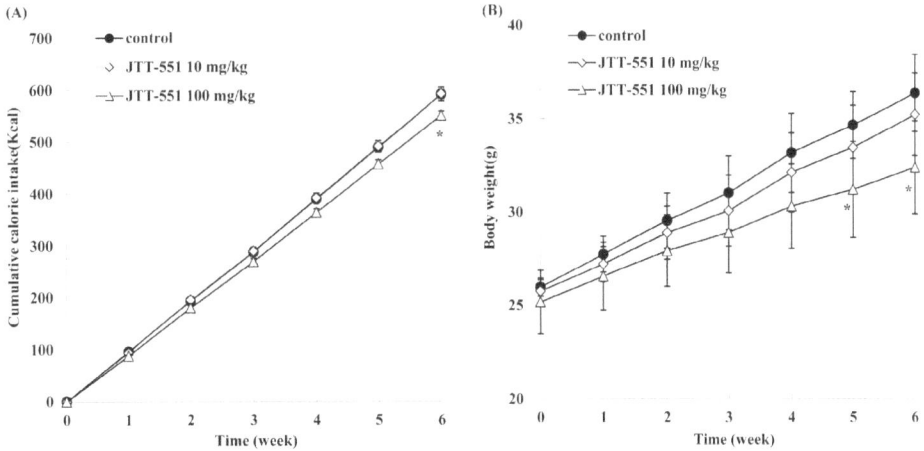

Fig. (25). Chronic effects of JTT-551 on food intake and body weight in C57BL/6J mice on a 35% fat diet.

In addition to the anorectic and the anti-obesity effects, JTT-551 chronic treatment resulted in improvements in glucose and lipid disorders, such as hyperglycemia, hyperlipidemia, hyperinsulinemia, and hyperleptinemia [20]. The anorectic and weight loss effects in DIO rats are shown in Fig. (**26**) Seven-wee- -old DIO rats were given 100 or 300 mg/kg JTT-551 contained in food for 9 weeks and effects were compared with pioglitazone treatment. The JTT-551 treatment group showed dose-dependent reductions in food intake and body weight gain, while the pioglitazone treatment group showed a tendency toward increases in food intake and body weight.

PTP1B is a unique target that shows not only improvements in glucose metabolism but also anti-obesity effects, possibly through the enhancement of leptin signaling.

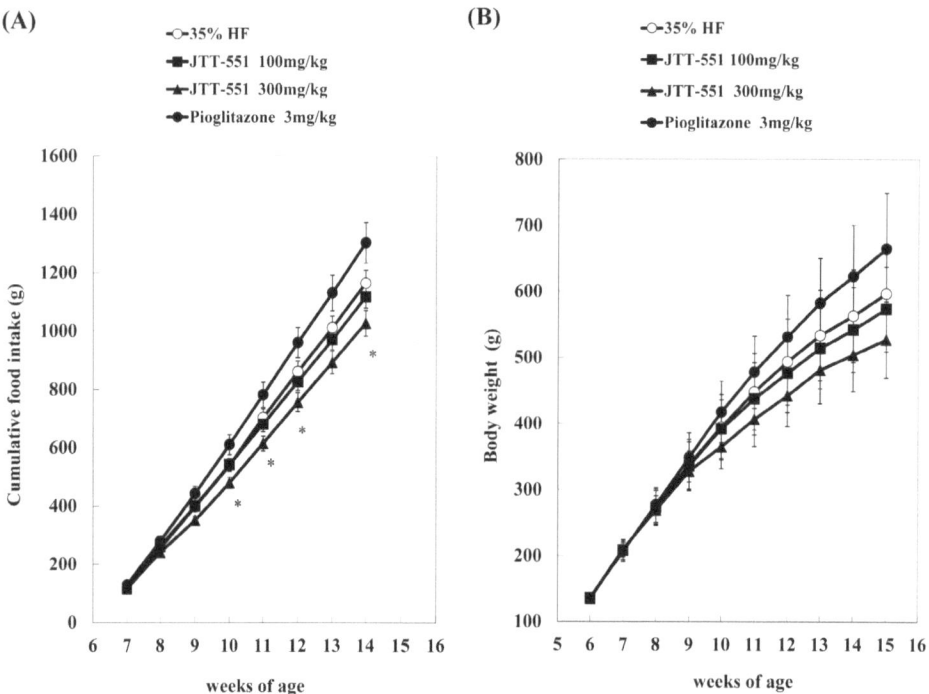

Fig. (26). Chronic effects of JTT-551 on food intake and body weight in Sprague-Dawley rats on a 35% fat diet.

SGLT2 Inhibitors

SGLT2 inhibitors are drugs for the treatment of type 2 diabetes, and canagliflozin became the first SGLT2 inhibitor to be approved in the U.S. in 2013 [225, 226]. SGLT2 is responsible for at least 90% of glucose reabsorption in the kidney and blocking this transporter causes about 50-80 g/day of blood glucose to be eliminated through urine, corresponding to 200-300 kcal. There are some clinical reports in which SGLT2 inhibitors, such as dapagliflozin and empagliflozin, showed anti-obesity effects [227 - 229]. Bolinder *et al.* reported results from a clinical study in which dapagliflozin at a dose of 10 mg/day or placebo was added to open-label metformin for 24 weeks. At 24 weeks, placebo-corrected changes with dapagliflozin were as follows: total body weight; -2.08 kg; waist circumference, -1.52 cm; total-body fat mass, -1.48 kg; visceral adipose tissue, -258.4 cm^3; subcutaneous adipose tissue, -184.9 cm^3. In dapagliflozin *vs.* placebo groups, serious adverse effects were reported in 6.6 *vs.* 1.1% of patients; events suggestive of vulvovaginitis, balanitis, and related genital infection in 3.3 *vs.* 0% of patients; and lower urinary tract infections in 6.6 *vs.* 2.2% of patients, respectively. Moreover, the anti-obesity effects of SGLT2 inhibitors, such as dapagliflozin, tofogliflozin, and canagliflozin, were investigated in basic research studies [230 - 232]. Dapagliflozin at doses of 0.5-5 mg/kg was administered to DIO rats with or without ad libitum access to food for 38 days. Along with inducing urinary glucose excretion, chronic treatment resulted in dose-dependent increases in food and water intake relative to control group. Despite this phenomenon, dapagliflozin treatment reduced body weight by 4% at the high dose group compared with the control group. These data suggest that, in rodents, persistent urinary glucose excretion induced by dapagliflozin was accompanied by compensatory hyperphagia, which attenuated the weight loss induced by SGLT2 inhibition. SGLT2 inhibitor-induced weight loss could be enhanced with dietary intervention.

Future Prospects

Obesity is the consequence of an imbalance between energy intake and energy expenditure, and basic therapies for obesity are appropriate dietary restriction to decrease energy intake and effective exercise to increase energy consumption. However, maintaining these lifestyle modifications, such as diet therapy and exercise, are difficult and therapeutic effects are limited. Medical therapy then becomes a pivotal step and several drug types that target various mechanisms, such as increased satiety with anorexia, inhibition of nutritional absorption, and acceleration of energy consumption, have been developed. Combination therapies, including Qsymia and Contrave, demonstrate the recent tendency for development of anti-obesity drugs. Advantages with combination therapy include the alleviation of side effects and the reinforcement of pharmacological effects and, in the future, the number of combination therapies are expected to increase further. MTP inhibitors reportedly not only suppress food intake but also reduce food preference for fat [233]. Developing a drug for modification of food preference in obesity patients is therefore an interesting concept. Moreover, obesity, in particular visceral obesity, is important for the development of metabolic syndromes, and drugs that can chiefly decrease visceral fat along with affecting weight loss are useful in the development of anti-obesity drugs. As such, a better understanding of the underlying molecular mechanisms in the regulation of obesity and distribution of body weight is essential. Brown adipose tissues are known to dissipate energy through heat and are known to function as protection against cold and obesity. Peroxisome proliferator-activated receptor (PPAR) γ ligands have been shown to induce browning of white adipose tissue. Ohno *et al.* recently reported that PPARγ agonist rosiglitazone induced a white-to-brown fat conversion through the stabilization of the PR domain containing (PRDM) 16 protein [234]. Identifying compounds that stabilize PRDM16 protein may represent a plausible therapeutic pathway for the treatment of obesity. Numerous anti-obesity drugs were withdrawn from the market because of adverse effects observed with treatment; however, a tremendous amount of research to develop novel anti-obesity drugs is still ongoing.

Obesity Animal Models

To help develop new anti-obesity therapies, including the discovery of novel drugs, it is important to elucidate the complex mechanisms of obesity. In particular, investigations using obese animal models are essential to clarify the pathophysiology and develop new anti-obesity drugs. We will first introduce the characteristics of genetic obese mouse models; Lep^{ob} mutant (ob/ob) mouse, $Lepr^{db}$ mutant (db/db) mouse, *kk-A^y* mouse, Tsumura Suzuki Obese Diabetes (TSOD) mouse, and obese rat models, as well as the Spontaneously Diabetic Torii (SDT) fatty rat, Zucker Fatty (ZF) rat, Zucker Diabetic Fatty (ZDF) rat, Spontaneously Hypertensive rats (SHR)/NDmcr-cp (cp/cp) rat (SHR/NDcp), and Wistar Bonn/Kobori (WBN/Kob) fatty rat (Table **4**). We will also introduce the characteristics of non-genetic animal models, such as diet-induced obese (DIO) models.

Table 4. Genetic obese models on the market.

	Commercial name	Notes
Mouse	ob/ob (Type 2 diabetes, obesity)	Lep^{ob} (Leptin deficiency)
	db/db (Type 2 diabetes, obesity)	$Lepr^{db}$ (Leptin receptor dysfunction)
	KKA^y (Type 2 diabetes, obesity)	A^y (Yellow obese gene)
	TSOD (Type 2 diabetes, obesity)	Established by Suzuki *et al.* in 1992

(Table 4) contd.....

	Commercial name	**Notes**
Rat	SDT fatty (Type 2 diabetes, obesity)	$Lepr^{fa}$ (Leptin receptor dysfunction) Established by Masuyama *et al.* in 2004
	ZF (Obesity)	$Lepr^{fa}$ (Leptin receptor dysfunction) Insulin resistance without hyperglycemia
	ZDF (Type 2 diabetes, obesity)	$Lepr^{fa}$ (Leptin receptor dysfunction)
	cp/cp (Obesity)	$Lepr^{fa}$ (Leptin receptor dysfunction), Hypertension
	WBN/Kob fatty (Type 2 diabetes, obesity)	$Lepr^{fa}$ (Leptin receptor dysfunction) Established by Akimoto *et al.*

ob/ob Mouse

The first ob/ob mouse was discovered at the Jackson laboratory in a multiple recessive stock in 1949, and the Lep^{ob} mutation was subsequently transferred to the B6 inbred strain background [235]. The gene affected by the Lep^{ob} mutation was identified by positional cloning [236], and the mutation was found to be recessive. Lep^{ob} mutations in B6 background (ob/ob) mice are phenotypically indistinguishable from their unaffected littermates at birth, but gain weight rapidly throughout their lives (body weights at 11 weeks of age; ob/ob mice, 55.1 ± 1.1 g *vs.* lean mice, 26.8 ± 0.7 g). ob/ob mice show obesity, hyperinsulinemia, and relatively mild hyperglycemia. Abnormal adipose tissue enlargement with hyperphagia is observed, *de novo* lipogenesis is markedly enhanced, and hepatic fatty acid synthesis is also increased. Lipolytic defects in adipose tissues are observed, and one of the reasons was considered to be β3-adrenergic receptor dysfunction in white adipose tissues [237].

db/db Mouse

The $Lepr^{db}$ mutation is a recessive mutation on chromosome 4 that was discovered in C57BL KS/J inbred strains in 1966 [238]. The $Lepr^{db}$ mutation was subsequently transferred to the C57BL KS/J inbred strain by backcrossing. db/db mice are similar to ob/ob mice in terms of rapid development of obesity after weaning (body weights at 11 weeks of age; ob/ob mice, 51.0 ± 3.3 g *vs.* lean mice, 31.3 ± 0.4 g); however, the diabetes syndrome is more severe.

KK-A^y Mouse

Kondo *et al.* selected and established numerous mouse strains from native Japanese mice. Among these inbred strains, Nakamura *et al.* found that the KK mouse is spontaneously diabetic. Since diabetes and obesity in KK mice were relatively moderate, Nishimura *et al.* transferred the yellow obese gene (A^y) into KK mice by crossing yellow obese mice with KK mice. The A^y allele was associated phenotypically with yellow fur, hyperphagia, and obesity [239]. This congenic strain of KK mice has been named KK-A^y mouse. In KK-A^y mice, diabetic characteristics, such as obesity, hyperinsulinemia, and hyperglycemia, are observed from a young age (6-8 weeks of age). KK-A^y mice are raised by isolated rearing to prevent injuries from fighting.

TSOD Mouse

By selectively breeding obese ddy strain male mice and using indices of heavy body weight and appearance of urinary glucose, Suzuki *et al.* established two inbred strains in 1992: one with obesity and urinary glucose (TSOD) and the other without (Tsumura Suzuki non obese: TSNO). Male TSOD mice showed diabetic symptoms, such as hyperphagia, polydipsia, obesity, hyperglycemia, hyperlipidemia, and hyperinsulinemia [240, 241].

SDT fatty Rat

In 2004, Masuyama *et al.* established the congenic type 2 diabetic model Spontaneously Diabetic Torii (SDT) fatty rats by introducing the fa allele of the Zucker Fatty rat into the genome of the original SDT rat [242]. SDT fatty rats were transferred to Central Pharmaceutical Research Institute, Japan Tobacco Inc. (Osaka, Japan) and were characterized in detail, such as the occurrence of diabetes and associated complications, by Ohta *et al* [243 - 246]. CLEA Japan (Tokyo, Japan) has received the rights for production and sales from Japan Tobacco Inc., and has distributed this animal model as SDT fatty rats from 2012. SDT fatty rats become overtly obese just after weaning and are distinguishable from normal or original SDT rats (body weights at 4 weeks of age; male SDT fatty rats, 157.8 ± 17.3 g *vs.* male SDT rats, 136.4 ± 12.9 g, body weights at 6 weeks of age; male SDT fatty rats, 282.7 ± 27.3 g *vs.* male SDT rats, 201.1 ± 13.0 g), and show significant polyphagia. SDT fatty rats show hyperglycemia much earlier than original SDT rats and show slightly higher blood glucose levels even after weaning. With the earlier onset of diabetes mellitus, diabetes-associated complications in SDT fatty rats are seen at younger ages. Furthermore, female SDT fatty rats show diabetes and its complications at young ages, and female rats are expected to become an important animal model of type 2 diabetes with obesity, especially for women, for which few models currently exist [247].

ZF Rat

Zucker rats were originally bred to be a genetic model for research on obesity and hypertension. Two types of Zucker rat: a lean Zucker rat, denoted as those with the dominant trait (Fa/Fa) or (Fa/fa); and the characteristically obese Zucker rat (ZF) rat, which is actually a recessive trait (fa/fa) of the leptin receptor [248, 249]. Zucker rats were originally bred to be a genetic model for research on obesity and hypertension. Two types of Zucker rat: a lean Zucker rat, denoted as those with the dominant trait (Fa/Fa) or (Fa/fa); and the characteristically obese Zucker rat (ZF) rat, which is actually a recessive trait (fa/fa) of the leptin receptor

ZDF Rat

ZDF rats derived from the ZF strain exhibit obesity with diabetes. Characteristics of the male ZDF rat maintained on Purina5008 diet include hyperinsulinemia, hyperglycemia, insulin resistance, and obesity beginning at 6-7 weeks of age [245, 250, 251]. By 10-12 weeks of age, blood glucose levels steadily increase, reaching an average of approximately 500 mg/dl. Since ZDF rats develop diabetes, the degree of obesity in ZDF rats is mild compared with that in ZF rats (body weights at 9 weeks of age; ZDF rats, 314.3 ± 10.7 g vs. ZF rats, 414.6 ± 19.2 g vs. lean rats, 277.6 ± 11.9 g, body weights at 13 weeks of age; ZDF rats, 388.3 ± 17.7 g vs. ZF rats, 572.5 ± 33.2 g vs. lean rats, 352.0 ± 15.8 g).

cp/cp Rat

cp/cp rats spontaneously develop obesity and hypertension, and show dyslipidemia and hyperglycemia, the body weight, systolic blood pressure, serum TG and blood glucose levels in cp/cp rats being 1.43, 1.65, 25.4 and 1.25-fold, respectively, of results in control rats, Wistar Kyoto rats at 19 or 20 weeks of age [252]. Hypertensive rats that spontaneously developed as a colony from normotensive Wistar Kyoto rats were named SHR [253]. By crossing SHR with Sprague-Dawley rats, obese and spontaneously hypertensive rats, the Koletsky strain, were obtained. This strain of rats is heterozygous for the *cp* gene [254]. To eliminate the noncorpulent genes of the Koletsky strain, rats were mated with SHR, and a congenic rat strain (SHR/National Institutes of Health (NIH)-corpulent) was developed [255]. In brief, cp/cp rats are a substrain of SHR/NIH-corpulent rats.

WBN/Kob fatty Rat

The WBN/Kob fatty rat is a new congenic strain for the fa allele of the leptin receptor gene, and the homozygous rat provides a model for type 2 diabetes with obesity [256 - 258]. At 7 weeks of age, both male and female WBN/Kob fatty rats show inflammatory cell infiltration of the pancreas, suggesting pan-pancreatitis and impaired glucose tolerance. At 3 months of age, both male and female rats develop overt diabetes associated with severe chronic pancreatitis.

DIO Models

The Diet-induced obesity (DIO) animal model was a model created to study obesity and associated co-morbidities, such as insulin resistance, type 2 diabetes, dyslipidemia, hypertension, and atherosclerosis. In this model, an animal is fed a high-fat diet or high-fat/high-sucrose or fructose diet for a longer period of time. Accordingly, the animals become obese and have several glucose and lipid metabolic abnormalities, such as impaired glucose tolerance, increased fasting glucose level, hyperlipidemia, and hyperinsulinemia. DIO models have become one of the most important tools for understanding the relationship between high-calorie Western diets and the development of obesity [259]. In recent years, Western diet-loaded genetic animal models have been investigated to elucidate the pathophysiology of obesity-related diseases, including nonalcoholic fatty liver disease (NAFLD)/nonalcoholic steatohepatitis (NASH) and pancreatic lesions with diabetes, as well as to develop new therapies for these diseases [260 - 263].

We have also investigated the pathophysiology of Western diet-loaded SDT fatty rats. Female SDT fatty rats (Torii, Tokyo, Japan) were divided into two groups at 5 weeks of age, a control group (CRF-1 group) and a high-fat/sucrose diet group (HFS group). Rats in the control group were fed a standard diet (CRF-1, Charles River Japan, Yokohama, Japan), and rats in the HFS group were fed a high-fat/sucrose diet (47.7% fat and 20.7% sucrose, based on the percentage of total calories, D12468, Research Diets Inc., New Brunswick, NJ), from 5 to 16 weeks of age. Consequently, we observed deterioration to diabetes, dyslipidemia, and visceral obesity in HFS diet-loaded SDT fatty rats. HFS group gained less weight compared to CRF-1group (Fig. **27A**). Calorie intake in the HFS group was higher than intake in the CRF-1 group at 8 and 12 weeks of age; however, intake at 16 weeks of age decreased (Fig. **27B**). Serum glucose level in the HFS group significantly increased at 8 weeks of age compared with results in the CRF-1 group (HFS group, 936.2 ± 45.7 mg/dl *vs*. CRF-1 group, 564.0 ± 101.4 mg/dl) (Fig. **27C**). Serum insulin levels in the HFS group significantly decreased at 8 weeks of age compared with results in the CRF-1 group (HFS group, 9.3 ± 3.2 ng/ml *vs*. CRF-1 group, 24.6 ± 4.2 ng/ml), and insulin levels tended to decrease from 12 to 16 weeks of age (Fig. **27D**). Serum TG levels in the HFS group significantly increased during the experimental period, and a sustained increase in TC levels was observed in the HFS group (Fig. **27E, F**).

Moreover, visceral and subcutaneous fat tissue weights in each rat were determined at 15 weeks of age by computed tomography (CT). Fat weight was measured using a laboratory X-ray CT device (LATheta, ALOKA Co., LTD., Osaka, Japan). Visceral fat tissue weight in the HFS group significantly increased compared with weight in the CRF-1 group (Table **5**). Total fat tissue weight in the

HFS group also significantly increased. Subcutaneous fat tissue weight and V/S ratio tended to increase in the HFS group, but this increase was not significant.

Table 5. Fat tissue weights in CRF-1 and HFS diets. Visceral and subcutaneous fat tissue weights were determined by computed tomography.

	Visceral fat (g)	Subcutaneous fat (g)	Total fat (g)	V/S ratio
CRF-1	75.6 ± 2.7	75.6 ± 7.7	151.3 ± 8.2	1.01 ± 0.11
HFS	88.8 ± 3.2**	81.5 ± 3.0	170.3 ± 5.1**	1.09 ± 0.05

Data represent the mean ± standard deviation (n=5). ** $p<0.01$ vs. CRF-1

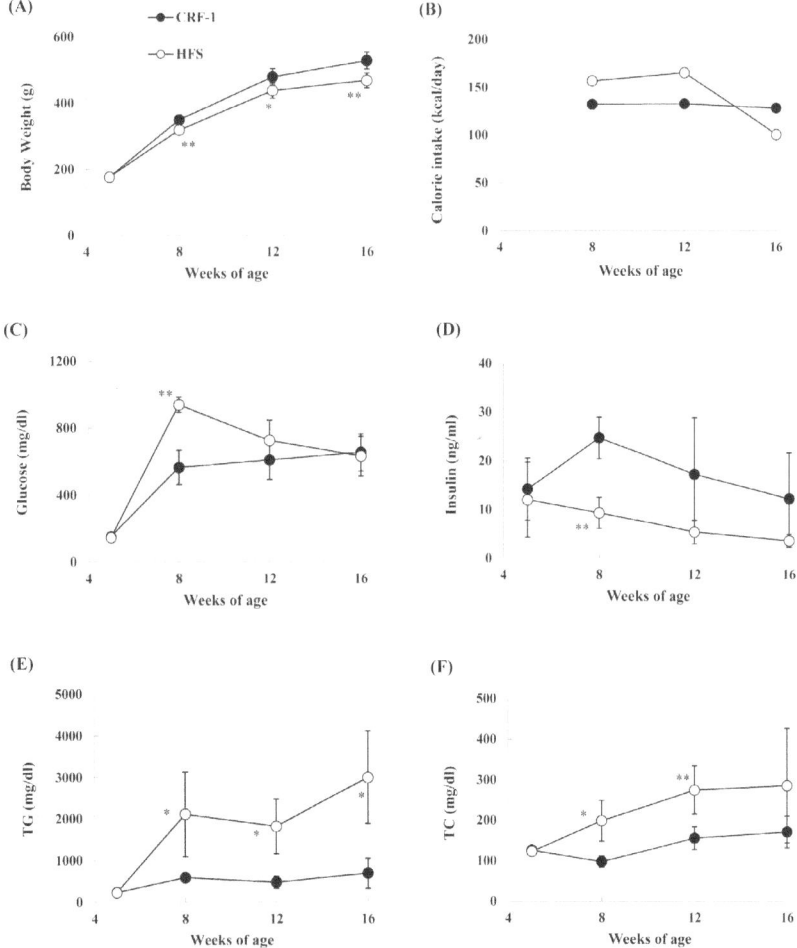

Fig. (27). Changes in body weight (**A**), caloric intake (**B**), and serum glucose (**C**), insulin (**D**), triglyceride (TG) (**E**), and total cholesterol (TC) (**F**) levels in SDT fatty rats fed a standard diet (CRF-1 group) or a high-fat/sucrose diet (HFS group).

A high-fat/sucrose diet in female SDT fatty rats accelerated hyperglycemia, hyperlipidemia, and fat storage. Western diet-loaded genetic models are considered useful for the investigation of the development of glucose and lipid metabolic abnormalities with obesity.

CONFLICT OF INTEREST

Chihiro Okuma, Yukihito Ishii, and Takeshi Ohta are employees of Japan Tobacco Inc.

ACKNOWLEDGEMENTS

Declared none.

REFERENCES

[1] Henry RR, Chilton R, Garvey WT. New options for the treatment of obesity and type 2 diabetes mellitus (narrative review). J Diabetes Complications 2013; 27(5): 508-18.
[http://dx.doi.org/10.1016/j.jdiacomp.2013.04.011] [PMID: 23726071]

[2] Boulghassoul-Pietrzykowska N, Franceschelli J, Still C. New medications for obesity management: changing the landscape of obesity treatment. Curr Opin Endocrinol Diabetes Obes 2013; 20(5): 407-11.
[http://dx.doi.org/10.1097/01.med.0000433059.78485.fa] [PMID: 23974768]

[3] Mahgerefteh B, Vigue M, Freestone Z, Silver S, Nguyen Q. New drug therapies for the treatment of overweight and obese patients. Am Health Drug Benefits 2013; 6(7): 423-30.
[PMID: 24991373]

[4] Millward DJ. Energy balance and obesity: a UK perspective on the gluttony v. sloth debate. Nutr Res Rev 2013; 26(2): 89-109.
[http://dx.doi.org/10.1017/S095442241300005X] [PMID: 23750809]

[5] Fock KM, Khoo J. Diet and exercise in management of obesity and overweight. J Gastroenterol Hepatol 2013; 28 (Suppl. 4): 59-63.
[http://dx.doi.org/10.1111/jgh.12407] [PMID: 24251706]

[6] Colquitt JL, Pickett K, Loveman E, Frampton GK. Surgery for weight loss in adults. Cochrane Database Syst Rev 2014; 8(8): CD003641.
[PMID: 25105982]

[7] Kushner RF. Weight loss strategies for treatment of obesity. Prog Cardiovasc Dis 2014; 56(4): 465-72.
[http://dx.doi.org/10.1016/j.pcad.2013.09.005] [PMID: 24438739]

[8] Kim GW, Lin JE, Blomain ES, Waldman SA. New advances in models and strategies for developing anti-obesity drugs. Expert Opin Drug Discov 2013; 8(6): 655-71.
[http://dx.doi.org/10.1517/17460441.2013.792804] [PMID: 23621300]

[9] Mori Y. Mazindol. Nihon Rinsho 2011; 69 (Suppl. 1): 683-6.
[PMID: 21766681]

[10] Finkelstein MS, Mandell GA, Tarbell KV. Hypertrophic pyloric stenosis: volumetric measurement of nasogastric aspirate to determine the imaging modality. Radiology 1990; 177(3): 759-61.
[http://dx.doi.org/10.1148/radiology.177.3.2243984] [PMID: 2243984]

[11] McClendon KS, Riche DM, Uwaifo GI. Orlistat: current status in clinical therapeutics. Expert Opin Drug Saf 2009; 8(6): 727-44.
[http://dx.doi.org/10.1517/14740330903321485] [PMID: 19998527]

[12] Simonyi G, Pados G, Medvegy M, Bedros JR. The pharmacological treatment of obesity: past, present and future. Orv Hetil 2012; 153(10): 363-73.
[http://dx.doi.org/10.1556/OH.2012.29317] [PMID: 22370224]

[13] Shyh G, Cheng-Lai A. New antiobesity agents: lorcaserin (Belviq) and phentermine/topiramate ER (Qsymia). Cardiol Rev 2014; 22(1): 43-50.
[http://dx.doi.org/10.1097/CRD.0000000000000001] [PMID: 24304809]

[14] Nigro SC, Luon D, Baker WL. Lorcaserin: a novel serotonin 2C agonist for the treatment of obesity. Curr Med Res Opin 2013; 29(7): 839-48.
[http://dx.doi.org/10.1185/03007995.2013.794776] [PMID: 23574263]

[15] Li J, Bronk BS, Dirlam JP, *et al.* In vitro and in vivo profile of 5-[(4-trifluoromethyl-biphen-l-2-carbonyl)-amino]-1H-indole-2-carboxylic acid benzylmethyl carbamoylamide (dirlotapide), a novel potent MTP inhibitor for obesity. Bioorg Med Chem Lett 2007; 17(7): 1996-9.
[http://dx.doi.org/10.1016/j.bmcl.2007.01.018] [PMID: 17276061]

[16] Yamamoto T, Yamaguchi H, Miki H, *et al.* Coenzyme A: diacylglycerol acyltransferase 1 inhibitor ameliorates obesity, liver steatosis, and lipid metabolism abnormality in KKAy mice fed high-fat or high-carbohydrate diets. Eur J Pharmacol 2010; 640(1-3): 243-9.
[http://dx.doi.org/10.1016/j.ejphar.2010.04.050] [PMID: 20478303]

[17] Birch AM, Buckett LK, Turnbull AV. DGAT1 inhibitors as anti-obesity and anti-diabetic agents. Curr Opin Drug Discov Devel 2010; 13(4): 489-96.
[PMID: 20597032]

[18] Hata T, Mera Y, Tadaki H, *et al.* JTT-130, a novel intestine-specific inhibitor of microsomal triglyceride transfer protein, suppresses high fat diet-induced obesity and glucose intolerance in Sprague-Dawley rats. Diabetes Obes Metab 2011; 13(5): 446-54.
[http://dx.doi.org/10.1111/j.1463-1326.2011.01368.x] [PMID: 21255216]

[19] Cho H. Protein tyrosine phosphatase 1B (PTP1B) and obesity. Vitam Horm 2013; 91: 405-24.
[http://dx.doi.org/10.1016/B978-0-12-407766-9.00017-1] [PMID: 23374726]

[20] Ito M, Fukuda S, Sakata S, Morinaga H, Ohta T. Pharmacological effects of JTT-551, a novel protein tyrosine phosphatase 1B inhibitor, in diet-induced obesity mice. J Diabetes Res 2014; 2014: 680348.
[http://dx.doi.org/10.1155/2014/680348]

[21] Bays H, Dujovne C. Pharmacotherapy of obesity: currently marketed and upcoming agents. Am J Cardiovasc Drugs 2002; 2(4): 245-53.
[http://dx.doi.org/10.2165/00129784-200202040-00004] [PMID: 14727970]

[22] Bray GA. Drug Insight: appetite suppressants. Nat Clin Pract Gastroenterol Hepatol 2005; 2(2): 89-95.
[http://dx.doi.org/10.1038/ncpgasthep0092] [PMID: 16265126]

[23] Barak LS, Salahpour A, Zhang X, *et al.* Pharmacological characterization of membrane-expressed human trace amine-associated receptor 1 (TAAR1) by a bioluminescence resonance energy transfer cAMP biosensor. Mol Pharmacol 2008; 74(3): 585-94.
[http://dx.doi.org/10.1124/mol.108.048884] [PMID: 18524885]

[24] Halpern A, Mancini MC. Treatment of obesity: an update on anti-obesity medications. Obes Rev 2003; 4(1): 25-42.
[http://dx.doi.org/10.1046/j.1467-789X.2003.00083.x] [PMID: 12608525]

[25] Ioannides-Demos LL, Proietto J, McNeil JJ. Pharmacotherapy for obesity. Drugs 2005; 65(10): 1391-418.
[http://dx.doi.org/10.2165/00003495-200565100-00006] [PMID: 15977970]

[26] Munro JF, MacCuish AC, Wilson EM, Duncan LJ. Comparison of continuous and intermittent anorectic therapy in obesity. BMJ 1968; 1(5588): 352-4.
[http://dx.doi.org/10.1136/bmj.1.5588.352] [PMID: 15508204]

[27] Inoue S. Clinical studies with mazindol. Obes Res 1995; 3 (Suppl. 4): 549S-52S.
[http://dx.doi.org/10.1002/j.1550-8528.1995.tb00226.x] [PMID: 8697057]

[28] Nakazato M. [Current status of medical therapy for obesity and the potential of novel anti-obesity drug development]. Nippon Rinsho 2013; 71(2): 324-8.
[PMID: 23631215]

[29] Sikdar SK, Oomura Y, Inokuchi A. Effects of mazindol on rat lateral hypothalamic neurons. Brain Res Bull 1985; 15(1): 33-8.
[http://dx.doi.org/10.1016/0361-9230(85)90058-9] [PMID: 2411361]

[30] Shiraishi T. [Mazindol effects on the salivary and gastric acid secretory mechanisms]. Nippon Yakurigaku Zasshi 1984; 83(2): 159-72.
[http://dx.doi.org/10.1254/fpj.83.159] [PMID: 6745806]

[31] Nagai K, Mori T, Ookura M, Tsujimoto H, Nakagawa H. Pharmacological action of mazindol on behaviors and metabolism. Nippon Yakurigaku Zasshi 1984; 83(2): 133-45.
[http://dx.doi.org/10.1254/fpj.83.133] [PMID: 6745804]

[32] Usami M, Seino Y, Nishi S, *et al.* Effect of mazindol on insulin and glucagon secretion in ventromedial hypothalamic obese rats. Nippon Yakurigaku Zasshi 1985; 85(4): 297-303.
[http://dx.doi.org/10.1254/fpj.85.297] [PMID: 3891549]

[33] Inoue S, Egawa M, Satoh S. Effects of an anorexiant, mazindol, on metabolic abnormalities of rats with ventromedial hypothalamic lesions. Nippon Yakurigaku Zasshi 1984; 83(5): 441-9.
[http://dx.doi.org/10.1254/fpj.83.441] [PMID: 6469133]

[34] Inoue S, Tsuchiya M, Takamura Y. Effects of mazindol on food intake in ventromedial hypothalamic lesioned rats and glucose absorption in rats. Int J Obes 1987; 11 (Suppl. 3): 63-9.
[PMID: 3440693]

[35] Ohminami K, Matsuoka E, Takahashi Y, Shimizu D, Okuda H. Effect of mazindol on obesity induced by administration of gold thioglucose. Nippon Yakurigaku Zasshi 1984; 83(2): 123-32.
[http://dx.doi.org/10.1254/fpj.83.123] [PMID: 6430760]

[36] Inoue S, Egawa M, Satoh S, *et al.* Clinical and basic aspects of an anorexiant, mazindol, as an antiobesity agent in Japan. Am J Clin Nutr 1992; 55(1) (Suppl.): 199S-202S.
[PMID: 1728834]

[37] Feeney S, Goodall E, Silverstone T. The effects of D- and L-fenfluramine (and their interactions with D-amphetamine) on psychomotor function and mood. Int Clin Psychopharmacol 1996; 11(2): 89-99.
[PMID: 8803646]

[38] Weir EK, Reeve HL, Huang JM, *et al.* Anorexic agents aminorex, fenfluramine, and dexfenfluramine inhibit potassium current in rat pulmonary vascular smooth muscle and cause pulmonary vasoconstriction. Circulation 1996; 94(9): 2216-20.
[http://dx.doi.org/10.1161/01.CIR.94.9.2216] [PMID: 8901674]

[39] Connolly HM, Crary JL, McGoon MD, *et al.* Valvular heart disease associated with fenfluramine-phentermine. N Engl J Med 1997; 337(9): 581-8.
[http://dx.doi.org/10.1056/NEJM199708283370901] [PMID: 9271479]

[40] Weissman NJ. Appetite suppressants and valvular heart disease. Am J Med Sci 2001; 321(4): 285-91.
[http://dx.doi.org/10.1097/00000441-200104000-00008] [PMID: 11307869]

[41] Chhina GS, Kang HK, Singh B, Anand BK. Effect of fenfluramine on the electrical activity of the hypothalamic feeding centers. Physiol Behav 1971; 7(3): 433-8.
[http://dx.doi.org/10.1016/0031-9384(71)90324-6] [PMID: 5000125]

[42] Ioannides-Demos LL, Proietto J, Tonkin AM, McNeil JJ. Safety of drug therapies used for weight loss and treatment of obesity. Drug Saf 2006; 29(4): 277-302.
[http://dx.doi.org/10.2165/00002018-200629040-00001] [PMID: 16569079]

[43] Roth BL. Drugs and valvular heart disease. N Engl J Med 2007; 356(1): 6-9.
[http://dx.doi.org/10.1056/NEJMp068265] [PMID: 17202450]

[44] Rothman RB, Baumann MH. Serotonergic drugs and valvular heart disease. Expert Opin Drug Saf 2009; 8(3): 317-29.
[http://dx.doi.org/10.1517/14740330902931524] [PMID: 19505264]

[45] Levitsky DA, Troiano R. Metabolic consequences of fenfluramine for the control of body weight. Am J Clin Nutr 1992; 55(1) (Suppl.): 167S-72S.
[PMID: 1728828]

[46] Levitsky DA, Schuster JA, Stallone D, Strupp BJ. Modulation of the thermic effect of food by fenfluramine. Int J Obes 1986; 10(3): 169-73.
[PMID: 3759326]

[47] Hudson KD. The anorectic and hypotensive effect of fenfluramine in obesity. J R Coll Gen Pract 1977; 27(181): 497-501.
[PMID: 616838]

[48] Craighead LW, Stunkard AJ, OBrien RM. Behavior therapy and pharmacotherapy for obesity. Arch Gen Psychiatry 1981; 38(7): 763-8.
[http://dx.doi.org/10.1001/archpsyc.1981.01780320043003] [PMID: 7247639]

[49] Sensi S, Della Loggia F, Del Ponte A, Guagnano MT. Long-term treatment with fenfluramine in obese subjects. Int J Clin Pharmacol Res 1985; 5(4): 247-53.
[PMID: 4055167]

[50] Stunkard AJ, Craighead LW, OBrien R. Controlled trial of behaviour therapy, pharmacotherapy, and their combination in the treatment of obesity. Lancet 1980; 2(8203): 1045-7.
[http://dx.doi.org/10.1016/S0140-6736(80)92272-2] [PMID: 6107677]

[51] Douglas JG, Gough J, Preston PG, *et al.* Long-term efficacy of fenfluramine in treatment of obesity. Lancet 1983; 1(8321): 384-6.
[http://dx.doi.org/10.1016/S0140-6736(83)91501-5] [PMID: 6130379]

[52] Guy-Grand B, Apfelbaum M, Crepaldi G, Gries A, Lefebvre P, Turner P. International trial of long-term dexfenfluramine in obesity. Lancet 1989; 2(8672): 1142-5.
[http://dx.doi.org/10.1016/S0140-6736(89)91499-2] [PMID: 2572857]

[53] Guy-Grand B, Apfelbaum M, Crepaldi G, Gries A, Lefebvre P, Turner P. [International study of the effect of dexfenfluramine in obesity (ISIS): 6 months results]. Rev Med Interne 1989; 10(3): 271-7. [International study of the effect of dexfenfluramine in obesity (ISIS): 6 months' results].
[http://dx.doi.org/10.1016/S0248-8663(89)80015-3] [PMID: 2669089]

[54] Finer N, Craddock D, Lavielle R, Keen H. Prolonged weight loss with dexfenfluramine treatment in obese patients. Diabete Metab 1987; 13(6): 598-602.
[PMID: 3329122]

[55] Derosa G, Mugellini A, Ciccarelli L, Fogari R. Randomized, double-blind, placebo-controlled comparison of the action of orlistat, fluvastatin, or both an anthropometric measurements, blood pressure, and lipid profile in obese patients with hypercholesterolemia prescribed a standardized diet. Clin Ther 2003; 25(4): 1107-22.
[http://dx.doi.org/10.1016/S0149-2918(03)80070-X] [PMID: 12809960]

[56] Sjöström L, Rissanen A, Andersen T, *et al.* Randomised placebo-controlled trial of orlistat for weight loss and prevention of weight regain in obese patients. Lancet 1998; 352(9123): 167-72.
[http://dx.doi.org/10.1016/S0140-6736(97)11509-4] [PMID: 9683204]

[57] Hogan S, Fleury A, Hadvary P, *et al.* Studies on the antiobesity activity of tetrahydrolipstatin, a potent and selective inhibitor of pancreatic lipase. Int J Obes 1987; 11 (Suppl. 3): 35-42.
[PMID: 3440690]

[58] Ueshima K, Akihisa-Umeno H, Nagayoshi A, Takakura S, Matsuo M, Mutoh S. A gastrointestinal lipase inhibitor reduces progression of atherosclerosis in mice fed a western-type diet. Eur J Pharmacol 2004; 501(1-3): 137-42.
[http://dx.doi.org/10.1016/j.ejphar.2004.08.014] [PMID: 15464072]

[59] Zaitone SA, Essawy S. Addition of a low dose of rimonabant to orlistat therapy decreases weight gain and reduces adiposity in dietary obese rats. Clin Exp Pharmacol Physiol 2012; 39(6): 551-9.
[http://dx.doi.org/10.1111/j.1440-1681.2012.05717.x] [PMID: 22524969]

[60] Li Z, Maglione M, Tu W, et al. Meta-analysis: pharmacologic treatment of obesity. Ann Intern Med 2005; 142(7): 532-46.
[http://dx.doi.org/10.7326/0003-4819-142-7-200504050-00012] [PMID: 15809465]

[61] Torgerson JS, Hauptman J, Boldrin MN, Sjöström L. XENical in the prevention of diabetes in obese subjects (XENDOS) study: a randomized study of orlistat as an adjunct to lifestyle changes for the prevention of type 2 diabetes in obese patients. Diabetes Care 2004; 27(1): 155-61.
[http://dx.doi.org/10.2337/diacare.27.1.155] [PMID: 14693982]

[62] Rucker D, Padwal R, Li SK, Curioni C, Lau DC. Long term pharmacotherapy for obesity and overweight: updated meta-analysis. BMJ 2007; 335(7631): 1194-9.
[http://dx.doi.org/10.1136/bmj.39385.413113.25] [PMID: 18006966]

[63] Heal DJ, Aspley S, Prow MR, Jackson HC, Martin KF, Cheetham SC. Sibutramine: a novel anti-obesity drug. A review of the pharmacological evidence to differentiate it from d-amphetamine and d-fenfluramine. Int J Obes Relat Metab Disord 1998; 22 (Suppl. 1): S18-28.
[PMID: 9758240]

[64] Hansen DL, Toubro S, Stock MJ, Macdonald IA, Astrup A. Thermogenic effects of sibutramine in humans. Am J Clin Nutr 1998; 68(6): 1180-6.
[PMID: 9846844]

[65] Colman E. Anorectics on trial: a half century of federal regulation of prescription appetite suppressants. Ann Intern Med 2005; 143(5): 380-5.
[http://dx.doi.org/10.7326/0003-4819-143-5-200509060-00013] [PMID: 16144896]

[66] Fernstrom JD, Choi S. The development of tolerance to drugs that suppress food intake. Pharmacol Ther 2008; 117(1): 105-22.
[http://dx.doi.org/10.1016/j.pharmthera.2007.09.001] [PMID: 17950459]

[67] Williams G. Withdrawal of sibutramine in Europe. BMJ 2010; 340: c824.
[http://dx.doi.org/10.1136/bmj.c824] [PMID: 20144986]

[68] Finer N. Sibutramine: its mode of action and efficacy. Int J Obes Relat Metab Disord 2002; 26 (Suppl. 4): S29-33.
[http://dx.doi.org/10.1038/sj.ijo.0802216] [PMID: 12457297]

[69] Garfield AS, Heisler LK. Pharmacological targeting of the serotonergic system for the treatment of obesity. J Physiol 2009; 587(1): 49-60.
[http://dx.doi.org/10.1113/jphysiol.2008.164152] [PMID: 19029184]

[70] Tziomalos K, Krassas GE, Tzotzas T. The use of sibutramine in the management of obesity and related disorders: an update. Vasc Health Risk Manag 2009; 5(1): 441-52.
[http://dx.doi.org/10.2147/VHRM.S4027] [PMID: 19475780]

[71] Schwartz MW, Woods SC, Porte D Jr, Seeley RJ, Baskin DG. Central nervous system control of food intake. Nature 2000; 404(6778): 661-71.
[http://dx.doi.org/10.1038/35007534] [PMID: 10766253]

[72] Jackson HC, Bearham MC, Hutchins LJ, Mazurkiewicz SE, Needham AM, Heal DJ. Investigation of the mechanisms underlying the hypophagic effects of the 5-HT and noradrenaline reuptake inhibitor, sibutramine, in the rat. Br J Pharmacol 1997; 121(8): 1613-8.
[http://dx.doi.org/10.1038/sj.bjp.0701311] [PMID: 9283694]

[73] Brown M, Bing C, King P, Pickavance L, Heal D, Wilding J. Sibutramine reduces feeding, body fat and improves insulin resistance in dietary-obese male Wistar rats independently of hypothalamic neuropeptide Y. Br J Pharmacol 2001; 132(8): 1898-904.
[http://dx.doi.org/10.1038/sj.bjp.0704030] [PMID: 11309262]

[74] Casado A, Rodríguez VM, Portillo MP, et al. Sibutramine decreases body weight gain and increases energy expenditure in obese Zucker rats without changes in NPY and orexins. Nutr Neurosci 2003; 6(2): 103-11.
[http://dx.doi.org/10.1080/1028415031000094264] [PMID: 12722985]

[75] Smith IG, Goulder MA. Sibutramine Clinical Study 1047 Team. Randomized placebo-controlled trial of long-term treatment with sibutramine in mild to moderate obesity. J Fam Pract 2001; 50(6): 505-12.
[PMID: 11407998]

[76] Nisoli E, Carruba MO. An assessment of the safety and efficacy of sibutramine, an anti-obesity drug with a novel mechanism of action. Obes Rev 2000; 1(2): 127-39.
[http://dx.doi.org/10.1046/j.1467-789x.2000.00020.x] [PMID: 12119986]

[77] James WP, Caterson ID, Coutinho W, et al. Effect of sibutramine on cardiovascular outcomes in overweight and obese subjects. N Engl J Med 2010; 363(10): 905-17.
[http://dx.doi.org/10.1056/NEJMoa1003114] [PMID: 20818901]

[78] Christensen R, Kristensen PK, Bartels EM, Bliddal H, Astrup A. Efficacy and safety of the weight-loss drug rimonabant: a meta-analysis of randomised trials. Lancet 2007; 370(9600): 1706-13.
[http://dx.doi.org/10.1016/S0140-6736(07)61721-8] [PMID: 18022033]

[79] Pagotto U, Marsicano G, Cota D, Lutz B, Pasquali R. The emerging role of the endocannabinoid system in endocrine regulation and energy balance. Endocr Rev 2006; 27(1): 73-100.
[http://dx.doi.org/10.1210/er.2005-0009] [PMID: 16306385]

[80] Pacher P, Bátkai S, Kunos G. The endocannabinoid system as an emerging target of pharmacotherapy. Pharmacol Rev 2006; 58(3): 389-462.
[http://dx.doi.org/10.1124/pr.58.3.2] [PMID: 16968947]

[81] de Kloet AD, Woods SC. Minireview: Endocannabinoids and their receptors as targets for obesity therapy. Endocrinology 2009; 150(6): 2531-6.
[http://dx.doi.org/10.1210/en.2009-0046] [PMID: 19372200]

[82] Giuffrida A, Désarnaud F, Piomelli D. Endogenous cannabinoid signaling and psychomotor disorders. Prostaglandins Other Lipid Mediat 2000; 61(1-2): 63-70.
[http://dx.doi.org/10.1016/S0090-6980(00)00055-1] [PMID: 10785542]

[83] Leite CE, Mocelin CA, Petersen GO, Leal MB, Thiesen FV. Rimonabant: an antagonist drug of the endocannabinoid system for the treatment of obesity. Pharmacol Rep 2009; 61(2): 217-24.
[http://dx.doi.org/10.1016/S1734-1140(09)70025-8] [PMID: 19443932]

[84] DiPatrizio NV, Astarita G, Schwartz G, Li X, Piomelli D. Endocannabinoid signal in the gut controls dietary fat intake. Proc Natl Acad Sci USA 2011; 108(31): 12904-8.
[http://dx.doi.org/10.1073/pnas.1104675108] [PMID: 21730161]

[85] Fride E, Bregman T, Kirkham TC. Endocannabinoids and food intake: newborn suckling and appetite regulation in adulthood. Exp Biol Med (Maywood) 2005; 230(4): 225-34.
[PMID: 15792943]

[86] Nogueiras R, Veyrat-Durebex C, Suchanek PM, et al. Peripheral, but not central, CB1 antagonism provides food intake-independent metabolic benefits in diet-induced obese rats. Diabetes 2008; 57(11): 2977-91.
[http://dx.doi.org/10.2337/db08-0161] [PMID: 18716045]

[87] Gelfand EV, Cannon CP. Rimonabant: a cannabinoid receptor type 1 blocker for management of multiple cardiometabolic risk factors. J Am Coll Cardiol 2006; 47(10): 1919-26.
[http://dx.doi.org/10.1016/j.jacc.2005.12.067] [PMID: 16697306]

[88] Rinaldi-Carmona M, Barth F, Héaulme M, *et al.* SR141716A, a potent and selective antagonist of the brain cannabinoid receptor. FEBS Lett 1994; 350(2-3): 240-4.
[http://dx.doi.org/10.1016/0014-5793(94)00773-X] [PMID: 8070571]

[89] Vickers SP, Webster LJ, Wyatt A, Dourish CT, Kennett GA. Preferential effects of the cannabinoid CB1 receptor antagonist, SR 141716, on food intake and body weight gain of obese (fa/fa) compared to lean Zucker rats. Psychopharmacology (Berl) 2003; 167(1): 103-11.
[http://dx.doi.org/10.1007/s00213-002-1384-8] [PMID: 12632249]

[90] Di Marzo V, Matias I. Endocannabinoid control of food intake and energy balance. Nat Neurosci 2005; 8(5): 585-9.
[http://dx.doi.org/10.1038/nn1457] [PMID: 15856067]

[91] Ravinet Trillou C, Delgorge C, Menet C, Arnone M, Soubrié P. CB1 cannabinoid receptor knockout in mice leads to leanness, resistance to diet-induced obesity and enhanced leptin sensitivity. Int J Obes Relat Metab Disord 2004; 28(4): 640-8.
[http://dx.doi.org/10.1038/sj.ijo.0802583] [PMID: 14770190]

[92] Liu YL, Connoley IP, Wilson CA, Stock MJ. Effects of the cannabinoid CB1 receptor antagonist SR141716 on oxygen consumption and soleus muscle glucose uptake in Lep(ob)/Lep(ob) mice. Int J Obes 2005; 29(2): 183-7.
[http://dx.doi.org/10.1038/sj.ijo.0802847] [PMID: 15558076]

[93] Després JP, Golay A, Sjöström L. Effects of rimonabant on metabolic risk factors in overweight patients with dyslipidemia. N Engl J Med 2005; 353(20): 2121-34.
[http://dx.doi.org/10.1056/NEJMoa044537] [PMID: 16291982]

[94] Van Gaal LF, Rissanen AM, Scheen AJ, Ziegler O, Rössner S. Effects of the cannabinoid-1 receptor blocker rimonabant on weight reduction and cardiovascular risk factors in overweight patients: 1-year experience from the RIO-Europe study. Lancet 2005; 365(9468): 1389-97.
[http://dx.doi.org/10.1016/S0140-6736(05)66374-X] [PMID: 15836887]

[95] Pi-Sunyer FX, Aronne LJ, Heshmati HM, Devin J, Rosenstock J. Effect of rimonabant, a cannabinoid-1 receptor blocker, on weight and cardiometabolic risk factors in overweight or obese patients: RIO-North America: a randomized controlled trial. JAMA 2006; 295(7): 761-75.
[http://dx.doi.org/10.1001/jama.295.7.761] [PMID: 16478899]

[96] Scheen AJ, Finer N, Hollander P, Jensen MD, Van Gaal LF. Efficacy and tolerability of rimonabant in overweight or obese patients with type 2 diabetes: a randomised controlled study. Lancet 2006; 368(9548): 1660-72.
[http://dx.doi.org/10.1016/S0140-6736(06)69571-8] [PMID: 17098084]

[97] Azebu LM. The FDAs risk/benefit calculus in the approvals of Qsymia and Belviq: treating an obesity epidemic while avoiding another fen-phen. Food Drug Law J 2014; 69(1): 87-111, ii-iii. [ii-iii.].
[PMID: 24772687]

[98] Verrotti A, Scaparrotta A, Agostinelli S, Di Pillo S, Chiarelli F, Grosso S. Topiramate-induced weight loss: a review. Epilepsy Res 2011; 95(3): 189-99.
[http://dx.doi.org/10.1016/j.eplepsyres.2011.05.014] [PMID: 21684121]

[99] Hottinger A, Sutter R, Marsch S, Rüegg S. Topiramate as an adjunctive treatment in patients with refractory status epilepticus: an observational cohort study. CNS Drugs 2012; 26(9): 761-72.
[http://dx.doi.org/10.2165/11633090-000000000-00000] [PMID: 22823481]

[100] French JA, Gazzola DM. Antiepileptic drug treatment: new drugs and new strategies 2013.
[http://dx.doi.org/10.1212/01.CON.0000431380.21685.75]

[101] Czapiński P, Blaszczyk B, Czuczwar SJ. Mechanisms of action of antiepileptic drugs. Curr Top Med Chem 2005; 5(1): 3-14.
[http://dx.doi.org/10.2174/1568026053386962] [PMID: 15638774]

[102] Aroniadou-Anderjaska V, Qashu F, Braga MF. Mechanisms regulating GABAergic inhibitory transmission in the basolateral amygdala: implications for epilepsy and anxiety disorders. Amino Acids 2007; 32(3): 305-15.
[http://dx.doi.org/10.1007/s00726-006-0415-x] [PMID: 17048126]

[103] Shank RP, Gardocki JF, Streeter AJ, Maryanoff BE. An overview of the preclinical aspects of topiramate: pharmacology, pharmacokinetics, and mechanism of action. Epilepsia 2000; 41 (Suppl. 1): S3-9.
[http://dx.doi.org/10.1111/j.1528-1157.2000.tb02163.x] [PMID: 10768292]

[104] York DA, Singer L, Thomas S, Bray GA. Effect of topiramate on body weight and body composition of osborne-mendel rats fed a high-fat diet: alterations in hormones, neuropeptide, and uncoupling-protein mRNAs. Nutrition 2000; 16(10): 967-75.
[http://dx.doi.org/10.1016/S0899-9007(00)00451-2] [PMID: 11054603]

[105] Smith SM, Meyer M, Trinkley KE. Phentermine/topiramate for the treatment of obesity. Ann Pharmacother 2013; 47(3): 340-9.
[http://dx.doi.org/10.1345/aph.1R501] [PMID: 23482732]

[106] Garvey WT. Phentermine and topiramate extended-release: a new treatment for obesity and its role in a complications-centric approach to obesity medical management. Expert Opin Drug Saf 2013; 12(5): 741-56.
[http://dx.doi.org/10.1517/14740338.2013.806481] [PMID: 23738843]

[107] Brashier DB, Sharma AK, Dahiya N, Singh SK, Khadka A. Lorcaserin: A novel antiobesity drug. J Pharmacol Pharmacother 2014; 5(2): 175-8.
[http://dx.doi.org/10.4103/0976-500X.130158] [PMID: 24799830]

[108] Thomsen WJ, Grottick AJ, Menzaghi F, *et al.* Lorcaserin, a novel selective human 5-hydroxytryptamine2C agonist: *in vitro* and *in vivo* pharmacological characterization. J Pharmacol Exp Ther 2008; 325(2): 577-87.
[http://dx.doi.org/10.1124/jpet.107.133348] [PMID: 18252809]

[109] Rezvani AH, Cauley MC, Levin ED. Lorcaserin, a selective 5-HT(2C) receptor agonist, decreases alcohol intake in female alcohol preferring rats. Pharmacol Biochem Behav 2014; 125: 8-14.
[http://dx.doi.org/10.1016/j.pbb.2014.07.017] [PMID: 25109272]

[110] Smith BM, Smith JM, Tsai JH, *et al.* Discovery and SAR of new benzazepines as potent and selective 5-HT(2C) receptor agonists for the treatment of obesity. Bioorg Med Chem Lett 2005; 15(5): 1467-70.
[http://dx.doi.org/10.1016/j.bmcl.2004.12.080] [PMID: 15713408]

[111] Smith BM, Smith JM, Tsai JH, *et al.* Discovery and structure-activity relationship of (1R)-8-chloro-2,3,4,5-tetrahydro-1-methyl-1H-3-benzazepine (Lorcaserin), a selective serotonin 5-HT2C receptor agonist for the treatment of obesity. J Med Chem 2008; 51(2): 305-13.
[http://dx.doi.org/10.1021/jm0709034] [PMID: 18095642]

[112] Burke LK, Doslikova B, DAgostino G, *et al.* 5-HT obesity medication efficacy *via* POMC activation is maintained during aging. Endocrinology 2014; 155(10): 3732-8.
[http://dx.doi.org/10.1210/en.2014-1223] [PMID: 25051442]

[113] Bai B, Wang Y. The use of lorcaserin in the management of obesity: a critical appraisal. Drug Des Devel Ther 2010; 5: 1-7.
[PMID: 21267355]

[114] Fleming JW, McClendon KS, Riche DM. New obesity agents: lorcaserin and phentermine/topiramate. Ann Pharmacother 2013; 47(7-8): 1007-16.
[http://dx.doi.org/10.1345/aph.1R779] [PMID: 23800750]

[115] Berlie HD, Hurren KM. Evaluation of lorcaserin for the treatment of obesity. Expert Opin Drug Metab Toxicol 2013; 9(8): 1053-9.
[http://dx.doi.org/10.1517/17425255.2013.798643] [PMID: 23802690]

[116] Smith SR, Weissman NJ, Anderson CM, *et al.* Multicenter, placebo-controlled trial of lorcaserin for weight management. N Engl J Med 2010; 363(3): 245-56.
[http://dx.doi.org/10.1056/NEJMoa0909809] [PMID: 20647200]

[117] Hurren KM, Berlie HD. Lorcaserin: an investigational serotonin 2C agonist for weight loss. Am J Health Syst Pharm 2011; 68(21): 2029-37.
[http://dx.doi.org/10.2146/ajhp100638] [PMID: 22011982]

[118] Adams D. Age changes in oral structures. Dent Update 1991; 18(1): 14-7.
[PMID: 1936425]

[119] Padwal R. Contrave, a bupropion and naltrexone combination therapy for the potential treatment of obesity. Curr Opin Investig Drugs 2009; 10(10): 1117-25.
[PMID: 19777400]

[120] Naltrexone/bupropion: Contrave(R); naltrexone SR/bupropion SR. Drugs R D 2010; 10(1): 25-32.
[http://dx.doi.org/10.2165/11537710-000000000-00000] [PMID: 20509712]

[121] Ornellas T, Chavez B. Naltrexone SR/Bupropion SR (Contrave): A New Approach to Weight Loss in Obese Adults. P&T 2011; 36(5): 255-62.
[PMID: 21785538]

[122] Verpeut JL, Bello NT. Drug safety evaluation of naltrexone/bupropion for the treatment of obesity. Expert Opin Drug Saf 2014; 13(6): 831-41.
[PMID: 24766397]

[123] Carpinacci JA. [General considerations on psychiatric interconsultation]. Acta Psiquiatr Psicol Am Lat 1975; 21(1): 64-70. [General considerations on psychiatric interconsultation].
[PMID: 1163271]

[124] Dwoskin LP, Rauhut AS, King-Pospisil KA, Bardo MT. Review of the pharmacology and clinical profile of bupropion, an antidepressant and tobacco use cessation agent. CNS Drug Rev 2006; 12(3-4): 178-207.
[http://dx.doi.org/10.1111/j.1527-3458.2006.00178.x] [PMID: 17227286]

[125] Fava M, Rush AJ, Thase ME, *et al.* 15 years of clinical experience with bupropion HCl: from bupropion to bupropion SR to bupropion XL. Prim Care Companion J Clin Psychiatry 2005; 7(3): 106-13.
[http://dx.doi.org/10.4088/PCC.v07n0305] [PMID: 16027765]

[126] Palamara KL, Mogul HR, Peterson SJ, Frishman WH. Obesity: new perspectives and pharmacotherapies. Cardiol Rev 2006; 14(5): 238-58.
[http://dx.doi.org/10.1097/01.crd.0000233903.57946.fd] [PMID: 16924165]

[127] Francis LP, Lennard R, Singh J. Mechanism of action of magnesium on acetylcholine-evoked secretory responses in isolated rat pancreas. Exp Physiol 1990; 75(5): 669-80.
[http://dx.doi.org/10.1113/expphysiol.1990.sp003445] [PMID: 1700913]

[128] Mooney ME, Sofuoglu M. Bupropion for the treatment of nicotine withdrawal and craving. Expert Rev Neurother 2006; 6(7): 965-81.
[http://dx.doi.org/10.1586/14737175.6.7.965] [PMID: 16831112]

[129] Moreira R. The efficacy and tolerability of bupropion in the treatment of major depressive disorder. Clin Drug Investig 2011; 31 (Suppl. 1): 5-17.
[http://dx.doi.org/10.2165/1159616-S0-000000000-00000] [PMID: 22015858]

[130] Stahl SM, Pradko JF, Haight BR, Modell JG, Rockett CB, Learned-Coughlin S. A Review of the Neuropharmacology of Bupropion, a Dual Norepinephrine and Dopamine Reuptake Inhibitor. Prim Care Companion J Clin Psychiatry 2004; 6(4): 159-66.
[http://dx.doi.org/10.4088/PCC.v06n0403] [PMID: 15361919]

[131] Serretti A, Chiesa A. Treatment-emergent sexual dysfunction related to antidepressants: a meta-analysis. J Clin Psychopharmacol 2009; 29(3): 259-66.
[http://dx.doi.org/10.1097/JCP.0b013e3181a5233f] [PMID: 19440080]

[132] Ryan DH, Bray GA. Pharmacologic treatment options for obesity: what is old is new again. Curr Hypertens Rep 2013; 15(3): 182-9.
[http://dx.doi.org/10.1007/s11906-013-0343-6] [PMID: 23625271]

[133] Latt NC, Jurd S, Houseman J, Wutzke SE. Naltrexone in alcohol dependence: a randomised controlled trial of effectiveness in a standard clinical setting. Med J Aust 2002; 176(11): 530-4.
[PMID: 12064984]

[134] Volpicelli JR. Naltrexone in alcohol dependence. Lancet 1995; 346(8973): 456.
[http://dx.doi.org/10.1016/S0140-6736(95)91316-5] [PMID: 7637475]

[135] Weinrieb RM, OBrien CP. Naltrexone in the treatment of alcoholism. Annu Rev Med 1997; 48: 477-87.
[http://dx.doi.org/10.1146/annurev.med.48.1.477] [PMID: 9046978]

[136] Kast RE. Use of FDA approved methamphetamine to allow adjunctive use of methylnaltrexone to mediate core anti-growth factor signaling effects in glioblastoma. J Neurooncol 2009; 94(2): 163-7.
[http://dx.doi.org/10.1007/s11060-009-9863-y] [PMID: 19322519]

[137] King A, de Wit H, Riley RC, Cao D, Niaura R, Hatsukami D. Efficacy of naltrexone in smoking cessation: a preliminary study and an examination of sex differences. Nicotine Tob Res 2006; 8(5): 671-82.
[http://dx.doi.org/10.1080/14622200600789767] [PMID: 17008194]

[138] Lobmaier PP, Kunøe N, Gossop M, Waal H. Naltrexone depot formulations for opioid and alcohol dependence: a systematic review. CNS Neurosci Ther 2011; 17(6): 629-36.
[http://dx.doi.org/10.1111/j.1755-5949.2010.00194.x] [PMID: 21554565]

[139] Caixàs A, Albert L, Capel I, Rigla M. Naltrexone sustained-release/bupropion sustained-release for the management of obesity: review of the data to date. Drug Des Devel Ther 2014; 8: 1419-27.
[http://dx.doi.org/10.2147/DDDT.S55587] [PMID: 25258511]

[140] Greenway FL, Fujioka K, Plodkowski RA, *et al.* Effect of naltrexone plus bupropion on weight loss in overweight and obese adults (COR-I): a multicentre, randomised, double-blind, placebo-controlled, phase 3 trial. Lancet 2010; 376(9741): 595-605.
[http://dx.doi.org/10.1016/S0140-6736(10)60888-4] [PMID: 20673995]

[141] Ueno H, Nakazato M. [Cutting-edge of medicine; the prospects of novel anti-obesity drugs]. Nippon Naika Gakkai Zasshi 2014; 103(3): 753-9. [Cutting-edge of medicine; the prospects of novel anti-obesity drugs].
[http://dx.doi.org/10.2169/naika.103.753] [PMID: 24796150]

[142] Yamada Y, Kato T, Ogino H, Ashina S, Kato K. Cetilistat (ATL-962), a novel pancreatic lipase inhibitor, ameliorates body weight gain and improves lipid profiles in rats. Horm Metab Res 2008; 40(8): 539-43.
[http://dx.doi.org/10.1055/s-2008-1076699] [PMID: 18500680]

[143] Kopelman P, Bryson A, Hickling R, *et al.* Cetilistat (ATL-962), a novel lipase inhibitor: a 12-week randomized, placebo-controlled study of weight reduction in obese patients. Int J Obes 2007; 31(3): 494-9.
[http://dx.doi.org/10.1038/sj.ijo.0803446] [PMID: 16953261]

[144] Kopelman P, Groot GdeH, Rissanen A, *et al.* Weight loss, HbA1c reduction, and tolerability of cetilistat in a randomized, placebo-controlled phase 2 trial in obese diabetics: comparison with orlistat (Xenical). Obesity (Silver Spring) 2010; 18(1): 108-15.
[http://dx.doi.org/10.1038/oby.2009.155] [PMID: 19461584]

[145] Ioannides-Demos LL, Piccenna L, McNeil JJ. Pharmacotherapies for obesity: past, current, and future therapies. J Obes 2011; 2011: 179674.

[146] Adan RA. Mechanisms underlying current and future anti-obesity drugs. Trends Neurosci 2013; 36(2): 133-40.
[http://dx.doi.org/10.1016/j.tins.2012.12.001] [PMID: 23312373]

[147] Cincâ D, Tomescu E, Sbenghe-Tetu L, Udrescu S. Experience of the Coltea ORL clinic in reconstructive surgery of the ear. Rev Chir Oncol Radiol O R L Oftalmol Stomatol Otorinolaringol 1976; 21(4): 247-52.
[PMID: 139647]

[148] Mimaki T, Suzuki Y, Tagawa T, Karasawa T, Yabuuchi H. Interaction of zonisamide with benzodiazepine and GABA receptors in rat brain. Med J Osaka Univ 1990; 39(1-4): 13-7.
[PMID: 1369646]

[149] Ueda Y, Doi T, Tokumaru J, Willmore LJ. Effect of zonisamide on molecular regulation of glutamate and GABA transporter proteins during epileptogenesis in rats with hippocampal seizures. Brain Res Mol Brain Res 2003; 116(1-2): 1-6.
[http://dx.doi.org/10.1016/S0169-328X(03)00183-9] [PMID: 12941455]

[150] Leppik IE. Zonisamide: chemistry, mechanism of action, and pharmacokinetics. Seizure 2004; 13 (Suppl. 1): S5-9.
[http://dx.doi.org/10.1016/j.seizure.2004.04.016] [PMID: 15511691]

[151] Gadde KM, Franciscy DM, Wagner HR II, Krishnan KR. Zonisamide for weight loss in obese adults: a randomized controlled trial. JAMA 2003; 289(14): 1820-5.
[http://dx.doi.org/10.1001/jama.289.14.1820] [PMID: 12684361]

[152] Gadde KM, Kopping MF, Wagner HR II, Yonish GM, Allison DB, Bray GA. Zonisamide for weight reduction in obese adults: a 1-year randomized controlled trial. Arch Intern Med 2012; 172(20): 1557-64.
[http://dx.doi.org/10.1001/2013.jamainternmed.99] [PMID: 23147455]

[153] Nguyen ML, Pirzada MH, Shapiro MA. Zonisamide for weight loss in adolescents. J Pediatr Pharmacol Ther 2013; 18(4): 311-4.
[http://dx.doi.org/10.5863/1551-6776-18.4.311] [PMID: 24719592]

[154] Jackson VM, Price DA, Carpino PA. Investigational drugs in Phase II clinical trials for the treatment of obesity: implications for future development of novel therapies. Expert Opin Investig Drugs 2014; 23(8): 1055-66.
[http://dx.doi.org/10.1517/13543784.2014.918952] [PMID: 25000213]

[155] Shin JH, Gadde KM, Østbye T, Bray GA. Weight changes in obese adults 6-months after discontinuation of double-blind zonisamide or placebo treatment. Diabetes Obes Metab 2014; 16(8): 766-8.
[http://dx.doi.org/10.1111/dom.12275] [PMID: 25123600]

[156] Doggrell SA. Tesofensinea novel potent weight loss medicine. Evaluation of: Astrup A, Breum L, Jensen TJ, Kroustrup JP, Larsen TM. Effect of tesofensine on bodyweight loss, body composition, and quality of life in obese patients: a randomised, double-blind, placebo-controlled trial. Lancet 2008;372:190613. Expert Opin Investig Drugs 2009; 18(7): 1043-6.
[http://dx.doi.org/10.1517/13543780902967632] [PMID: 19548858]

[157] Bello NT, Zahner MR. Tesofensine, a monoamine reuptake inhibitor for the treatment of obesity. Curr Opin Investig Drugs 2009; 10(10): 1105-16.
[PMID: 19777399]

[158] Bara-Jimenez W, Dimitrova T, Sherzai A, Favit A, Mouradian MM, Chase TN. Effect of monoamine reuptake inhibitor NS 2330 in advanced Parkinsons disease. Mov Disord 2004; 19(10): 1183-6.
[http://dx.doi.org/10.1002/mds.20124] [PMID: 15390018]

[159] Hauser RA, Salin L, Juhel N, Konyago VL. Randomized trial of the triple monoamine reuptake inhibitor NS 2330 (tesofensine) in early Parkinsons disease. Mov Disord 2007; 22(3): 359-65.
[http://dx.doi.org/10.1002/mds.21258] [PMID: 17149725]

[160] Rascol O, Poewe W, Lees A, *et al.* Tesofensine (NS 2330), a monoamine reuptake inhibitor, in patients with advanced Parkinson disease and motor fluctuations: the ADVANS Study. Arch Neurol 2008; 65(5): 577-83.
[http://dx.doi.org/10.1001/archneur.65.5.577] [PMID: 18474731]

[161] Astrup A, Meier DH, Mikkelsen BO, Villumsen JS, Larsen TM. Weight loss produced by tesofensine in patients with Parkinsons or Alzheimers disease. Obesity (Silver Spring) 2008; 16(6): 1363-9.
[http://dx.doi.org/10.1038/oby.2008.56] [PMID: 18356831]

[162] Larsen MH, Rosenbrock H, Sams-Dodd F, Mikkelsen JD. Expression of brain derived neurotrophic factor, activity-regulated cytoskeleton protein mRNA, and enhancement of adult hippocampal neurogenesis in rats after sub-chronic and chronic treatment with the triple monoamine re-uptake inhibitor tesofensine. Eur J Pharmacol 2007; 555(2-3): 115-21.
[http://dx.doi.org/10.1016/j.ejphar.2006.10.029] [PMID: 17112503]

[163] Axel AM, Mikkelsen JD, Hansen HH. Tesofensine, a novel triple monoamine reuptake inhibitor, induces appetite suppression by indirect stimulation of alpha1 adrenoceptor and dopamine D1 receptor pathways in the diet-induced obese rat. Neuropsychopharmacology 2010; 35(7): 1464-76.
[http://dx.doi.org/10.1038/npp.2010.16] [PMID: 20200509]

[164] Hansen HH, Hansen G, Tang-Christensen M, *et al.* The novel triple monoamine reuptake inhibitor tesofensine induces sustained weight loss and improves glycemic control in the diet-induced obese rat: comparison to sibutramine and rimonabant. Eur J Pharmacol 2010; 636(1-3): 88-95.
[http://dx.doi.org/10.1016/j.ejphar.2010.03.026] [PMID: 20385125]

[165] Astrup A, Madsbad S, Breum L, Jensen TJ, Kroustrup JP, Larsen TM. Effect of tesofensine on bodyweight loss, body composition, and quality of life in obese patients: a randomised, double-blind, placebo-controlled trial. Lancet 2008; 372(9653): 1906-13.
[http://dx.doi.org/10.1016/S0140-6736(08)61525-1] [PMID: 18950853]

[166] Knauf C, Cani PD, Perrin C, *et al.* Brain glucagon-like peptide-1 increases insulin secretion and muscle insulin resistance to favor hepatic glycogen storage. J Clin Invest 2005; 115(12): 3554-63.
[http://dx.doi.org/10.1172/JCI25764] [PMID: 16322793]

[167] Komatsu R, Matsuyama T, Namba M, *et al.* Glucagonostatic and insulinotropic action of glucagonlike peptide I-(736)-amide. Diabetes 1989; 38(7): 902-5.
[http://dx.doi.org/10.2337/diab.38.7.902] [PMID: 2661287]

[168] Dunning BE, Foley JE, Ahrén B. Alpha cell function in health and disease: influence of glucagon-like peptide-1. Diabetologia 2005; 48(9): 1700-13.
[http://dx.doi.org/10.1007/s00125-005-1878-0] [PMID: 16132964]

[169] Kielgast U, Asmar M, Madsbad S, Holst JJ. Effect of glucagon-like peptide-1 on alpha- and beta-cell function in C-peptide-negative type 1 diabetic patients. J Clin Endocrinol Metab 2010; 95(5): 2492-6.
[http://dx.doi.org/10.1210/jc.2009-2440] [PMID: 20207828]

[170] Kinzig KP, DAlessio DA, Seeley RJ. The diverse roles of specific GLP-1 receptors in the control of food intake and the response to visceral illness. J Neurosci 2002; 22(23): 10470-6.
[PMID: 12451146]

[171] Schick RR, Zimmermann JP. vorm Walde T, Schusdziarra V. Peptides that regulate food intake: glucagon-like peptide 1-(736) amide acts at lateral and medial hypothalamic sites to suppress feeding in rats. Am J Physiol Regul Integr Comp Physiol 2003; 284(6): R1427-35.
[http://dx.doi.org/10.1152/ajpregu.00479.2002] [PMID: 12776726]

[172] Imeryüz N, Yeğen BC, Bozkurt A, Coşkun T, Villanueva-Peñacarrillo ML, Ulusoy NB. Glucagon-like peptide-1 inhibits gastric emptying *via* vagal afferent-mediated central mechanisms. Am J Physiol

1997; 273(4 Pt 1): G920-7.
[PMID: 9357836]

[173] Hayes MR, Skibicka KP, Grill HJ. Caudal brainstem processing is sufficient for behavioral, sympathetic, and parasympathetic responses driven by peripheral and hindbrain glucagon-like-peptie-1 receptor stimulation. Endocrinology 2008; 149(8): 4059-68.
[http://dx.doi.org/10.1210/en.2007-1743] [PMID: 18420740]

[174] Elliott RM, Morgan LM, Tredger JA, Deacon S, Wright J, Marks V. Glucagon-like peptide-1 (736)amide and glucose-dependent insulinotropic polypeptide secretion in response to nutrient ingestion in man: acute post-prandial and 24-h secretion patterns. J Endocrinol 1993; 138(1): 159-66.
[http://dx.doi.org/10.1677/joe.0.1380159] [PMID: 7852887]

[175] Deacon CF, Johnsen AH, Holst JJ. Degradation of glucagon-like peptide-1 by human plasma *in vitro* yields an N-terminally truncated peptide that is a major endogenous metabolite *in vivo*. J Clin Endocrinol Metab 1995; 80(3): 952-7.
[PMID: 7883856]

[176] Vilsbøll T, Agersø H, Krarup T, Holst JJ. Similar elimination rates of glucagon-like peptide-1 in obese type 2 diabetic patients and healthy subjects. J Clin Endocrinol Metab 2003; 88(1): 220-4.
[http://dx.doi.org/10.1210/jc.2002-021053] [PMID: 12519856]

[177] Göke R, Larsen PJ, Mikkelsen JD, Sheikh SP. Distribution of GLP-1 binding sites in the rat brain: evidence that exendin-4 is a ligand of brain GLP-1 binding sites. Eur J Neurosci 1995; 7(11): 2294-300.
[http://dx.doi.org/10.1111/j.1460-9568.1995.tb00650.x] [PMID: 8563978]

[178] Baggio LL, Drucker DJ. Biology of incretins: GLP-1 and GIP. Gastroenterology 2007; 132(6): 2131-57.
[http://dx.doi.org/10.1053/j.gastro.2007.03.054] [PMID: 17498508]

[179] Madsen K, Knudsen LB, Agersoe H, *et al.* Structure-activity and protraction relationship of long-acting glucagon-like peptide-1 derivatives: importance of fatty acid length, polarity, and bulkiness. J Med Chem 2007; 50(24): 6126-32.
[http://dx.doi.org/10.1021/jm070861j] [PMID: 17975905]

[180] Garber A, Henry R, Ratner R, *et al.* Liraglutide *versus* glimepiride monotherapy for type 2 diabetes (LEAD-3 Mono): a randomised, 52-week, phase III, double-blind, parallel-treatment trial. Lancet 2009; 373(9662): 473-81.
[http://dx.doi.org/10.1016/S0140-6736(08)61246-5] [PMID: 18819705]

[181] Hansen G, Jelsing J, Vrang N. Effects of liraglutide and sibutramine on food intake, palatability, body weight and glucose tolerance in the gubra DIO-rats. Acta Pharmacol Sin 2012; 33(2): 194-200.
[http://dx.doi.org/10.1038/aps.2011.168] [PMID: 22301859]

[182] Larsen PJ, Wulff EM, Gotfredsen CF, *et al.* Combination of the insulin sensitizer, pioglitazone, and the long-acting GLP-1 human analog, liraglutide, exerts potent synergistic glucose-lowering efficacy in severely diabetic ZDF rats. Diabetes Obes Metab 2008; 10(4): 301-11.
[http://dx.doi.org/10.1111/j.1463-1326.2008.00865.x] [PMID: 18333889]

[183] Jeon WS, Park CY. Antiobesity pharmacotherapy for patients with type 2 diabetes: focus on long-term management. Endocrinol Metab (Seoul) 2014; 29(4): 410-7.
[http://dx.doi.org/10.3803/EnM.2014.29.4.410] [PMID: 25559569]

[184] Larrabee JA, Leung CH, Moore RL, Thamrong-nawasawat T, Wessler BS. Magnetic circular dichroism and cobalt(II) binding equilibrium studies of Escherichia coli methionyl aminopeptidase. J Am Chem Soc 2004; 126(39): 12316-24.
[http://dx.doi.org/10.1021/ja0485006] [PMID: 15453765]

[185] Johansson FB, Bond AD, Nielsen UG, *et al.* Dicobalt II-II, II-III, and III-III complexes as spectroscopic models for dicobalt enzyme active sites. Inorg Chem 2008; 47(12): 5079-92.
[http://dx.doi.org/10.1021/ic7020534] [PMID: 18494467]

[186] Folkman J. Angiogenesis in cancer, vascular, rheumatoid and other disease. Nat Med 1995; 1(1): 27-31.
[http://dx.doi.org/10.1038/nm0195-27] [PMID: 7584949]

[187] Kim YM, An JJ, Jin YJ, *et al.* Assessment of the anti-obesity effects of the TNP-470 analog, CKD-732. J Mol Endocrinol 2007; 38(4): 455-65.
[http://dx.doi.org/10.1677/jme.1.02165] [PMID: 17446235]

[188] Joharapurkar AA, Dhanesha NA, Jain MR. Inhibition of the methionine aminopeptidase 2 enzyme for the treatment of obesity. Diabetes Metab Syndr Obes 2014; 7: 73-84.
[http://dx.doi.org/10.2147/DMSO.S56924] [PMID: 24611021]

[189] Lin MC, Gordon D, Wetterau JR. Microsomal triglyceride transfer protein (MTP) regulation in HepG2 cells: insulin negatively regulates MTP gene expression. J Lipid Res 1995; 36(5): 1073-81.
[PMID: 7658155]

[190] Wetterau JR, Gregg RE, Harrity TW, *et al.* An MTP inhibitor that normalizes atherogenic lipoprotein levels in WHHL rabbits. Science 1998; 282(5389): 751-4.
[http://dx.doi.org/10.1126/science.282.5389.751] [PMID: 9784135]

[191] Olofsson SO, Asp L, Borén J. The assembly and secretion of apolipoprotein B-containing lipoproteins. Curr Opin Lipidol 1999; 10(4): 341-6.
[http://dx.doi.org/10.1097/00041433-199908000-00008] [PMID: 10482137]

[192] Xie Y, Newberry EP, Young SG, *et al.* Compensatory increase in hepatic lipogenesis in mice with conditional intestine-specific Mttp deficiency. J Biol Chem 2006; 281(7): 4075-86.
[http://dx.doi.org/10.1074/jbc.M510622200] [PMID: 16354657]

[193] Shiomi M, Ito T. MTP inhibitor decreases plasma cholesterol levels in LDL receptor-deficient WHHL rabbits by lowering the VLDL secretion. Eur J Pharmacol 2001; 431(1): 127-31.
[http://dx.doi.org/10.1016/S0014-2999(01)01419-4] [PMID: 11716851]

[194] Burnett JR, Watts GF. MTP inhibition as a treatment for dyslipidaemias: time to deliver or empty promises? Expert Opin Ther Targets 2007; 11(2): 181-9.
[http://dx.doi.org/10.1517/14728222.11.2.181] [PMID: 17227233]

[195] Hata T, Mera Y, Ishii Y, *et al.* JTT-130, a novel intestine-specific inhibitor of microsomal triglyceride transfer protein, suppresses food intake and gastric emptying with the elevation of plasma peptide YY and glucagon-like peptide-1 in a dietary fat-dependent manner. J Pharmacol Exp Ther 2011; 336(3): 850-6.
[http://dx.doi.org/10.1124/jpet.110.176560] [PMID: 21139060]

[196] Mera Y, Odani N, Kawai T, *et al.* Pharmacological characterization of diethyl-2-(3-dimethyl-carbamoyl-4-[(4-trifluoromethylbiphenyl-2-carbonyl)amino]phenylacetyloxymethyl)-2-phenyl-malonate (JTT-130), an intestine-specific inhibitor of microsomal triglyceride transfer protein. J Pharmacol Exp Ther 2011; 336(2): 321-7.
[http://dx.doi.org/10.1124/jpet.110.173807] [PMID: 20974698]

[197] Hata T, Mera Y, Kawai T, *et al.* JTT-130, a novel intestine-specific inhibitor of microsomal triglyceride transfer protein, ameliorates impaired glucose and lipid metabolism in Zucker diabetic fatty rats. Diabetes Obes Metab 2011; 13(7): 629-38.
[http://dx.doi.org/10.1111/j.1463-1326.2011.01387.x] [PMID: 21362121]

[198] Cases S, Smith SJ, Zheng YW, *et al.* Identification of a gene encoding an acyl CoA:diacylglycerol acyltransferase, a key enzyme in triacylglycerol synthesis. Proc Natl Acad Sci USA 1998; 95(22): 13018-23.
[http://dx.doi.org/10.1073/pnas.95.22.13018] [PMID: 9789033]

[199] Neulen J, Williams RF, Hodgen GD. RU 486 (mifepristone): induction of dose dependent elevations of estradiol receptor in endometrium from ovariectomized monkeys. J Clin Endocrinol Metab 1990; 71(4): 1074-5.

[http://dx.doi.org/10.1210/jcem-71-4-1074] [PMID: 2401709]

[200] Buhman KK, Smith SJ, Stone SJ, *et al.* DGAT1 is not essential for intestinal triacylglycerol absorption or chylomicron synthesis. J Biol Chem 2002; 277(28): 25474-9.
[http://dx.doi.org/10.1074/jbc.M202013200] [PMID: 11959864]

[201] Smith SJ, Cases S, Jensen DR, *et al.* Obesity resistance and multiple mechanisms of triglyceride synthesis in mice lacking Dgat. Nat Genet 2000; 25(1): 87-90.
[http://dx.doi.org/10.1038/75651] [PMID: 10802663]

[202] Tomimoto D, Okuma C, Ishii Y, *et al.* Pharmacological characterization of [trans-5-(4-amino-7,7-dimethyl-2-trifluoromethyl-7H-pyrimido[4,5-b][1,4]oxazin-6-yl)-2,3-dihydrospiro(cyclohexane-1,1-inden)-4-yl]acetic acid monobenzenesulfonate (JTT-553), a novel acyl CoA:diacylglycerol transferase (DGAT) 1 inhibitor. Biol Pharm Bull 2015; 38(2): 263-9.
[http://dx.doi.org/10.1248/bpb.b14-00655] [PMID: 25747985]

[203] Ables GP, Yang KJ, Vogel S, *et al.* Intestinal DGAT1 deficiency reduces postprandial triglyceride and retinyl ester excursions by inhibiting chylomicron secretion and delaying gastric emptying. J Lipid Res 2012; 53(11): 2364-79.
[http://dx.doi.org/10.1194/jlr.M029041] [PMID: 22911105]

[204] Denison H, Nilsson C, Kujacic M, *et al.* Proof of mechanism for the DGAT1 inhibitor AZD7687: results from a first-time-in-human single-dose study. Diabetes Obes Metab 2013; 15(2): 136-43.
[http://dx.doi.org/10.1111/dom.12002] [PMID: 22950654]

[205] Dow RL, Andrews MP, Li JC, *et al.* Defining the key pharmacophore elements of PF-04620110: discovery of a potent, orally-active, neutral DGAT-1 inhibitor. Bioorg Med Chem 2013; 21(17): 5081-97.
[http://dx.doi.org/10.1016/j.bmc.2013.06.045] [PMID: 23871442]

[206] Denison H, Nilsson C, Löfgren L, *et al.* Diacylglycerol acyltransferase 1 inhibition with AZD7687 alters lipid handling and hormone secretion in the gut with intolerable side effects: a randomized clinical trial. Diabetes Obes Metab 2014; 16(4): 334-43.
[http://dx.doi.org/10.1111/dom.12221] [PMID: 24118885]

[207] Yen CL, Farese RV Jr. MGAT2, a monoacylglycerol acyltransferase expressed in the small intestine. J Biol Chem 2003; 278(20): 18532-7.
[http://dx.doi.org/10.1074/jbc.M301633200] [PMID: 12621063]

[208] Senior JR, Isselbacher KJ. Direct esterification of monoglycerides with palmityl coenzyme A by intestinal epithelial subcellular fractions. J Biol Chem 1962; 237: 1454-9.
[PMID: 13910673]

[209] Yen CL, Stone SJ, Cases S, Zhou P, Farese RV Jr. Identification of a gene encoding MGAT1, a monoacylglycerol acyltransferase. Proc Natl Acad Sci USA 2002; 99(13): 8512-7.
[http://dx.doi.org/10.1073/pnas.132274899] [PMID: 12077311]

[210] Cao J, Cheng L, Shi Y. Catalytic properties of MGAT3, a putative triacylgycerol synthase. J Lipid Res 2007; 48(3): 583-91.
[http://dx.doi.org/10.1194/jlr.M600331-JLR200] [PMID: 17170429]

[211] Tsuchida T, Fukuda S, Aoyama H, *et al.* MGAT2 deficiency ameliorates high-fat diet-induced obesity and insulin resistance by inhibiting intestinal fat absorption in mice. Lipids Health Dis 2012; 11: 75.
[http://dx.doi.org/10.1186/1476-511X-11-75] [PMID: 22698140]

[212] Okawa M, Fujii K, Ohbuchi K, *et al.* Role of MGAT2 and DGAT1 in the release of gut peptides after triglyceride ingestion. Biochem Biophys Res Commun 2009; 390(3): 377-81.
[http://dx.doi.org/10.1016/j.bbrc.2009.08.167] [PMID: 19732742]

[213] Yen CL, Cheong ML, Grueter C, *et al.* Deficiency of the intestinal enzyme acyl CoA:monoacylglycerol acyltransferase-2 protects mice from metabolic disorders induced by high-fat feeding. Nat Med 2009; 15(4): 442-6.

[http://dx.doi.org/10.1038/nm.1937] [PMID: 19287392]

[214] Nelson DW, Gao Y, Spencer NM, Banh T, Yen CL. Deficiency of MGAT2 increases energy expenditure without high-fat feeding and protects genetically obese mice from excessive weight gain. J Lipid Res 2011; 52(9): 1723-32.
[http://dx.doi.org/10.1194/jlr.M016840] [PMID: 21734185]

[215] Gao Y, Nelson DW, Banh T, Yen MI, Yen CL. Intestine-specific expression of MOGAT2 partially restores metabolic efficiency in Mogat2-deficient mice. J Lipid Res 2013; 54(6): 1644-52.
[http://dx.doi.org/10.1194/jlr.M035493] [PMID: 23536640]

[216] Nelson DW, Gao Y, Yen MI, Yen CL. Intestine-specific deletion of acyl-CoA:monoacylglycerol acyltransferase (MGAT) 2 protects mice from diet-induced obesity and glucose intolerance. J Biol Chem 2014; 289(25): 17338-49.
[http://dx.doi.org/10.1074/jbc.M114.555961] [PMID: 24784138]

[217] Okuma C, Ohta T, Tadaki H, *et al.* JTP-103237, a novel monoacylglycerol acyltransferase inhibitor, modulates fat absorption and prevents diet-induced obesity. Eur J Pharmacol 2015; 758: 72-81.
[http://dx.doi.org/10.1016/j.ejphar.2015.03.072] [PMID: 25857225]

[218] Tonks NK, Neel BG. Combinatorial control of the specificity of protein tyrosine phosphatases. Curr Opin Cell Biol 2001; 13(2): 182-95.
[http://dx.doi.org/10.1016/S0955-0674(00)00196-4] [PMID: 11248552]

[219] Wu X, Hardy VE, Joseph JI, *et al.* Protein-tyrosine phosphatase activity in human adipocytes is strongly correlated with insulin-stimulated glucose uptake and is a target of insulin-induced oxidative inhibition. Metabolism 2003; 52(6): 705-12.
[http://dx.doi.org/10.1016/S0026-0495(03)00065-9] [PMID: 12800095]

[220] Zabolotny JM, Bence-Hanulec KK, Stricker-Krongrad A, *et al.* PTP1B regulates leptin signal transduction *in vivo*. Dev Cell 2002; 2(4): 489-95.
[http://dx.doi.org/10.1016/S1534-5807(02)00148-X] [PMID: 11970898]

[221] Cheng A, Uetani N, Simoncic PD, *et al.* Attenuation of leptin action and regulation of obesity by protein tyrosine phosphatase 1B. Dev Cell 2002; 2(4): 497-503.
[http://dx.doi.org/10.1016/S1534-5807(02)00149-1] [PMID: 11970899]

[222] Elchebly M, Payette P, Michaliszyn E, *et al.* Increased insulin sensitivity and obesity resistance in mice lacking the protein tyrosine phosphatase-1B gene. Science 1999; 283(5407): 1544-8.
[http://dx.doi.org/10.1126/science.283.5407.1544] [PMID: 10066179]

[223] Klaman LD, Boss O, Peroni OD, *et al.* Increased energy expenditure, decreased adiposity, and tissue-specific insulin sensitivity in protein-tyrosine phosphatase 1B-deficient mice. Mol Cell Biol 2000; 20(15): 5479-89.
[http://dx.doi.org/10.1128/MCB.20.15.5479-5489.2000] [PMID: 10891488]

[224] Fukuda S, Ohta T, Sakata S, *et al.* Pharmacological profiles of a novel protein tyrosine phosphatase 1B inhibitor, JTT-551. Diabetes Obes Metab 2010; 12(4): 299-306.
[http://dx.doi.org/10.1111/j.1463-1326.2009.01162.x] [PMID: 20380650]

[225] Katsi VK, Michalakeas CA, Grassos CE, *et al.* Canagliflozin: a new hope in the antidiabetic armamentarium. Recent Patents Cardiovasc Drug Discov 2013; 8(3): 216-20.
[http://dx.doi.org/10.2174/1574890108666131213100613] [PMID: 24359233]

[226] Kaushal S, Singh H, Thangaraju P, Singh J. Canagliflozin: A Novel SGLT2 Inhibitor for Type 2 Diabetes Mellitus. N Am J Med Sci 2014; 6(3): 107-13.
[http://dx.doi.org/10.4103/1947-2714.128471] [PMID: 24741548]

[227] Bolinder J, Ljunggren Ö, Kullberg J, *et al.* Effects of dapagliflozin on body weight, total fat mass, and regional adipose tissue distribution in patients with type 2 diabetes mellitus with inadequate glycemic control on metformin. J Clin Endocrinol Metab 2012; 97(3): 1020-31.
[http://dx.doi.org/10.1210/jc.2011-2260] [PMID: 22238392]

[228] Ferrannini E, Seman L, Seewaldt-Becker E, Hantel S, Pinnetti S, Woerle HJ. A Phase IIb, randomized, placebo-controlled study of the SGLT2 inhibitor empagliflozin in patients with type 2 diabetes. Diabetes Obes Metab 2013; 15(8): 721-8.
[http://dx.doi.org/10.1111/dom.12081] [PMID: 23398530]

[229] Grandy S, Hashemi M, Langkilde AM, Parikh S, Sjöström CD. Changes in weight loss-related quality of life among type 2 diabetes mellitus patients treated with dapagliflozin. Diabetes Obes Metab 2014; 16(7): 645-50.
[http://dx.doi.org/10.1111/dom.12263] [PMID: 24443876]

[230] Liang Y, Arakawa K, Ueta K, et al. Effect of canagliflozin on renal threshold for glucose, glycemia, and body weight in normal and diabetic animal models. PLoS One 2012; 7(2): e30555.
[http://dx.doi.org/10.1371/journal.pone.0030555] [PMID: 22355316]

[231] Devenny JJ, Godonis HE, Harvey SJ, Rooney S, Cullen MJ, Pelleymounter MA. Weight loss induced by chronic dapagliflozin treatment is attenuated by compensatory hyperphagia in diet-induced obese (DIO) rats. Obesity (Silver Spring) 2012; 20(8): 1645-52.
[http://dx.doi.org/10.1038/oby.2012.59] [PMID: 22402735]

[232] Suzuki M, Takeda M, Kito A, et al. Tofogliflozin, a sodium/glucose cotransporter 2 inhibitor, attenuates body weight gain and fat accumulation in diabetic and obese animal models. Nutr Diabetes 2014; 4: e125.
[http://dx.doi.org/10.1038/nutd.2014.20] [PMID: 25000147]

[233] Mera Y, Hata T, Ishii Y, et al. JTT-130, a novel intestine-specific inhibitor of microsomal triglyceride transfer protein, reduces food preference for fat. J Diabetes Res 2014; 2014: 583752.
[http://dx.doi.org/10.1155/2014/583752]

[234] Ohno H, Shinoda K, Spiegelman BM, Kajimura S. PPARγ agonists induce a white-to-brown fat conversion through stabilization of PRDM16 protein. Cell Metab 2012; 15(3): 395-404.
[http://dx.doi.org/10.1016/j.cmet.2012.01.019] [PMID: 22405074]

[235] Ingalls AM, Dickie MM, Snell GD. Obese, a new mutation in the house mouse. J Hered 1950; 41(12): 317-8.
[PMID: 14824537]

[236] Zhang Y, Proenca R, Maffei M, Barone M, Leopold L, Friedman JM. Positional cloning of the mouse obese gene and its human homologue. Nature 1994; 372(6505): 425-32.
[http://dx.doi.org/10.1038/372425a0] [PMID: 7984236]

[237] Bégin-Heick N. Beta-adrenergic receptors and G-proteins in the ob/ob mouse. Int J Obes Relat Metab Disord 1996; 20 (Suppl. 3): S32-5.
[PMID: 8680474]

[238] Hummel KP, Dickie MM, Coleman DL. Diabetes, a new mutation in the mouse. Science 1966; 153(3740): 1127-8.
[http://dx.doi.org/10.1126/science.153.3740.1127] [PMID: 5918576]

[239] Michaud EJ, Bultman SJ, Klebig ML, et al. A molecular model for the genetic and phenotypic characteristics of the mouse lethal yellow (Ay) mutation. Proc Natl Acad Sci USA 1994; 91(7): 2562-6.
[http://dx.doi.org/10.1073/pnas.91.7.2562] [PMID: 8146154]

[240] Hirayama I, Yi Z, Izumi S, et al. Genetic analysis of obese diabetes in the TSOD mouse. Diabetes 1999; 48(5): 1183-91.
[http://dx.doi.org/10.2337/diabetes.48.5.1183] [PMID: 10331427]

[241] Suzuki W, Iizuka S, Tabuchi M, et al. A new mouse model of spontaneous diabetes derived from ddY strain. Exp Anim 1999; 48(3): 181-9.
[http://dx.doi.org/10.1538/expanim.48.181] [PMID: 10480023]

[242] Masuyama T, Katsuda Y, Shinohara M. A novel model of obesity-related diabetes: introgression of the Lepr(fa) allele of the Zucker fatty rat into nonobese Spontaneously Diabetic Torii (SDT) rats. Exp Anim 2005; 54(1): 13-20.
[http://dx.doi.org/10.1538/expanim.54.13] [PMID: 15725677]

[243] Matsui K, Ohta T, Oda T, *et al.* Diabetes-associated complications in Spontaneously Diabetic Torii fatty rats. Exp Anim 2008; 57(2): 111-21.
[http://dx.doi.org/10.1538/expanim.57.111] [PMID: 18421173]

[244] Sasase T, Ohta T, Masuyama T, Yokoi N, Kakehashi A, Shinohara M. 2013.

[245] Katsuda Y, Ohta T, Miyajima K, *et al.* Diabetic complications in obese type 2 diabetic rat models. Exp Anim 2014; 63(2): 121-32.
[http://dx.doi.org/10.1538/expanim.63.121] [PMID: 24770637]

[246] Ohta T, Katsuda Y, Miyajima K, *et al.* 2014.

[247] Ishii Y, Ohta T, Sasase T, *et al.* Pathophysiological analysis of female Spontaneously Diabetic Torii fatty rats. Exp Anim 2010; 59(1): 73-84.
[http://dx.doi.org/10.1538/expanim.59.73] [PMID: 20224171]

[248] Kurtz TW, Morris RC, Pershadsingh HA. The Zucker fatty rat as a genetic model of obesity and hypertension. Hypertension 1989; 13(6 Pt 2): 896-901.
[http://dx.doi.org/10.1161/01.HYP.13.6.896] [PMID: 2786848]

[249] Takaya K, Ogawa Y, Isse N, *et al.* Molecular cloning of rat leptin receptor isoform complementary DNAsidentification of a missense mutation in Zucker fatty (fa/fa) rats. Biochem Biophys Res Commun 1996; 225(1): 75-83.
[http://dx.doi.org/10.1006/bbrc.1996.1133] [PMID: 8769097]

[250] Shiota M, Printz RL. Diabetes in Zucker diabetic fatty rat. Methods Mol Biol 2012; 933: 103-23.
[PMID: 22893404]

[251] Yokoi N, Hoshino M, Hidaka S, *et al.* A Novel Rat Model of Type 2 Diabetes: The Zucker Fatty Diabetes Mellitus ZFDM Rat. J Diabetes Res 2013; 2013: 103731.
[http://dx.doi.org/10.1155/2013/103731]

[252] Kawai K, Sakairi T, Harada S, *et al.* Diet modification and its influence on metabolic and related pathological alterations in the SHR/NDmcr-cp rat, an animal model of the metabolic syndrome. Exp Toxicol Pathol 2012; 64(4): 333-8.
[http://dx.doi.org/10.1016/j.etp.2010.09.006] [PMID: 20965707]

[253] Okamoto K, Aoki K. Development of a strain of spontaneously hypertensive rats. Jpn Circ J 1963; 27: 282-93.
[http://dx.doi.org/10.1253/jcj.27.282] [PMID: 13939773]

[254] Koletsky S. Obese spontaneously hypertensive rats a model for study of atherosclerosis. Exp Mol Pathol 1973; 19(1): 53-60.
[http://dx.doi.org/10.1016/0014-4800(73)90040-3] [PMID: 4721724]

[255] Michaelis OE IV, Ellwood KC, Judge JM, Schoene NW, Hansen CT. Effect of dietary sucrose on the SHR/N-corpulent rat: a new model for insulin-independent diabetes. Am J Clin Nutr 1984; 39(4): 612-8.
[PMID: 6369957]

[256] Akimoto T, Nakama K, Katsuta Y, *et al.* Characterization of a novel congenic strain of diabetic fatty (WBN/Kob-Lepr(fa)) rat. Biochem Biophys Res Commun 2008; 366(2): 556-62.
[http://dx.doi.org/10.1016/j.bbrc.2007.12.003] [PMID: 18068663]

[257] Akimoto T, Terada M, Shimizu A, Sawai N, Ozawa H. The influence of dietary restriction on the development of diabetes and pancreatitis in female WBN/Kob-fatty rats. Exp Anim 2010; 59(5): 623-30.

[http://dx.doi.org/10.1538/expanim.59.623] [PMID: 21030790]

[258] Akimoto T, Terada M, Shimizu A. Progression of pancreatitis prior to diabetes onset in WBN/Kob-Lepr(fa) rats. J Vet Med Sci 2012; 74(1): 65-70.
[http://dx.doi.org/10.1292/jvms.11-0168] [PMID: 21836382]

[259] Wang CY, Liao JK. A mouse model of diet-induced obesity and insulin resistance. Methods Mol Biol 2012; 821: 421-33.
[http://dx.doi.org/10.1007/978-1-61779-430-8_27] [PMID: 22125082]

[260] Ikarashi N, Toda T, Okaniwa T, Ito K, Ochiai W, Sugiyama K. Anti-Obesity and Anti-Diabetic Effects of Acacia Polyphenol in Obese Diabetic KKAy Mice Fed High-Fat Diet 2011.
[http://dx.doi.org/10.1093/ecam/nep241]

[261] Kubo K, Shimada T, Onishi R, *et al.* Puerariae flos alleviates metabolic diseases in Western diet-loaded, spontaneously obese type 2 diabetic model mice. J Nat Med 2012; 66(4): 622-30.
[http://dx.doi.org/10.1007/s11418-012-0629-z] [PMID: 22350143]

[262] Matsuda A, Makino N, Tozawa T, *et al.* Pancreatic fat accumulation, fibrosis, and acinar cell injury in the Zucker diabetic fatty rat fed a chronic high-fat diet. Pancreas 2014; 43(5): 735-43.
[http://dx.doi.org/10.1097/MPA.0000000000000129] [PMID: 24717823]

[263] Takahashi Y, Soejima Y, Kumagai A, Watanabe M, Uozaki H, Fukusato T. Japanese herbal medicines shosaikoto, inchinkoto, and juzentaihoto inhibit high-fat diet-induced nonalcoholic steatohepatitis in db/db mice. Pathol Int 2014; 64(10): 490-8.
[http://dx.doi.org/10.1111/pin.12199] [PMID: 25229199]

CHAPTER 2

Unravelling Potential Anorexigen Effects of Nesfatin-1: How Homeostatic Mechanisms Help Balance Excess Calories

Carmine Finelli[*]

Department of Emergency and Internal Medicine, S. Maria della Pietà Nola's Hospital, Via della Repubblica 1, 80035 Nola (Na), Italy

Abstract: In this chapter, we review the current concepts about Nesfatin-1 as a new anti-obesity treatment and evaluate the existing issues about this knowledge and the available literature. The intent is to inform clinicians about Nesfatin-1 as a new kind of anti-obesity treatment and make a rational decision based on this perspective as possible clinical application. It can be potentially helpful in the therapy of metabolic disorders and obesity of various origins. In fact, the details of nesfatin-1 physiology could be clarified, and it may be considered suitable in the future as a potential drug in the pharmacotherapy of obesity, due to its anorexigenic effects, and as a new potential modulator of appetite in the therapy of eating disorders such as anorexia nervosa by using selective nesfatin-1 antagonists. Therefore, further progress of pharmacological researches in this field is still very limited. Further research on this topic certainly merit attention.

Keywords: Drug treatment, Eating disorders, Feeding behaviour, Nesfatin-1, Obesity.

INTRODUCTION

Nesfatin-1 is an 82-amino-acid peptide originated from post-translational processing of the terminal fragment of nucleobindin 2 (NUCB2), a 396-amino-acid protein exceptionally conserved across mammalian species [1]. The structure of NUCB2 appears to predict the post-translational cleavage by nesfatin-2 fragment (85–163) and nesfatin-3 fragment (166–396) in addition to nesfatin-1 [1]. Pharmacological studies in rats [1] suggest that nesfatin-1 (named as acronym for NEFA/nucleobindin2-encoded satiety- and fat-influencing protein) might have physiological importance in regulating food intake.

---

[*] **Corresponding author Carmine Finelli:** Department of Emergency and Internal Medicine, S. Maria della Pietà Nola's Hospital, *Via* della Repubblica 1, ASL Napoli 3 Sud, 80035 Nola (Na), Italy; Tel: +39 349/8667338; Fax: +39 081/0322199; E-mail: carminefinelli74@yahoo.it

Atta-ur-Rahman and M. Iqbal Choudhary (Eds.)
All rights reserved-© 2017 Bentham Science Publishers

In fact, nesfatin-1 injected into the third brain ventricle reduced food intake during the dark phase, while nesfatin-2 or nesfatin-3 had no effect [1]. In the same way, continuous infusion of nesfatin-1 (5 pmol/day for 10 days into the third brain ventricle) decreased food intake significantly and body weight gain. Conversely, third ventricle infusion of a NUCB-2 antisense oligonucleotide increased food intake and body weight gain compared with a mis-sense NUCB-2 oligonucleotide [1]. Additionally, a 24-h fast decreased the expression of NUCB-2 in the paraventricular nucleus (PVN) [1].

Some studies [2 - 4] showed high expression level of nesfatin-1/NUCB-2 in hypothalamic and medullary sites implicated in feeding regulation in rats. The localisation on arcuate nucleus, PVN, and the nucleus of the solitary tract (NTS) further support the evidence that nesfatin-1 is involved in food intake regulation.

Nesfatin-1, a neuropeptide produced in the hypothalamus of mammals, is co-expressed with Melanin-Concentrating Hormone (MCH) in neurons from the tuberal hypothalamic area (THA), being both recruited during sleep states, especially paradoxical sleep [5]. To help decipher the contribution of this contingent of THA neurons to sleep regulatory mechanisms, Jego *et al.* investigated whether the co-factor Nesfatin-1 is also endowed with sleep-modulating properties in rats [5]. Jego *et al.* found that disruption of the brain Nesfatin-1 signaling, achieved by intracerecroventricular administration of Nesfatin-1 antiserum or antisense against the nucleobindin2 (NUCB2) prohormone, suppressed PS with little, if any alteration of slow wave sleep (SWS) [5]. Additionally, the infusion of Nesfatin-1 antiserum after a selective PS deprivation, designed for elevating PS needs, severely prevented the ensuing expected PS recovery [5]. Strengthening these pharmacological data, Jergo *et al.* demonstrated by using c-Fos as an index of neuronal activation that the recruitment of Nesfatin-1-immunoreactive neurons within THA is positively correlated to PS but not to SWS amounts experienced on rats previously to sacrifice [5]. In conclusion, this work supports a functional contribution of the Nesfatin-1 effects, which are managed by THA neurons, to PS regulatory mechanisms [5]. Jergo *et al.* proposed that these neurons, maybe releasing MCH as a synergistic factor, constitute an appropriate lever trough which the hypothalamus may integrate endogenous signals to adapt the ultradian rhythm and maintenance of PS in a manner dictated by homeostatic needs [5]. This could be done through the inhibition of downstream targets comprised primarily of the local hypothalamic wake-active orexin- and histamine-containing neurons [5].

The corticotropin-releasing factor (CRF)/urocortin family of neuropeptides and receptors constitute an affective regulatory system due to the integral role it plays in controlling neural substrates of arousal, emotionality, and aversive processes

[6]. Activation of brain CRF signaling pathways by CRF acting on CRF1 and CRF2 receptors and by selective endogenous CRF2 agonists urocortin 2 or 3 [6] inhibits food intake [7]. Nesfatin-1 injected intracerebroventricularly significantly decreased gastric emptying [8]. Goebel-Stengel *et al.* showed that NUCB2/nesfatin-1 immunoreactivity is distributed in mouse brain areas involved in the regulation of stress response and visceral functions are activated by an acute psychological stressor, suggesting that nesfatin-1 might play a role in the efferent component of the stress response [8].

Nesfatin-1/NUCB-2 and Anorexigenic Effect

Peptides that often regulate food intake act in concert or in series with other neurotransmitters to exert their actions [9]. Nesfatin-1/NUCB-2 is co-localized with a number of hypothalamic peptides regulating food intake [10 - 16]. Several interactions have been described to underlie the central anorexic effect of nesfatin-1 [17]. In situ hybridization and immunohistochemical researches have evaluated the expression of nesfatin-1 throughout the brain and, particularly, in the medullary autonomic gateway known as NTS [18].

Two proteins have been localized in the arcuate nucleus (ARC) and implicated in the regulation of food intake: the serine-threonine-kinase mammalian target of rapamycin (mTOR) as part of the TOR signaling complex 1 (TORC1) that integrates signals from multiple pathways, including nutrients (*e.g.*, amino acids and glucose), growth factors (*e.g.*, insulin and insulin like growth factor 1), hormones (*e.g.*, leptin), and stresses (*e.g.*, starvation, hypoxia, and DNA damage) to regulate a wide variety of eukaryotic cellular functions, such as translation, transcription, protein turnover, cell growth, differentiation, cell survival, metabolism, energy balance, and stress response, and nesfatin-1 derived from the precursor protein nucleobindin2, as reported by Inhoff *et al.* [19]. In fact, nesfatin-1 is not only intracellularly co-localized with cocaine- and amphetamine-regulated transcript (CART) peptide as reported before, but also with phospho-mTOR (pmTOR) and neuropeptide Y (NPY) in ARC neurons [19]. This data could also confirm results from previous studies, showing that the majority of nesfatin-1 neurons are also positive for CART peptide, whereas most of the pmTOR is co-localized with NPY and only to a lesser extent with CART [19].

The Oxytocin Pathway in Nesfatin-1's Inhibitory Effect on Food Intake

Oxytocin is a hormone secreted by the posterior lobe of the pituitary gland, a pea-sized structure at the base of the brain. The oxytocin injected into the 3v reduces food intake *via* a leptin-independent mechanism [12] and nesfatin-1 injected into the 3v activates oxytocin-positive neurons in the magnocellular part of the PVN as assessed by double labelling for Fos/oxytocin immunoreactivity. Furthermore, *in vitro* it stimulates the release of oxytocin from PVN neurons [12]. In addition, there is pharmacologic and anatomical support for the involvement of oxytocinergic projections from the PVN to the nucleus of the solitary tract in the anorexigenic signalling of nesfatin-1 [12]. Injection of an oxytocin receptor antagonist into the hindbrain at the level of the 4v blocked the anorexigenic effect of nesfatin-1 injected into the PVN. Furthermore, tracing studies showed synaptic contacts between oxytocinergic nerve terminals and pro-opiomelanocortin (POMC) neurons in the nucleus of the solitary tract. An oxytocin antagonist injected in intracerebroventricular blocks suppresses the food intake effects of intracerebroventricular nesfatin-1 and α-melanocyte-stimulating hormone (α-MSH) [20]. Therefore, nesfatin-1 acts through serial neuronal circuits in which it activates the central melanocortin system that in turn acts through the central oxytocin system, leading to an inhibition of food and water intake and an increase in mean arterial pressure [20]. Future research should try to clarify whether the hypothalamic/nesfatin-1-oxytocinbrainstem/POMC signalling is the predominant pathway or an intrahypothalamic nesfatin-1 POMC/oxytocin network exists.

Nesfatin-1 and CRF

Over time anorexigenic effect, following intracerebroventricular injection of nesfatin-1 mimics the characteristics of the food intake reducing the effect of CRF2 receptor agonists, urocortins [6, 21]. Therefore, involvement of the CRF2 receptors in mediation of the nesfatin-1's effect was investigated. The CRF2 antagonist, astressin2-B [22], injected intracerebroventricular completely abolished the dark phase. Consequently, food intake reduction is induced by intracerebroventricular nesfatin-1 [23]. By contrast, a control peptide of similar structure as astressin2-B but without affinity to the CRF2 receptor did not influence intracerebroventricular nesfatin-1's action [23]. However, astressin2-B injected intracerebroventricular did not modulate the rapid onset reduction of food intake observed after intracerebroventricular injection of nesfatin-1 [23]. In contrast to the effect on food intake, the CRF2 antagonist, astressin2-B injected intracerebroventricular did not alter the intracerebroventricular nesfatin-1 induced delayed gastric emptying [23] suggesting different downstream signalling pathways mediating intracerebroventricular nesfatin-1's inhibitory effects on food intake and gastric transit. The melanocortin 3/4 receptor antagonist, SHU9119 injected intracerebroventricular diminished, and into the 3v abolished [1], the anorexigenic effect of nesfatin-1 [20]. Nesfatin-1 probably acts in series through the recruitment of the central melanocortin and CRF2's pathways to reduce food intake.

Intracerebroventricular administration of nesfatin-1 lead to c-Fos expression in CRF neurons, and nesfatin-1 increased cytosolic Ca^{2+} concentrations in single

CRF neurons in the PVN [24]. It is now well established that the brain CRF/CRF1 signaling system modulates pain responses [24]. These observations suggest that nesfatin-1 may be involved in the autonomic regulation of visceral sensation [24].

Nesfatin-1 and Anti-Obesity Treatment

It has also been postulated that nesfatin-1/NUCB-2 may be produced by the hypothalamus [16]; the relatively high CerebroSpinalFluid (CSF)/plasma nesfatin-1/NUCB-2 ratios suggest that a substantial amount of CSF nesfatin-1/NUCB-2 may originate from central neurons. The possible discrepancy in the production of nesfatin-1/NUCB-2, by these central neurons may account for the differences in CSF/plasma nesfatin-1/NUCB-2 ratio between obese and lean subjects observed by Tan et al [14]. Finally, it is possible that the efficiency of nesfatin-1/NUCB-2 uptake into CSF is reduced in obese individuals, possibly due to saturation of transporters [14]. Further studies could be useful to elucidate this hypothesis. Some data demonstrated that nesfatin-1/NUCB-2 is a novel depot specific adipokine preferentially expressed in subcutaneous adipose tissue/adipocytes. Adipose tissue nesfatin-1/NUCB-2 expression increases with obesity and is altered in states of feeding and malnutrition [25].

A reduced leptin sensitivity or leptin resistance is a common phenomenon in obesity. Because central and peripheral injection of nesfatin-1 exert its food uptake reducing effects *via* a leptin-independent mechanism [1, 11], targeting nesfatin-1 may be a promising approach in the treatment of obesity and its complications. Over time pre-clinical data suggest the possible use of subcutaneous and intranasal routes of nesfatin-1 administration [26], which needs to be further explored.

Another important aspect to be unraveled is the weight loss upon chronic administration of nesfatin-1 [27 - 30] and possible related changes in energy balance and/or basal metabolic rate [31 - 36]. In fact, nesfatin-1 has a remarkably prolonged effect on food intake and body temperature [37]. Time course of nesfatin-1's effects may be varied depending on the time applied [37]. Many of the nesfatin1/NUCB2 neurones are cold sensitive, and are positioned in key centres of thermoregulation [37]. Nesfatin-1 regulates energy expenditure making it a preferable candidate anti-obesity drug [37].

Moreover, bariatric surgery produces differential influences with regards to circulating nesfatin-1 and in particular the receptor involved in the peptide's actions and the processing of NUCB2 to nesfatin-1 in hypothalamic or gut tissues still remain elusive [38].

Nesfatin-1 and Food Behaviour Control

The central nervous system regulates feeding behaviour; in particular, the regulation of appetite is managed by the ventromedial nucleus (VMH), the PVN, ARC and suprachiasmatic nucleus (SCN) of the hypothalamus and the lateral hypothalamic area (LHA) [39 - 41]. Hypothalamic and brainstem neuronal circuits are critically involved in the sensing of circulating and local factors conveying information about food intake, energy status of the organism and environmental stimuli through the integration and the modulation of peripheral and central orexigenic or anorexigenic signals [41]. The integration of these signals culminates in the generation of specific and coordinated physiological responses aimed at regulating energy balance through the modulation of appetite/food intake and energy expenditure [41].

Several neuropeptides are implicated in the hypothalamic control of feeding behaviour [42]. Of those, neuropeptide Y (NPY), a potent orexigenic factor whose expression increases during negative states of energy balance, is one of the major substances stimulating populations of neurons during conditions of low leptin levels, hypoglycemia, hypoinsulinemia, and conditions of negative energy balance, showing an elevated mRNA expression in ARC [40, 41]. Also, POMC is the precursor of various molecules including α-melanocyte-stimulating hormone (α-MSH), which produces an anorexigenic effect [40, 41]. The other peptide is cocaine- and amphetamine-regulated transcript (CART) that it is particularly abundant in the hypothalamus (co-localizing for more than 95% with POMC in the ARC). The axons of these hypothalamic neurons extending to "second order neurons" probably influence the anorexigenic effects of leptin, likely caused by the mid-segment of nesfatin-1 [11, 40, 41]. Therefore, anorexigenic peptides have direct action through a catabolic circuit, when signals of adiposity excess reach ARC.

After intracerebroventricular injection, nesfatin-1 had a half-time disappearance of 23.8 min, which was not significantly different from that of albumin, indicating that nesfatin-1 exited the brain by bulk absorption of cerebrospinal fluid without a specific efflux transport system [43]. Some studies [43, 44] showed that the permeation of nesfatin-1 is a non-saturable process in either the blood-to-brain or brain-to-blood direction.

Nesfatin-1, when centrally administered, inhibits feeding behaviour and gastroduodenal motility in mice [45]. In addition, feeding behaviour is stimulated from intracerebroventricular injection of the antibody neutralizing nesfatin-1, but not of the other fragments [1, 17].

Nesfatin-1 and Signaling Pathway

The leptin-melanocortin signaling pathway does not appear to influence nesfatin signalling [1, 11, 12, 17]. As previously emphasised, nesfatin-1 inhibits feeding behaviour and gastroduodenal motility when centrally administered in mice [45]; vice versa, peripherally administered in the same animal model, it reduces food intake with a leptin-independent action [11]. Therefore, the loss of appetite is stimulated, through a leptin-independent melanocortin mechanism, by nesfatin--regulated oxytocinergic signalling originated in the paraventricular nucleus [12], suggesting that, in the hypothalamus, melanocortin signalling mechanism might be associated with nesfatin-1 signalling pathway. The POMC and CART genes expression, on nucleus of the solitary tract, is increased from an intra-peritoneal injection of M30 nesfatin-1 fragment, suggesting that M30 may induce anorexia [32]. Inhoff *et al.* [19] showed that the majority of nesfatin-1 neurons are also positive for CART peptide, whereas most of the phospho-mTOR (pmTOR), a newly identified protein that functions regulating food intake, is co-localized with NPY and only to a lesser extent with CART. Therefore, the inhibition of orexigenic NPY neurons could mediate nesfatin-1-induced inhibition of feeding [46].

Iwasaki *et al.* [47] showed that nesfatin-1 evokes $Ca2^+$ signalling in isolated vagal afferent neurons *via* $Ca2^+$ influx through N-type channels, demonstrating from one side through which mechanisms it conveys signals to the brain and from the other that feeding behaviour can be suppressed by peripheral nesfatin-1. Regarding researches about nesfatin-1 brain expression, some studies found nesfatin-1 immuno-reactivity in the rat gastric mucosa, the major part of nesfatin-1 immunoreactive cells simultaneously expressing ghrelin [48 - 51]. It has been evidenced an important role of gastric X/A-like cells in the food intake regulation through the expression of the orexigenic peptide ghrelin along with des-acyl ghrelin and nesfatin-1, all capable of reducing food intake upon exogenous injection, although their mechanisms of action and functional significance remain to be established [52].

A marked increase in intracellular nesfatin-1 levels is not derived by stimulation of only subcutaneous adipose tissue with inflammatory cytokines (TNF-a and IL-6), but also because of insulin and dexamethasone [26]. Moreover, in high-fat-fed mice higher circulating levels of nesfatin-1 have been observed, while in human a positive correlation to body mass index has been evidenced [26].

In addition, after abdominal surgery, Stengel *et al.* [52] found nesfatin-1 immunoreactive neurons in specific nuclei of the hypothalamus and brainstem, hypothesizing that nesfatin-1 could be implicated in the alterations of food intake and gastric transit correlated to such a trauma.

It is known that the central regulation of food intake is up-regulated or down regulated in diabetic patients according to plasma the levels of some of the brain-gut peptides. On this basis, some researchers highlighted the association between nesfatin-1 and diabetes mellitus or simple hyperglycemia, hypothesizing firstly a possible role for pro-nesfatin-derived peptides in islet biology and glucose homeostasis in rats, secondly a function of beta-cell mechanism for NUCB2, and finally a possible implication in diabetic pathology [53, 54]. Su *et al.* [55] also showed that, in hyperglycemic rats, the intravenous administration of nesfatin-1 has an anti-hyperglycemic effect. Li *et al.* [28] found that patients with type 2 diabetes mellitus presented significantly lower values of fasting nesfatin-1 compared to healthy subjects, hypothesizing that, in diabetic hyperphagia, nesfatin-1 could represent one of the appetite-related hormones, being characterized by low values in fasting.

Bonnet *et al.* [56] showed that peripheral inflammatory signals could act on a portion of nesfatin-1 neurons of both hypothalamus and brainstem, and provided the first clues that the endotoxaemic anorexia could be caused, through neural mechanisms, by centrally released nesfatin-1.

Nesfatin-1 and Eating Disorders

Nesfatin-1 shows some anorexigenic properties, therefore there is a need to conduct further research studies analysing its potential role in pathogenesis of psychogenic eating disorders.

Ogiso *et al.* [57] showed that although anorexia nervosa (AN-R) is associated with emaciation for a prolonged period, results suggested that nesfatin-1 levels might be regulated by nutrition status and response to starvation. This may indicate a negative correlation with ghrelin and des-acyl ghrelin levels [57]. In contrast, a positive correlation between nesfatin-1 levels and BMI was demonstrated [57].

However, low nesfatin-1 levels may be related to generalized anxiety disorder [58], while NUCB2/nesfatin-1 is associated with elevated scores of anxiety in female obese patients [59], but there is still not convincing evidence that the low nesfatin-1 level underlies anxiety disorders in AN-R. Probably, during periods of extreme starvation, the reduced nesfatin-1 level may decrease "worries", "tension", "demands", "anxiety" or "fear" and stimulate food-intake. Unfortunately, few research papers on this topic do not allow us to precisely interpret these phenomena. Therefore, there is a need that some valuable data, contributing to this debate, could be provided by brain imaging studies (PET,

SPECT), using radiolabelled nesfatin-1.

CONCLUSIVE REMARKS

Nesfatin-1 is a neuropeptide that is active in the CNS. Nesfatin-1 could play a role as regulator of food intake and body weight. Kuksis and Ferguson [60] showed that nesfatin-1 has the ability to influence the membrane potential of subfornical organ neurones, and thus identifies the subfornical organ as a potential site at which nesfatin-1 may act to regulate ingestive behaviour and cardiovascular control.

Future research should seek to clarify whether nesfatin-1/NUCB-2 would be beneficial in the management of obesity. Furthermore, bariatric surgery produces differential influences with regards to circulating nesfatin-1. In particular the receptor involved in the peptide's action, and the processing of NUCB2 to nesfatin-1 in hypothalamic or gut tissues still remain elusive [38].

Albayrak *et al.* [4] showed that the central nesfatin-1 system should be taken into consideration, rather than the peripheral nesfatin-1 system, when considering the regulation of appetite in a with burns and particularly those accompanied by infection.

Anik *et al.* [61] showed that there was no significant increase in the postprandial level of nesfatin1. This observation suggested that oral glucose load in obese children may not be sufficient for nesfatin-1 response and that nesfatin-1 may not have an effect as a short-term regulator of food intake, as reported by Anik et al [61].

Endogenous GLP-1 acts on paraventricular nucleus to suppress the food intake [62]. Glucagon-like peptide-1 (GLP-1) receptor agonists have been used to treat type 2 diabetic patients and shown to reduce food intake and body weight, as reported by Katsurada *et al.* [62]. The anorexigenic effects of GLP-1 and GLP-1 receptor agonists are thought to be mediated primarily *via* the hypothalamic PVN [62]. GLP-1, an intestinal hormone, is also localized in the NTS of the brain stem. The majority of GLP-1-responsive neurons were immunoreactive predominantly to corticotropin releasing hormone (CRH) and nesfatin-1, and less frequently to oxytocin, as showed by Katsurada *et al.* [62]. Katsurada et. al [62] indicate that endogenous GLP-1 targets PVN to restrict feeding behaviour, in which the projection from NTS GLP-1 neurons and activation of CRH and nesfatin-1 neurons might be implicated. Recently, Darambazar *et al.* [63] showed that paraventricular NUCB2/nesfatin-1 is directly targeted by leptin and mediates its anorexigenic effect. Leptin is an adipokine that plays a central role in the regulation of feeding and energy homeostasis *via* acting on the hypothalamus.

Darambazar *et al.* [63] showed that peripheral and central injections of leptin failed to significantly inhibit food intake in mice receiving adeno-associated virus (AAV) NUCB2. Therefore, Darambazar *et al.* [63] showed that PVN NUCB2/nesfatin-1 is directly targeted by leptin, and mediates its anorexigenic effect.

The data obtained in basic experiments of nesfatin-1 should be useful for the development of a new anti-obesity treatment [64]. However, the mechanisms of endocrine and metabolic effects of nesfatin-1 have not been elucidated until now, and the influences of nesfatin-1 administered peripherally should be much more clarified *in vivo* before starting controlled clinical trials in the future. In fact, the details of nesfatin-1 physiology ought to be clarified, and it may be considered suitable in the future, as a potential drug in the pharmacotherapy of obesity, due to its anorexigenic effects, and as a new potential modulator of appetite in therapy of eating disorders such as anorexia nervosa by using selective nesfatin-1 antagonists. Therefore, the further progress of pharmacological researches in this field is still very limited. Further research on this topic certainly merits attention.

CONFLICT OF INTEREST

The authors confirm that they have no conflict of interest to declare for this publication.

ACKNOWLEDGEMENTS

Declared none.

ABBREVIATIONS

α-MSH	=	α-melanocyte-stimulating hormone
AgRP	=	Agouti-related peptide
AN-R	=	anorexia nervosa
ARC	=	arcuate nucleus
CART	=	cocaine- and amphetamine-regulated transcript
CRH	=	corticotropin-releasing hormone
CSF	=	Cerebro Spinal Fluid
GLP-1	=	Glucagon-like peptide-1
LHA	=	lateral hypothalamic area
MCH	=	Melanin-Concentrating Hormone
mTOR	=	mammalian target of rapamycin
NPY	=	neuropeptide Y
NTS	=	nucleus of the solitary tract
NUCB2	=	nucleobindin 2
pmTOR	=	phospho-mTOR
POMC	=	pro-opiomelanocortin
PVN	=	paraventricular nucleus
SCN	=	suprachiasmatic nucleus
SWS	=	slow wave sleep
THA	=	tuberal hypothalamic area
VMH	=	ventromedial nucleus

REFERENCES

[1] Oh-I S, Shimizu H, Satoh T, *et al.* Identification of nesfatin-1 as a satiety molecule in the hypothalamus. Nature 2006; 443(7112): 709-12.
[http://dx.doi.org/10.1038/nature05162] [PMID: 17036007]

[2] Zheng H, Lenard NR, Shin AC, Berthoud HR. Appetite control and energy balance regulation in the modern world: reward-driven brain overrides repletion signals. Int J Obes 2009; 33(2) (Suppl. 2): S8-S13.
[http://dx.doi.org/10.1038/ijo.2009.65] [PMID: 19528982]

[3] Ishida E, Hashimoto K, Shimizu H, *et al.* Nesfatin-1 induces the phosphorylation levels of cAMP response element-binding protein for intracellular signaling in a neural cell line. PLoS One 2012; 7(12): e50918.
[http://dx.doi.org/10.1371/journal.pone.0050918] [PMID: 23236405]

[4] Albayrak A, Demiryilmaz I, Albayrak Y, *et al.* The role of diminishing appetite and serum nesfatin-1 level in patients with burn wound infection. Iran Red Crescent Med J 2013; 15(5): 389-92.
[http://dx.doi.org/10.5812/ircmj.4198] [PMID: 24349725]

[5] Jego S, Salvert D, Renouard L, *et al.* Tuberal hypothalamic neurons secreting the satiety molecule Nesfatin-1 are critically involved in paradoxical (REM) sleep homeostasis. PLoS One 2012; 7(12): e52525.
[http://dx.doi.org/10.1371/journal.pone.0052525] [PMID: 23300698]

[6] Chen P, Hover CV, Lindberg D, Li C. Central urocortin 3 and type 2 corticotropin-releasing factor receptor in the regulation of energy homeostasis: critical involvement of the ventromedial hypothalamus. Front Endocrinol (Lausanne) 2013; 3: 180.
[http://dx.doi.org/10.3389/fendo.2012.00180] [PMID: 23316185]

[7] Doyon C, Moraru A, Richard D. The corticotropin-releasing factor system as a potential target for antiobesity drugs. Drug News Perspect 2004; 17(8): 505-17.
[http://dx.doi.org/10.1358/dnp.2004.17.8.863694] [PMID: 15605110]

[8] García-Galiano D, Pineda R, Ilhan T, *et al.* Cellular distribution, regulated expression, and functional role of the anorexigenic peptide, NUCB2/nesfatin-1, in the testis. Endocrinology 2012; 153(4): 1959-71.
[http://dx.doi.org/10.1210/en.2011-2032] [PMID: 22334726]

[9] Perry B, Wang Y. Appetite regulation and weight control: the role of gut hormones. Nutr Diabetes 2012; 2: e26.
[http://dx.doi.org/10.1038/nutd.2011.21] [PMID: 23154682]

[10] Fort P, Salvert D, Hanriot L, *et al.* The satiety molecule nesfatin-1 is co-expressed with melanin concentrating hormone in tuberal hypothalamic neurons of the rat. Neuroscience 2008; 155(1): 174-81.
[http://dx.doi.org/10.1016/j.neuroscience.2008.05.035] [PMID: 18573315]

[11] Shimizu H, Oh-I S, Hashimoto K, *et al.* Peripheral administration of nesfatin-1 reduces food intake in mice: the leptin-independent mechanism. Endocrinology 2009; 150(2): 662-71.
[http://dx.doi.org/10.1210/en.2008-0598] [PMID: 19176321]

[12] Maejima Y, Sedbazar U, Suyama S, *et al.* Nesfatin-1-regulated oxytocinergic signaling in the paraventricular nucleus causes anorexia through a leptin-independent melanocortin pathway. Cell Metab 2009; 10(5): 355-65.
[http://dx.doi.org/10.1016/j.cmet.2009.09.002] [PMID: 19883614]

[13] Yoshida N, Maejima Y, Sedbazar U, *et al.* Stressor-responsive central nesfatin-1 activates corticotropin-releasing hormone, noradrenaline and serotonin neurons and evokes hypothalamic-pituitary-adrenal axis. Aging (Albany, NY) 2010; 2(11): 775-84.
[http://dx.doi.org/10.18632/aging.100207] [PMID: 20966530]

[14] Tan BK, Hallschmid M, Kern W, Lehnert H, Randeva HS. Decreased cerebrospinal fluid/plasma ratio of the novel satiety molecule, nesfatin-1/NUCB-2, in obese humans: evidence of nesfatin-1/NUCB-2 resistance and implications for obesity treatment. J Clin Endocrinol Metab 2011; 96(4): E669-73.
[http://dx.doi.org/10.1210/jc.2010-1782] [PMID: 21252251]

[15] Kerbel B, Unniappan S. Nesfatin-1 suppresses energy intake, co-localises ghrelin in the brain and gut, and alters ghrelin, cholecystokinin and orexin mRNA expression in goldfish. J Neuroendocrinol 2012; 24(2): 366-77.
[http://dx.doi.org/10.1111/j.1365-2826.2011.02246.x] [PMID: 22023656]

[16] Goebel-Stengel M, Wang L. Central and peripheral expression and distribution of NUCB2/nesfatin-1. Curr Pharm Des 2013; 19(39): 6935-40.
[http://dx.doi.org/10.2174/1381612819391311271248141] [PMID: 23537079]

[17] Shimizu H, Ohsaki A, Oh-I S, Okada S, Mori M. A new anorexigenic protein, nesfatin-1. Peptides 2009; 30(5): 995-8.
[http://dx.doi.org/10.1016/j.peptides.2009.01.002] [PMID: 19452636]

[18] Mimee A, Smith PM, Ferguson AV. Nesfatin-1 influences the excitability of neurons in the nucleus of the solitary tract and regulates cardiovascular function. Am J Physiol Regul Integr Comp Physiol 2012; 302(11): R1297-304.
[http://dx.doi.org/10.1152/ajpregu.00266.2011] [PMID: 22442196]

[19] Inhoff T, Stengel A, Peter L, *et al.* Novel insight in distribution of nesfatin-1 and phospho-mTOR in the arcuate nucleus of the hypothalamus of rats. Peptides 2010; 31(2): 257-62.
[http://dx.doi.org/10.1016/j.peptides.2009.11.024] [PMID: 19961888]

[20] Yosten GL, Samson WK. The anorexigenic and hypertensive effects of nesfatin-1 are reversed by pretreatment with an oxytocin receptor antagonist. Am J Physiol Regul Integr Comp Physiol 2010; 298(6): R1642-7.
[http://dx.doi.org/10.1152/ajpregu.00804.2009] [PMID: 20335376]

[21] Yakabi K, Noguchi M, Ohno S, *et al.* Urocortin 1 reduces food intake and ghrelin secretion *via* CRF(2) receptors. Am J Physiol Endocrinol Metab 2011; 301(1): E72-82.
[http://dx.doi.org/10.1152/ajpendo.00695.2010] [PMID: 21540451]

[22] Wang L, Stengel A, Goebel-Stengel M, Shaikh A, Yuan PQ, Taché Y. Intravenous injection of urocortin 1 induces a CRF2 mediated increase in circulating ghrelin and glucose levels through distinct mechanisms in rats. Peptides 2013; 39: 164-70.
[http://dx.doi.org/10.1016/j.peptides.2012.11.009] [PMID: 23183626]

[23] Stengel A, Goebel M, Wang L, *et al.* Central nesfatin-1 reduces dark-phase food intake and gastric emptying in rats: differential role of corticotropin-releasing factor2 receptor. Endocrinology 2009; 150(11): 4911-9.
[http://dx.doi.org/10.1210/en.2009-0578] [PMID: 19797401]

[24] Jia FY, Li XL, Li TN, Wu J, Xie BY, Lin L. Role of nesfatin-1 in a rat model of visceral hypersensitivity. World J Gastroenterol 2013; 19(22): 3487-93.
[http://dx.doi.org/10.3748/wjg.v19.i22.3487] [PMID: 23801843]

[25] Ramanjaneya M, Chen J, Brown JE, *et al.* Identification of nesfatin-1 in human and murine adipose tissue: a novel depot-specific adipokine with increased levels in obesity. Endocrinology 2010; 151(7): 3169-80.
[http://dx.doi.org/10.1210/en.2009-1358] [PMID: 20427481]

[26] Shimizu H, Oh-I S, Okada S, Mori M. Nesfatin-1: an overview and future clinical application. Endocr J 2009; 56(4): 537-43.
[http://dx.doi.org/10.1507/endocrj.K09E-117] [PMID: 19461159]

[27] Li QC, Wang HY, Chen X, Guan HZ, Jiang ZY. Fasting plasma levels of nesfatin-1 in patients with type 1 and type 2 diabetes mellitus and the nutrient-related fluctuation of nesfatin-1 level in normal

humans. Regul Pept 2010; 159(1-3): 72-7.
[http://dx.doi.org/10.1016/j.regpep.2009.11.003] [PMID: 19896982]

[28] Gonzalez R, Shepperd E, Thiruppugazh V, *et al.* Nesfatin-1 regulates the hypothalamo-pituitary-ovarian axis of fish. Biol Reprod 2012; 87(4): 84.
[http://dx.doi.org/10.1095/biolreprod.112.099630] [PMID: 22895855]

[29] Li Z, Gao L, Tang H, *et al.* Peripheral effects of nesfatin-1 on glucose homeostasis. PLoS One 2013; 8(8): e71513.
[http://dx.doi.org/10.1371/journal.pone.0071513] [PMID: 23967220]

[30] Dong J, Xu H, Xu H, *et al.* Nesfatin-1 stimulates fatty-acid oxidation by activating AMP-activated protein kinase in STZ-induced type 2 diabetic mice. PLoS One 2013; 8(12): e83397.
[http://dx.doi.org/10.1371/journal.pone.0083397] [PMID: 24391760]

[31] Foo KS, Brismar H, Broberger C. Distribution and neuropeptide coexistence of nucleobindin-2 mRNA/nesfatin-like immunoreactivity in the rat CNS. Neuroscience 2008; 156(3): 563-79.
[http://dx.doi.org/10.1016/j.neuroscience.2008.07.054] [PMID: 18761059]

[32] García-Galiano D, Navarro VM, Roa J, *et al.* The anorexigenic neuropeptide, nesfatin-1, is indispensable for normal puberty onset in the female rat. J Neurosci 2010; 30(23): 7783-92.
[http://dx.doi.org/10.1523/JNEUROSCI.5828-09.2010] [PMID: 20534827]

[33] Gonzalez R, Perry RL, Gao X, *et al.* Nutrient responsive nesfatin-1 regulates energy balance and induces glucose-stimulated insulin secretion in rats. Endocrinology 2011; 152(10): 3628-37.
[http://dx.doi.org/10.1210/en.2010-1471] [PMID: 21828181]

[34] Pałasz A, Krzystanek M, Worthington J, *et al.* Nesfatin-1, a unique regulatory neuropeptide of the brain. Neuropeptides 2012; 46(3): 105-12.
[http://dx.doi.org/10.1016/j.npep.2011.12.002] [PMID: 22225987]

[35] Ghanbari Niaki A, Mohammadi Joojadeh F, Zare Kookandeh N, *et al.* Liver and plasma nesfatin-1 responses to 6 weeks of treadmill running with or without zizyphus jujuba liquid extract in female rat. Int J Endocrinol Metab 2013; 11(2): 95-101.
[http://dx.doi.org/10.5812/ijem.8438] [PMID: 23825980]

[36] Vas S, Ádori C, Könczöl K, *et al.* Nesfatin-1/NUCB2 as a potential new element of sleep regulation in rats. PLoS One 2013; 8(4): e59809.
[http://dx.doi.org/10.1371/journal.pone.0059809] [PMID: 23560056]

[37] Könczöl K, Pintér O, Ferenczi S, *et al.* Nesfatin-1 exerts long-term effect on food intake and body temperature. Int J Obes 2012; 36(12): 1514-21.
[http://dx.doi.org/10.1038/ijo.2012.2] [PMID: 22290539]

[38] Finelli C, Padula MC, Martelli G, Tarantino G. Could the improvement of obesity-related co-morbidities depend on modified gut hormones secretion? World J Gastroenterol 2014; 20(44): 16649-64.
[http://dx.doi.org/10.3748/wjg.v20.i44.16649] [PMID: 25469034]

[39] Karatsoreos IN, Thaler JP, Borgland SL, Champagne FA, Hurd YL, Hill MN. Food for thought: hormonal, experiential, and neural influences on feeding and obesity. J Neurosci 2013; 33(45): 17610-6.
[http://dx.doi.org/10.1523/JNEUROSCI.3452-13.2013] [PMID: 24198352]

[40] Rui L. Brain regulation of energy balance and body weight. Rev Endocr Metab Disord 2013; 14(4): 387-407.
[http://dx.doi.org/10.1007/s11154-013-9261-9] [PMID: 23990408]

[41] Schneeberger M, Gomis R, Claret M. Hypothalamic and brainstem neuronal circuits controlling homeostatic energy balance. J Endocrinol 2014; 220(2): T25-46.
[http://dx.doi.org/10.1530/JOE-13-0398] [PMID: 24222039]

[42] Baldo BA, Pratt WE, Will MJ, Hanlon EC, Bakshi VP, Cador M. Principles of motivation revealed by the diverse functions of neuropharmacological and neuroanatomical substrates underlying feeding behavior. Neurosci Biobehav Rev 2013; 37 (9 Pt A): 1985-98.
[http://dx.doi.org/10.1016/j.neubiorev.2013.02.017] [PMID: 23466532]

[43] Pan W, Hsuchou H, Kastin AJ. Nesfatin-1 crosses the blood-brain barrier without saturation. Peptides 2007; 28(11): 2223-8.
[http://dx.doi.org/10.1016/j.peptides.2007.09.005] [PMID: 17950952]

[44] Price TO, Samson WK, Niehoff ML, Banks WA. Permeability of the blood-brain barrier to a novel satiety molecule nesfatin-1. Peptides 2007; 28(12): 2372-81.
[http://dx.doi.org/10.1016/j.peptides.2007.10.008] [PMID: 18006117]

[45] Atsuchi K, Asakawa A, Ushikai M, et al. Centrally administered nesfatin-1 inhibits feeding behaviour and gastroduodenal motility in mice. Neuroreport 2010; 21(15): 1008-11.
[PMID: 20827224]

[46] Price CJ, Samson WK, Ferguson AV. Nesfatin-1 inhibits NPY neurons in the arcuate nucleus. Brain Res 2008; 1230: 99-106.
[http://dx.doi.org/10.1016/j.brainres.2008.06.084] [PMID: 18625211]

[47] Iwasaki Y, Nakabayashi H, Kakei M, Shimizu H, Mori M, Yada T. Nesfatin-1 evokes Ca2+ signaling in isolated vagal afferent neurons via Ca2+ influx through N-type channels. Biochem Biophys Res Commun 2009; 390(3): 958-62.
[http://dx.doi.org/10.1016/j.bbrc.2009.10.085] [PMID: 19852938]

[48] Inhoff T, Mönnikes H, Noetzel S, et al. Desacyl ghrelin inhibits the orexigenic effect of peripherally injected ghrelin in rats. Peptides 2008; 29(12): 2159-68.
[http://dx.doi.org/10.1016/j.peptides.2008.09.014] [PMID: 18938204]

[49] Stengel A, Goebel M, Wang L, Taché Y. Ghrelin, des-acyl ghrelin and nesfatin-1 in gastric X/A-like cells: role as regulators of food intake and body weight. Peptides 2010; 31(2): 357-69.
[http://dx.doi.org/10.1016/j.peptides.2009.11.019] [PMID: 19944123]

[50] Stengel A, Goebel M, Yakubov I, et al. Identification and characterization of nesfatin-1 immunoreactivity in endocrine cell types of the rat gastric oxyntic mucosa. Endocrinology 2009; 150(1): 232-8.
[http://dx.doi.org/10.1210/en.2008-0747] [PMID: 18818289]

[51] Stengel A, Taché Y. Regulation of food intake: the gastric X/A-like endocrine cell in the spotlight. Curr Gastroenterol Rep 2009; 11(6): 448-54.
[http://dx.doi.org/10.1007/s11894-009-0069-4] [PMID: 19903420]

[52] Stengel A, Goebel M, Wang L, Taché Y. Abdominal surgery activates nesfatin-1 immunoreactive brain nuclei in rats. Peptides 2010; 31(2): 263-70.
[http://dx.doi.org/10.1016/j.peptides.2009.11.015] [PMID: 19944727]

[53] Foo KS, Brauner H, Ostenson CG, Broberger C. Nucleobindin-2/nesfatin in the endocrine pancreas: distribution and relationship to glycaemic state. J Endocrinol 2010; 204(3): 255-63.
[http://dx.doi.org/10.1677/JOE-09-0254] [PMID: 20032201]

[54] Gonzalez R, Tiwari A, Unniappan S. Pancreatic beta cells colocalize insulin and pronesfatin immunoreactivity in rodents. Biochem Biophys Res Commun 2009; 381(4): 643-8.
[http://dx.doi.org/10.1016/j.bbrc.2009.02.104] [PMID: 19248766]

[55] Su Y, Zhang J, Tang Y, Bi F, Liu JN. The novel function of nesfatin-1: anti-hyperglycemia. Biochem Biophys Res Commun 2010; 391(1): 1039-42.
[http://dx.doi.org/10.1016/j.bbrc.2009.12.014] [PMID: 19995555]

[56] Bonnet MS, Pecchi E, Trouslard J, Jean A, Dallaporta M, Troadec JD. Central nesfatin-1-expressing neurons are sensitive to peripheral inflammatory stimulus. J Neuroinflammation 2009; 6: 27.
[http://dx.doi.org/10.1186/1742-2094-6-27] [PMID: 19778412]

[57] Ogiso K, Asakawa A, Amitani H, *et al.* Plasma nesfatin-1 concentrations in restricting-type anorexia nervosa. Peptides 2011; 32(1): 150-3.
[http://dx.doi.org/10.1016/j.peptides.2010.10.004] [PMID: 20937336]

[58] Gunay H, Tutuncu R, Aydin S, Dag E, Abasli D. Decreased plasma nesfatin-1 levels in patients with generalized anxiety disorder. Psychoneuroendocrinology 2012; 37(12): 1949-53.
[http://dx.doi.org/10.1016/j.psyneuen.2012.04.007] [PMID: 22595767]

[59] Hofmann T, Stengel A, Ahnis A, Buße P, Elbelt U, Klapp BF. NUCB2/nesfatin-1 is associated with elevated scores of anxiety in female obese patients. Psychoneuroendocrinology 2013; 38(11): 2502-10.
[http://dx.doi.org/10.1016/j.psyneuen.2013.05.013] [PMID: 23796625]

[60] Kuksis M, Ferguson AV. Cellular actions of nesfatin-1 in the subfornical organ. J Neuroendocrinol 2014; 26(4): 237-46.
[http://dx.doi.org/10.1111/jne.12143] [PMID: 24612143]

[61] Anık A, Çatlı G, Abacı A, Küme T, Bober E. Fasting and postprandial levels of a novel anorexigenic peptide nesfatin in childhood obesity. J Pediatr Endocrinol Metab 2014; 27(7-8): 623-8.
[http://dx.doi.org/10.1515/jpem-2013-0475] [PMID: 24825087]

[62] Katsurada K, Maejima Y, Nakata M, *et al.* Endogenous GLP-1 acts on paraventricular nucleus to suppress feeding: projection from nucleus tractus solitarius and activation of corticotropin-releasing hormone, nesfatin-1 and oxytocin neurons. Biochem Biophys Res Commun 2014; 451(2): 276-81.
[http://dx.doi.org/10.1016/j.bbrc.2014.07.116] [PMID: 25089000]

[63] Darambazar G, Nakata M, Okada T, *et al.* Paraventricular NUCB2/nesfatin-1 is directly targeted by leptin and mediates its anorexigenic effect. Biochem Biophys Res Commun 2015; 456(4): 913-8.
[http://dx.doi.org/10.1016/j.bbrc.2014.12.065] [PMID: 25534851]

[64] Finelli C, Martelli G, Rossano R, *et al.* Nesfatin–1: role as possible new anti-obesity treatment. EXCLI J 2014; 13: 586-91.
[PMID: 26417285]

CHAPTER 3

Proteomics in the Characterization of New Target Therapies in Pediatric Obesity Treatment

Gillian E. Walker[1,*], Marilisa De Feudis[1], Marta Roccio[1], Gianni Bona[2] and Flavia Prodam[2]

[1] *Laboratory of Clinical Pediatrics, Department of Health Sciences, Università Del Piemonte Orientale, Novara, Italy*

[2] *Division of Pediatrics, Department of Health Sciences, Università Del Piemonte Orientale, Novara, Italy*

Abstract: Adipose tissue (AT) with a central role in body weight homeostasis, inflammation and insulin resistance, is a highly orchestrated tissue involving receptor and second messenger pathways with steps and passes that influence hyperplasia, hypertrophy, adipocyte differentiation, turnover, lipolysis, free-fatty acid (FFA) metabolism, lipogenesis and the secretome profile. Due to the limitations of the classical molecular biological methods only pieces of the puzzle have been studied, with studies failing to consider the global, time-resolved changes that are evident in this highly plastic organ. "Proteomics", first coined in 1995 is a large-scale characterization of the entire protein profile of a cell line, tissue, or organism not only from the perspective of expression but also post-translational modifications. As such proteomic technologies offer powerful tools for identifying key components of the adipose proteome, which may contribute to the pathogenesis of adipose tissue dysfunction in obesity. In this review, we plan to address the recent advances in the proteomic characterization of pediatric obesity, in particular the newly identified proteins that potentially play relevant roles and offer targets for novel therapies.

Keywords: Adipose tissue, Biomarkers, Circulation, Lifestyle, Obesity, Pediatric, Proteomic, Secretome, Therapy.

INTRODUCTION

According to the World Health Organization (WHO), obesity is now the most important contributor to ill health and expenditure worldwide, with the pediatric population paralleling adults. In 2014, WHO estimated that globally over 2 billion people were overweight, with 43 million children < 5 years overweight or obese.

---

[*] **Corresponding author Gillian E. Walker:** Department of Health Sciences, Università del Piemonte Orientale, *Via* Solaroli, 17 Novara, 28100 Italy; Tel: +39 0321 660 647; Fax: +39 0321 3733598; E-mail: gillian.walker@med.uniupo.it

Atta-ur-Rahman and M. Iqbal Choudhary (Eds.)
All rights reserved-© 2017 Bentham Science Publishers

While the prevalence rates are highly variable between countries, a clear growth has been seen in developed countries [http://www.who.int/topics/obesity/en/]. The most recent OECD "Health Behavior in School Children Survey" demonstrates overweight prevalence rates based on measured height and weight in children in the European Union of approximately 23% and 21% for 15 year old boys and girls, respectively, with a steady increase observed from the year 2000 [http://www.oecd.org/els/health-systems/Health-at-a-Glance-2013]. To address these alarming statistics, a growing number of countries have adopted and invested in health and awareness policies such as "Fit not Fat", with obesity trends in recent years stabilizing [1; http://www.who.int/topics/obesity/en/]. It remains, however, that in countries such as Greece, Italy, Slovenia, New Zealand and the United States, over 30% of the pediatric population are overweight or obese [http://www.oecd.org/health/obesity-update.htm]. The WHO estimates that if current trends continue the number of overweight or obese children globally will increase to 70 million by 2025.

Because obesity is a chronic disorder requiring continuous management, the impact of these statistics highlights a more important issue: the economic stress to National Health Care Systems. Obesity has been shown to decrease life expectancy by 7 years by the age of 40, if subjects were obese during their childhood [2]. This is because obesity in adults is closely associated with type 2 diabetes mellitus (T2D), cardiovascular disease (CVD), hypertension, non-alcoholic fatty liver disease (NAFLD), vitamin D deficiency, degenerative joint disease and certain types of cancer [3]. Further, obesity has also been demonstrated to impact an individual's functional capacity, with a higher prevalence of disability observed in obese as opposed to normal-weight individuals [4]. Even in early infancy, obesity has been demonstrated to be most strongly associated to insulin resistance [5], with childhood obesity predicting the long-term risk of adult diabetes [6]. Most alarming is the high likelihood that without intervention an obese child at puberty will likely remain obese into adulthood, further compounding the economic burden with obesity-related problems [7, 8].

The cause of obesity is a chronic imbalance between energy input and output, with a long-term energy imbalance inducing an accumulation of adipose tissue (AT) [9]. Energy homeostasis is critical for survival, where species have evolved highly complex mechanisms integrating AT, the central nervous system (CNS) and peripheral organs and tissues to maintain a tight energy balance. Simply put the accumulation of energy during periods of "feast" to be used during periods of "famine" for survival. In humans, however, this balance is easily influenced not only by our genotype but also by exogenous stimuli [9]. Known risk factors in pediatric obesity which can tip the balance include genetics, environmental and neighborhood factors, increased intake of sugar-sweetened beverages, fast-food and processed snacks, decreased physical activity, a shorter sleep duration, parental obesity and prenatal events, as well as increased individual stress [10]. While genetic alterations and the "thrifty gene hypothesis" may be the basis of obesity [11 - 13], it is now well accepted that obesity has a multifactorial etiology with diet, lifestyle and environmental factors key players in its development [13 - 15].

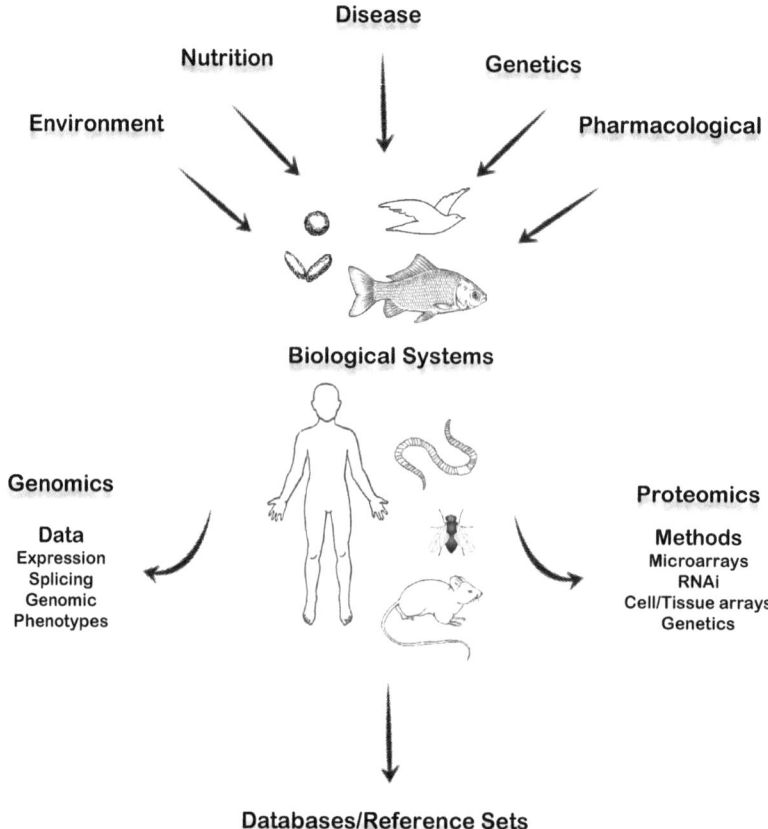

Fig. (1). Proteomics in hand with genomics offer global perspectives to complex biological systems.

Investigations in monogenic models of obesity and studies evaluating the molecular mechanisms of energy homeostasis [16 - 20], as well as the recognition that AT is an endocrine organ that secretes "adipokines" into the circulation which can impact peripheral tissues [21, 22], have improved our understanding of body weight control at the central and peripheral level [23, 24]. Despite these findings, however, no clear "central regulators" of metabolism, energy homeostasis and insulin sensitivity have been identified to date suggesting that obesity has a more complex basis. For the prevention and treatment of pediatric obesity, comprehension of the pathological-mechanisms at a global level whereby molecular and environmental interactions can be investigated, is necessary. Proteomics in hand with genomics offer global perspectives to complex pathologies, such obesity. Proteomics is the study of the proteome, all proteins in a given cell type or fluid, including isoforms and modifications as well as their interactions and higher order complexes at a given point in time. Simply put, proteomics is a major part of everything "post-genomic" and is considered the bridge between genomics and biology [25-30] (Fig. **1**). In the present review, we will address the recent advances in the proteomic characterization of obesity, with particular attention to pediatric obesity, as well as newly identified proteins which offer targets for novel therapies.

CHILDHOOD OBESITY: PATHOLOGICAL BASIS

Obesity is defined by an increase in body weight, or more specifically an increase in AT, which can result in adverse health consequences [31]. Childhood obesity is most strongly associated to insulin resistance [6], however an important array of medical conditions have been linked to this pathology [32] (Fig. **2**). Most alarming is the high likelihood that an obese child at puberty will remain obese into adulthood compounding the economic burden of obesity-related problems [7, 8]. The thresholds that define whether a child is overweight or obese is by being 110% or 120% of ideal weight for height, weight-for-height Z scores >1 or >2 and a body mass index (BMI) at the 85th, 90th, 95th and 97th percentile, based on international or country-specific references [33, 34]. While there is a genetic basis to explain the alarming global statistics for childhood obesity [15, 35], parental obesity as well as a child's environment has been demonstrated to have a strong impact on his/her risk of developing obesity [15]. Clear demonstrations of environmental involvement include prenatal events such as gestational diabetes and an unhealthy maternal diet [36, 37], duration of breast feeding [38], unhealthy diet such as increased consumption of sugar-sweetened beverages and fast foods [39, 40], a shorter sleep duration [41], stress [42] and sedentary activities [43], with transgenerational effects seen recently for endocrine-disrupting compounds [44] and adenoviruses [45, 46]. While national programs focused on obesity prevention have stabilized the exponential rise in childhood obesity, it remains however that in many developed/undeveloped countries more than a third of the pediatric population are over-weight or obese. Understanding the pathological basis of pediatric obesity is essential for developing more focused prevention programs.

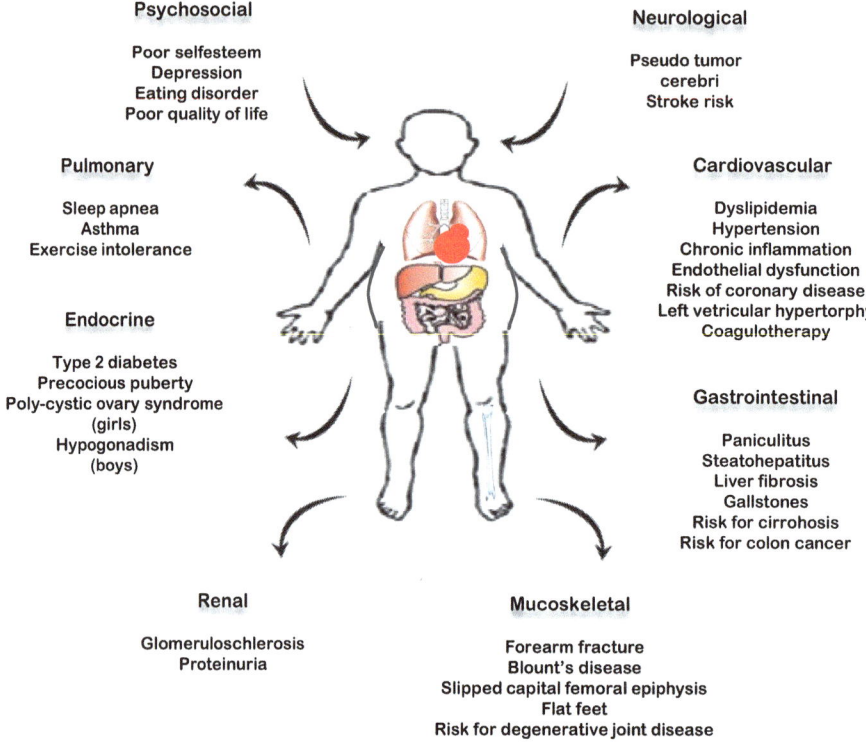

Fig. (2). Pediatric obesity and its associated complications.

Genetic Considerations for Childhood Obesity

Monogenic obesity is obesity attributable to single-gene mutations which are estimated to account for approximately 5% of the population [35, 47, 48]. While rare, to date there are more than 200 types of human obesity associated to single homozygous mutations with most characterized with an early onset and extreme phenotype of obesity [35, 49]. Monogenic obesity has been also further subcategorized as either syndromic or non-syndromic based on the presence or absence of additional phenotypic characteristics in addition to obesity, including mental retardation, organ-specific malformations and neuroendocrine abnormalities that affect the brain's appetite center. The best-known examples of syndromic obesity are Prader-Willi, Bardet-Biedl, Alström, Carpenter, Rubenstein-Taybi and Chen syndromes [13, 48]. With respects to non-syndromic monogenic obesity, 8 susceptibility genes have been identified, all of which code for proteins involved in the hypothalamic leptin/melanocortin satiety signaling pathway [13, 48]. The best characterized of these to date is the LEP mutation which blocks the production leptin, with leptin administration restoring satiety and promoting weight loss in affected subjects and mouse models [13, 48]. While these monogenic forms of obesity are rare, they have in turn expanded our knowledge of the pathways involved in satiety regulation.

Monogenic obesity does not explain the exponential rise in global obesity trends or the differences that exist between nations in both children and adults [50, 51]. One explanation is our current modern lifestyle which focuses on the rapid consumption of energy-dense foods as well as our sedentary work and recreational activities. Despite a clear obesogenic environment, there are clear genetic components as highlighted in early studies of twins, families and adoptions [52 - 54]. Collectively, they have demonstrated that there is a high heritability of obesity phenotypes which account for a 40-70% population variation in BMI [52 - 54]. The more recent genome-wide association studies (GWAS), exome array genotyping and copy number variation (CNV) studies which study a large number of genetic markers (SNPs) and sequence repeats spanning the entire genome and their association to specific phenotypic characteristics, combined with powerful technologies such as next generation sequencing (NGS) and highly advanced statistical modelling, have now identified 58 loci associated to obesity [55 - 57]. These findings demonstrate that obesity is largely a polygenic condition which can explain inter-individual sensibilities. When examined individually, SNPs in these loci have a limited phenotypic effect, yet the effect of multiple SNPs in the same and more loci, is phenotypically additive. The products of the loci identified to date include components of the neuroendocrine satiety signaling pathways, upregulation of the melanocortin pathway and the expression of the fat mass and obesity-associated gene (FTO) [58]. While the loci identified to date have opened the door to understanding polygenic obesity and the susceptibility across global populations, the data collected thus far explains only a small percentage of the heritability. Unravelling the complex genetic orchestra of polygenic obesity remains a challenging task.

Energy Homeostasis Dysregulation

Essential for the life of all organisms is energy homeostasis, the terminology used to describe the tight balance between energy input and energy expenditure [9]. When energy intake equals energy expenditure, the body is in energy balance and body weight remains stable. Obesity emerges when this balance is disrupted [59, 60]. Childhood and adolescence represent dynamic periods of rapid growth and weight gain [61]. The modernization of our current lifestyle, the sedentary activities of children as well as a chronic intake of excess energy rich foods, promotes a state of positive energy balance, the accumulation of AT beyond what is anticipated for normal development, and the emergence of obesity [62]. Understanding the pathways which regulate energy homeostasis is essential for prevention and therapeutical approaches for childhood obesity.

The "drivers" which effect energy balance are integrated and centralized by the CNS. Lesioning experiments performed in the 1940s confirmed the role of the CNS and established a central role for the hypothalamus and specific neuronal circuits in the regulation of energy homeostasis [63]. The hypothalamus is now regarded as the "hub" for the integration of key sensory inputs such as body temperature, circadian rhythms, electrolyte balance and energy homeostasis, and regulating a panel of responses including autonomic, endocrine and behavioral, all of which are aimed at maintaining the balance [reviewed by 64]. Body weight regulation is a complex orchestra involving not only the CNS but also the interaction between peripheral organs and tissues such as AT, gastrointestinal system and the pancreas, which transmit to the brain the individual nutritional and metabolic status [65]. The transmission of these signals to the brain comes from the vagas afferent nerves which provide sensory information as to the status of the body's organs, as well as from circulating peptides and hormones of peripheral origins, including AT [65 - 68]. The peripheral metabolic signals which regulate energy homeostasis are numerous and are often categorized as long-acting adiposity signals or short-acting, with the best characterized signals to date being insulin, leptin, ghrelin, glucagon like peptide-1 (GLP-1), glucocorticoids, cholecystokinin, peptide YY (PYY), amylin, oxyntomodulin, and somatostatin [65 - 67].

In every individual's life, the programming set for the regulation of energy balance is established early in life. In addition to a genetic basis, it has been demonstrated in a large number of epidemiological and animal studies, that environmental influences during the highly plastic developmental period, such as pregnancy and lactation, can have lasting influences on a child's body weight regulation [62, 69 - 71]. In particular, the hypothalamic neuronal circuits which control appetite and energy expenditure are set very early in life. Numerous models have demonstrated that a range of early life environmental drivers can upset these circuits [72]. Environmental drivers such as maternal obesity and undernutrition have been said to regulate epigenetic events including DNA methylation, miRNA as well as histone modifications of key adipokines such as leptin [73, 74]. Perinatal epigenetic analyses have been proposed to identify susceptible individuals [75, 76], however to date numerous questions remain as to therapeutic usefulness. Despite these advances, the mechanisms by which a child's environment can affect his/her energy homeostasis remain to be clearly understood.

Pathophysiology of Adipose Tissue

Originally viewed as a connective tissue central to energy homeostasis regulation through the storage of excess triglycerides and the release of free fatty acids (FFAs) for fuel, AT is now considered as an organized endocrine organ, both vascularized and innervated, with a clear anatomy and a high degree of plasticity responding to both corporeal and environmental drivers [reviewed by 77, 78]. Mammals have two distinct types of AT: white AT (WAT) and brown/beige (BAT), whose metabolic activity and endocrine function/s are crucial for immune responses, thermogenesis, fertility and lactation [79 - 82].

In the human body, AT can range from 5% to 60% of total body weight [reviewed by 78]. Evidence suggests at the population level, that childhood obesity increases the long-term risk of obesity-associated co-morbidities, such as T2D, CVD and cancer [31]. Interestingly, however, at an individual level the metabolic consequences of childhood obesity may vary considerably, with some children developing an early impaired glucose tolerance (IGT), while others maintain a normal glucose homeostasis [83]. One explanation for this, as Vague alluded to in 1956 [84], is the variation in the anatomical distribution of AT depots. In fact, AT is not a homogenous organ, but is made up of distinct anatomical depots, each demonstrated to have a clear metabolic diversity [77, 78, 85]. The principal depots of WAT include visceral adipose tissue (VAT), centrally located around the internal organs and enclosed by the peritoneum, the subcutaneous adipose tissue (SAT) located directly below the skin and finally ectopic AT, which are AT depots in localities not directly associated to storage [77, 78, 85, 86]. The largest depot is SAT, which comprises >80% of the total body fat and consists of gluteal, femoral and abdominal AT, with the abdominal AT further sub-divided by the scarpa's fascia into superficial-SAT (sSAT) located below the epidermis and deep-SAT (dSAT) adjacent to the peritoneum [87] (Fig. 3). Both VAT and SAT show subject-to-subject variation with respect to age, nutrition, race and gender [88]. Between the two, however, VAT accumulation is central to android obesity and is an independent risk factor for obesity-related metabolic and cardiovascular disorders, in particular insulin resistance, T2D, high triglycerides, high density lipoprotein (HDL) cholesterol, hypertension, and cancer in adults [89], while SAT has been viewed to have a protective role [90]. Emerging now, as key to child's long-term outcomes, are the ectopic AT depots, which include intrahepatic or" fatty liver", epicardial AT localized around the heart, perinephric or renal sinus linked to the kidney, pancreatic, intramuscular and perivascular AT [87]. These depots are thought to arise as a result of the metabolic disarrangement of VAT, however the more supported hypothesis is that these depots occur as a result of the restricted capacity of SAT to store excess lipids; in effect a "spillover" from SAT to VAT and eventually to other organs and tissues [86, 91 - 93]. To support this concept, it has been demonstrated that obese children with IGT have a reduced SAT and increased VAT depot with respect to those with a normal glucose homeostasis [94], with a further relationship observed between body composition, ectopic fat and insulin resistance in children prior to puberty [95]. As such, interventions aimed at reducing adiposity should have the potential to decrease ectopic fat accumulation, which in theory will delay the onset of insulin resistance and decrease the risk for development of T2D in children.

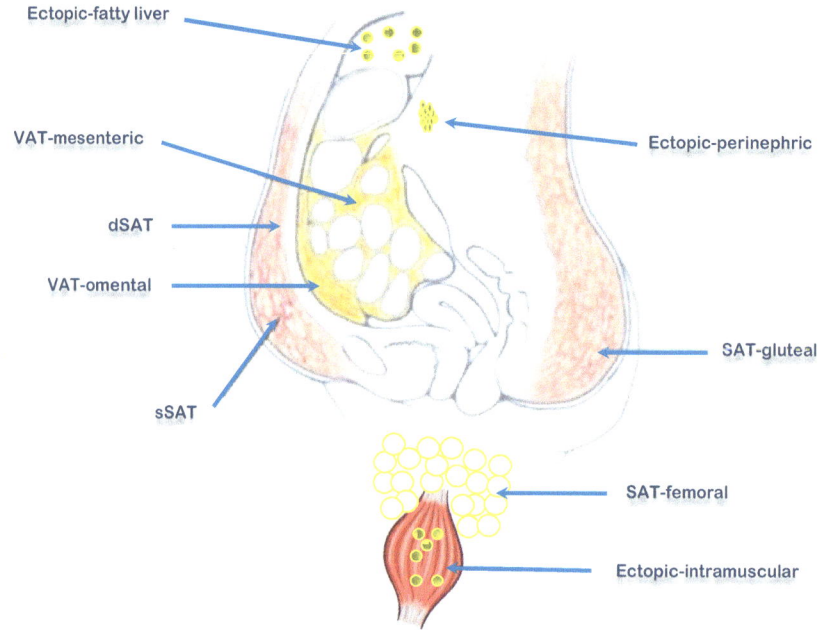

Fig. (3). The major adipose tissue depots in humans. The figure is a modified version obtained from Walker et al. [78].

To understand the disproportionate accumulation of AT which defines an obese phenotype, it is necessary to understand the cellular composition and the remodeling of AT. Adipose tissue is divided into two broad categories of cells: adipocytes and the remaining cellular components collectively termed the stromal vascular fraction (SVF). While conceptually it seems that adipocytes make up the majority of cells in the AT, there are in fact more cells from the SVF, which include preadipocytes, fibroblasts, endothelial cells, multipotent stem cells and immune cells [96]. This is explained by the fact the adipocytes take up a larger volume due to their unique morphology; a single large lipid droplet occupying

90% of the cell volume [96]. The accumulation of AT tissue is dependent on the proliferation of preadipocytes or hyperplasia, their differentiation into new adipocytes and the hypertrophy of existing adipocytes. The hyperplastic growth of AT occurs in the early stages of AT development and has been demonstrated to generally have a genetic foundation [97, 98], with hypertrophy occurring prior to hyperplasia to meet the need for an increased storage of triglycerides [98, 99]. Recent evidence also highlights the high degree of AT plasticity, where adipocytes have the ability to transdifferentiate as a result of extreme cold and physical activity, turning from a storage tissue to one that burns energy [100, 101]. It has been demonstrated in rat models that the sympathetic activation *via* treatment with 3-adrenergic receptor (3-AR) agonists, an extreme cold stress or the knockdown of orexigenic NPY in the dorsomedial hypothalamus, causes transdifferentiation in various WAT depots in rats [102, 103]. As such, white-t--brown adipocyte transdifferentiation has become a therapeutic interest for the treatment of obesity. Brown-like adipocytes have been identified in SAT depots 10.3% of lean children (0.3-10.7 years) and absent in obese children [104]. Animal model studies have demonstrated that a higher BAT content has a positive association to obesity resistance as well as obesity-associated co-morbidities [105], and that the "browning" of WAT, in particular VAT, is able to reduce these co-morbidities in both animal models [106 - 108] and humans [79, 109].

PROTEOMICS

Obesity is highly complex condition with no simple explanation. Comprehension of the pathological-mechanisms at a global level, whereby molecular and environmental interactions can be investigated is necessary for preventative and therapeutic strategies. "Proteomics" offers the technical approach to this global question (Fig. **4**).

Almost two decades ago the term "Proteome" was introduced to describe all the proteins encoded by the genome [25]. To date, the Encyclopedia of DNA Elements (ENCODE) project aimed at mapping transcription regions, transcription factor association, chromatin structure and histone modifications, has identified >20,000 protein coding genes in humans [110]. While the genome of an organism remains relatively constant, its resulting protein profile is highly dynamic, exhibiting differential patterns according to locality and environmental stimuli. Further, the number of proteins is expected to be substantially greater than the number of genes due to not only alternative splice variants but also the potential of >200 post translational modifications (PTMs), such as phosphorylation, glycosylation, sulfonation and acetylation [111], which reflect the functional state of the biological material under question. As such in the last 20 years a more precise definition for the proteome has emerged and now describes all proteins and their isoforms, PTMs and their interactions in higher order complexes in tissues, cells and biological fluids at an individual point in time [26].

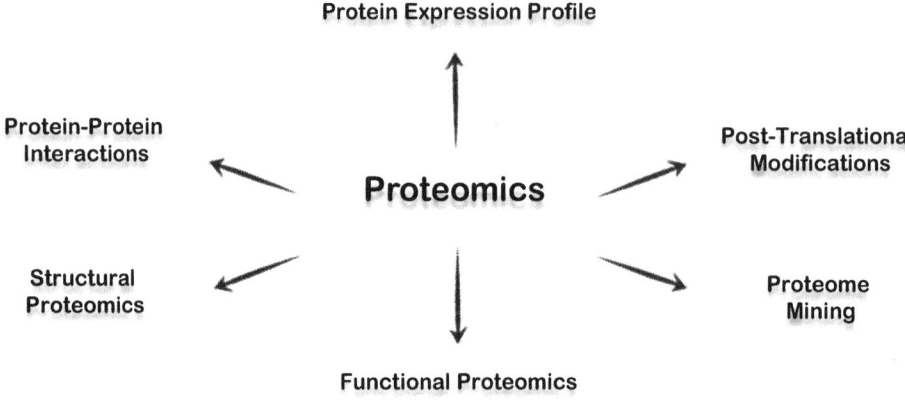

Fig. (4). Simplified schematic of the numerous strands of proteomic methodologies.

Proteomics is the term used to describe all methodologies and technologies that are used to study an organism's proteomes [25]. Three main proteomic strategies are currently applied: 1). Gel-based protein separation by 1- and 2-dimensional electrophoresis (2-DE) [112 - 114], 2). Liquid chromatography coupled to tandem mass spectrometry (LC-MS/MS) [115 - 117], 3). Array-based technologies [118, 119] (Fig. **5**).

Gel Based Methods

Due to protein modifications and alterations that reflect the dynamic state of cells, highly resolving, sensitive identification methodologies are required. At present, 2DE in combination with mass spectrometry (MS) is one of the most powerful methods used to address proteome studies [120 - 122]. In addition to its applicability and general low cost for most laboratories, 2DE also offers a visual picture of the profile intact proteins, enabling a quantitative evaluation between conditions and a control of the experimental quality and reproducibility.

The methodologies, technicalities and caveats of 2DE are well described in numerous articles [113, 114, 123, 124]. In brief, the basic principal of 2DE is to apply a two-step separation to give a 2D perspective of the proteome. The first step is isoelectric focusing (IEF), which is a charge separation employing the isoelectric point (pI) properties of proteins. This is followed by a second separation based on the molecular weight (MW) of proteins using SDS-PAGE. While 2DE involves a 2-step separation, the method itself involves 6-steps including: 1). Sample preparation/solubilization, 2). IEF, 3). Interfacing for SDS-

PAGE, 4). SDS-PAGE, 5). Protein detection and, 6). Image analysis (Fig. **5**).

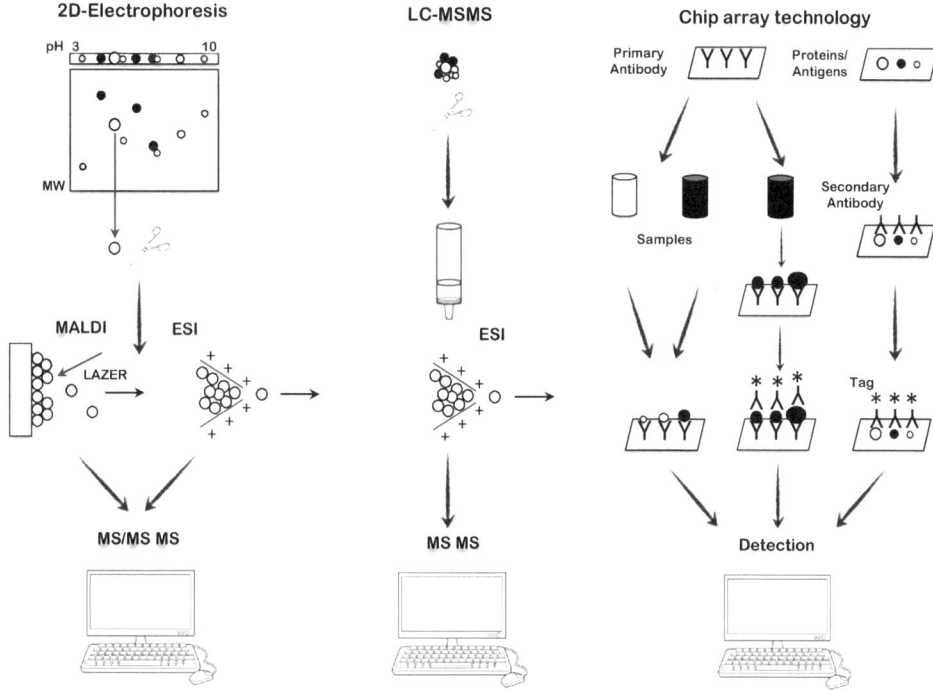

Fig. (5). Strategies in proteomic studies: 2DE; LC-MSMS; Chip array technologies.

The key and most problematic consideration for a good 2DE analysis is step 1, the ability to solubilize proteins in buffers suitable for IEF from the starting material of choice such as tissue and cell lines, membrane and nuclear proteins to plasma, urine and so forth. This is achieved by using optimized buffers that contain different combinations and concentrations of the chaotropic agents urea and thiourea, detergents such as 3-[3-cholamidopropyl) dimethylammonio]-1-propanesulfonate (CHAPS), reducing agents like dithiothreitol (DTT) and ampholytes [113, 114, 123, 124]. Unlike the sample preparation, problem solving is more straightforward for the IEF step, where the most important considerations are the voltage profile and isoelectric precipitation. Two different IEF methodologies are currently employed which use broad or narrow range immobilized pH gradient (IPG) strips, or non-equilibrium pH gel electrophoresis (NEPHGE), with IPG considered the method of choice for acidic proteins, and NEPHGE for basic proteins [125]. The interfacing step between IEF and SDS-PAGE involves the reduction/alkylation of the proteins followed by a coating with sodium-dodecyl sulphate (SDS) so that they are mobilized for SDS-PolyAcrylamide Gel Electrophoresis (SDS-PAGE).

Detection of proteins and image analysis, steps 5 and 6 are also critical points for the experimental question posed, as the quantitative differences observed will be the basis for protein spot identifications and future investigations. Crucial parameter includes the positional reproducibility, particularly for experimental designs that involve multiple gels that can't be performed in parallel. Marker proteins of known pI and MW are used to position all gels. Stained gels are digitized using conventional scanners/CCD-cameras and the image data is processed using image analysis software designed according to the instrumentation used. A "master gel" is created from multiple gels and is used as a standard gel to which all other gels obtained from the same starting material, can be correlated. Combined with strict statistical considerations and the reproductions, this will reduce the identification of false positives, which will only reveal themselves in later population or functional studies. The key demands for protein detection include sensitivity, linearity, homogeneity and compatibility with MS. The classic gold standard stain is the organic dye colloidal Coomassie Blue. Coomassie stains in the range 10-200ng/mm^2 and meets all demands; however, with respect to the newer stains it has a moderate sensitivity [126]. A more sensitive detection system is silver staining which stains 0.04-2ng/mm^2, however it is a complicated procedure and due to the presence of glutaraldehyde/formaldehyde it is incompatible for MS identifications, thus making it a second line choice [127]. While expensive, stains which meet all the demands of detection and have up to a 100-fold higher sensitivity than Coomassie, thus allowing for less sample to be used, are the fluorescent stains [128]. Examples of fluorescent stains used to date are oriole, flamingo and the most widely used, sypro ruby.

Another application of fluorescent staining of proteins which should be mentioned, is 2D-difference gel electrophoresis (2D-DIGE) which involves the fluorescent labelling of proteins with distinct fluorophores such as Cy2 and Cy3, which are then multiplexed on the same 2DE [129]. This methodology profits from the fluorescent properties of the different excitation and emission spectra using multi-wave imagers designed for this purpose and enables the user to see real-time changes in intact proteins and their PTMs with respect to conditions studied. Compared to the standard 2DE, DIGE has a better reproducibility and a greater statistical confidence.

Non Gel Based Methods: Mass Spectrometry (MS)

While 2DE allows a simultaneous, comparative and visual interpretation of the protein profile at a given point in time including PTMs, the drawbacks of this methodology are the reproducibility, a limited sensitivity, interference of abundantly expressed proteins and presently no high throughput automation. With the evolution that DNA sequence information could be combined with MW determinations via MS to identify proteins, MS has now evolved as a major analytical platform for protein identifications and quantitative proteomic studies due to its sensitivity (50-500fM), accuracy, speed and applicability for automation [115, 117, 130].

Early electron spray ionization (ESI) [131] or matrix-assisted laser desorption ionization (MALDI) [132] MS were the earliest and are the most broadly used methods which used a "bottom-up" approach to determine a protein identities. This approach involves the enzymatic digestion with trypsin or alternative enzymes of individual proteins [133 - 135] such as spots for identification from 2DE [136] or simple protein mixtures, into smaller peptides. The digests are then separated and analyzed by liquid chromatography MS (LC/MS) which determines the MW of the peptides or LC/MS/MS which combines MW of the peptides with sequence information [137]. The digested peptides are then compared to protein databases (Swiss-Prot http://web.expasy.org/) using programs such as MASCOT (http://www.matrixscience.com/), MS-FIT (http://prospector.ucsf.edu/) or Profound (http://omictools.com/) for protein identification or PMF. Where identified, proteins can then be confirmed by standard methods such as western immunoblot (WIB), WIB directly of 2DE gels or Enzyme-Linked Immuno Sorbent Assay (ELISA), dependent on the protein identified. If the protein is unable to be identified, the sequence can then be used as for oligonucleotide probing to identify the gene. Another common approach is "shotgun" proteomics where proteomics starts firstly with the enzymatic digestion to generate a complex mixture followed by 2DE and LC/MS or directly LC/MS/MS [138]. In the case of complex protein mixtures, additional pre-fractionation methodologies are generally applied prior to 2DE or MS, such as ion-exchange and affinity chromatography [139]. There are now numerous MS systems that have been used for proteomic studies, including amongst others Orbitrap [140], 3D and linear ion trap [141] and Fourier-transform ion-cyclotron resonance (FTICR) MS [142].

Despite being the current method of choice in proteomic studies and protein identifications, an important drawback for the "bottom-up" MS approach and shotgun proteomics is that analyses are not of intact proteins, unlike the 2DE and DIGE and as such they do not allow the quantitative measurement of changes in protein expression between different states, such as lean versus obese adipocyte secretome. Metabolic labeling and chemical derivatization are the early quantitative MS-based approaches that attempted to address these issues. A common metabolic labelling approach is stable-isotope labeling by amino acids in cell culture (SILAC), where cells are exposed to a medium containing specific isotopically labelled amino acids where in turn MS is able to separate heavy and light labeled peptides [143, 144]. A disadvantage of this method is that it is only applicable for *in vitro* cell models and not tissues or body fluids. Chemical derivatization alternatively depends on the incorporation of isotopically labelled functional groups to peptides which are then separated according to their different masses via MS. Examples of chemical derivatization strategies include isotope-coded affinity tags (ICAT) [145] and isobaric tags for relative and absolute quantification (iTRAQ) [146]. The strengths and weaknesses as well as the large array of both isotopic and label-free strategies that are presently available, are reviewed by Charour *et al.* [144]. Another approach which has been developed by a small number of labs and deals with a quantitative approach of intact proteins by MS is the "top-down" approach [147, 148]. With this methodology, intact proteins are analyzed directly by MS and are then dissociated subsequently by tandem MS, such as collision induced dissociation (CID) or electron capture dissociation (ECD) [147]. This methodology while powerful in its concept, is limited to proteins <30kDa in size [147, 148]. With the development of enrichment techniques and combinations of top and bottom-down approaches, these are now being applied to study an area which to date has been a limitation of MS, the PTMs [149, 150]. This is an important development due to the importance of PTMs in disease states and their potential role as drug targets. This area to date has been slow in its development, largely due to the absence of high-throughput methods such as MS.

Chips

Arrays are microscopic spots of immobilized biomolecules spatially arranged on glass slides, membranes, gels, beads or chips for the study of interactions [151]. A widely used methodology is the DNA microarray which has played a key role in evaluating organisms' genomes and expression patterns with respect to the conditions under question, whether it be healthy versus a pathology, or treatment with specific agents such as drugs [151]. Despite the impact of DNA microarrays, they do not address biological functions, which are essentially performed by proteins. Moreover, the mRNA expression does not always correspond to the protein expression and/or activity. As such protein biochips have developed as the protein addition of DNA microarrays, emerging as a relevant technology in the mid-1980s [152]. From their advent until now, biochips offer in addition to quantitative proteomic discoveries, a "system-orientated" approach which focuses on specific clusters of proteins with the same pathway/function/family [118, 119]. With these two approaches, biochips can be used to dissect not only a disease pathobiology with the potential to be used as a diagnostic tool, but can also be used to identify biological functions. Current biochip technologies are able to now consider one of the limitations of the bottom-up MS methods, the PTMs, and further they can determine biomolecular interactions essential for protein function [119, 153, 154].

Due to the significant possibilities for protein arrays, the technological advances over the last decade have created a large number of high-throughput protein based arrays, which have either an "analytical" or "functional" role. Analytical arrays have known biomolecular materials imprinted on the support material, including specific antibodies, proteins, peptides or aptamers. In brief, these arrays are incubated with a biological material for specific interactions, captured, amplified, detected and analyzed with secondary antibodies with an integrated data analysis. Analytical protein array methods have been applied to biomarker discoveries [155], diagnostics [153], autoimmune diseases [156], antibody profiles [157] as well as environmental [158] and food safety analyses [159]. Functional protein microarrays work in the opposite sense to analytical arrays, where the protein/s of interest are immobilized to study protein-protein interactions, the kinetics of PTMs and enzyme activities. Recombinant proteins synthesized from *E.Coli* or *S.cerevisiae,* or synthetic peptides, are incubated with crude cell lysates, conditioned medium or purified enzymes [160]. While technical limitations are relevant with this technology, such as protein synthesis and purification, immobilization so as to not mask the active regions, non-specific binding, cross-reactivity, a limited number of highly specific antibodies as well as the costs associated in miniaturizing a large quantity if data, array-based proteomics still offers a valuable resource for future proteomic studies. State-of-the art advancements in a still developing field have been recently well reviewed [119, 161, 162].

Challenges

For the moment there is no "gold standard" methodology for proteome studies based on the high complexity of the proteome and the limitations of the current proteomic methodologies. The 2DE based methods described are limited by their reduced sensitivity and reproducibility, with relevant problems associated to hydrophobic proteins, those with pIs in the extreme pH range as well as the separation of proteins with a MW >250kDa and <5kDa. Despite these limitations, it is not a method to shelve being that it gives a visual interpretation of the results and it allows an investigation of PTMs and alternatively spliced products, which methods such LC-MS/MS do not allow. Despite these limitations for LC-MS/MS in addition to the high costs, it is a highly popular methodology offering a high sensitivity, high throughput, quantitative approach to proteome studies. Chip technologies are an exploding field, offering quantitative and reproducible methods that are able to study small concentrations of samples. Chip approaches, like 2DE, are able to study PTMs, however an incomplete library of highly specific antibodies to cover all proteins and their PTMs, remains a challenge for this technology. In essence, proteome investigations must be designed with these challenges in mind.

PROTEOMIC STUDIES OF ADIPOSE TISSUE

An alarming sign for worldwide national healthcare systems is that pediatric obesity parallels adults [7, 8]. While national prevention programs have focused on obese children, where in some countries growth has slowed [1; http://www.who.int/topics/obesity/en/], it remains unlikely that these programs will resolve the problems of pediatric obesity and the long term health consequences for these children. Based on this picture, it is important to understand the cause/s of the disproportionate accumulation of AT and from these discoveries, develop novel strategies for resolving this problem. Adipose tissue is a highly orchestrated tissue involving receptor and second messenger pathways with steps and passes that influence hyperplasia, hypertrophy, differentiation, turnover, lipolysis, FFA metabolism and lipogenesis as well as the secretome profile [reviewed by 78]. Due to the limitations of the classical molecular biological methods, only pieces of the puzzle have been studied, with investigations failing to consider the global, time-resolved changes that are evident in this highly plastic organ. The advancement in proteomic technologies addresses these limitations enabling researchers to consider the pathophysiology of AT as a whole or according to its heterogeneous cell population. We will discuss some of the current AT-specific proteomic based discoveries how they may impact the obese pediatric population.

WAT Depots

Despite the publication of the first proteome evaluation in 1979, investigating adipocyte differentiation in murine 3T3-L1 preadipocytes [163], the first 2DE study of WAT was performed two decades later [164]. This study identified 140 2DE spots by MS and formed the basis of the current murine WAT 2D proteome map present to this day in the Swiss-Prot database [165; http://web.expasy.org/]. Despite the potential of proteomics, studies regarding pediatric obesity are still in their infancy, with 500+ articles present for obesity/proteomics, excluding pediatrics and childhood as tags in the search engine [http://www.ncbi.nlm.nih.gov/pubmed/]. Proteomic studies investigating WAT from children/adolescents are to our knowledge absent due to the obvious ethical issues of performing an invasive procedure on children to obtain biopsies. This means that current investigations are focused on animal models or adult subjects which in turn must be extrapolated for children and adolescents, where possible. Regardless, proteomic studies have remained slow likely due to the physiological characteristics of WAT. Apart from the obvious demands associated to extracting proteins from tissues, WAT has a very high lipid content which compromises efficient protein isolation. Successful rehydration buffers for AT from human and animal models used to date, are 7M urea with 2M thiourea, 2-4% CHAPS, 1-2%

ampholyte buffers and 20-50mM DTT [166, 167]. Further, the inclusion of hydroxyethyl disulphide (HED) in the place of DTT in the rehydration buffer has also been demonstrated to improve the resolution of the 2DE WAT proteome [168].

As a result of procedural advances, the first human WAT 2DE map was published in 2004 coming from VAT obtained during bariatric surgery of obese females with polycystic ovary syndrome (PCOS), where 16 proteins were identified by MS [168]. As described, WAT is composed of distinct anatomical depots, each demonstrated to have a clear metabolic diversity with VAT accumulation detrimental and key for obesity-associated co-morbidities [77, 78, 85]. In fact from this pioneering study to the present day, most proteome profiling of WAT have been done between healthy and/or obese subjects analyzing SAT and/or VAT depots. Cortón et al., [169] went onto to perform a more comprehensive study using 2D-DIGE and identified 1840 spots, of which 15 were significantly different between obese females with or without PCOS [169]. Independent of obesity, the most relevant findings were the identification of target proteins involved in oxidative stress and cell toxicity [171, 170], as well as cholesterol metabolism with the downregulation of proapolipoprotein A-1 (ApoA1), the major component of HDL [169, 171]. While this proteome profiling was performed in adult subjects, the study is relevant for the pediatric population as PCOS is a common endocrine disorder in adolescent girls, with long term reproductive, metabolic and psychological implications [172]. As in adults, PCOS adolescents also have increased cardiovascular risk factors, which include an irregular ApoB/ApoA1 ratio [173]. This ratio has been further demonstrated to be a good predictor of metabolic syndrome in adolescent Chinese girls [173]. In that ApoA1 plays an important role in many of the antiatherogenic functions of HDL, novel therapies currently under investigation include the administration of ApoA1 and the development mutated variants or mimetic peptides designed to mimic the positive functions of ApoA1 [174].

The first most comprehensively characterized human adipocyte proteome study was performed by Xie et al. [175], who performed 1D HPLC-ESI-MS/MS identifying 1493 proteins from adipocytes isolated from SAT biopsies of healthy lean subjects. A part from identifying proteins involved in lipid metabolism and storage, lipolysis and oxidative stress amongst others, they identified that 22% of all adipocyte proteins were mitochondrial in origin, as opposed to 4.8% in the human proteome, hypothesizing an important role for the mitochondria in adipocyte function [175]. In fact mitochondrial dysfunction in adipose tissue was implicated at the same to be a pathogenic step in the development of insulin resistance and T2D [176]. From these early observations to present day it is now known that the chronic nutrient overload in AT causes a mitochondria driven increase in reactive oxygen species leading to carbonylation of proteins that impair mitochondrial function [177]. A key carbonylated adipokine is fatty acid binding protein 4 (FABP4), which has gained a large degree of interest for the treatment of T2D [178, 179]. Elevated serum FABP4 levels have been demonstrated to be associated with obesity and insulin resistance not only in adults but also children [180, 181], where FABP4 knockout mouse models are protected from diet-induced insulin resistance and hyperglycemia [182]. It has been demonstrated that FABP4 is released from adipocytes under obesogenic conditions, such as hypoxia, to augment insulin secretion, thus regulating the β-cell response to obesity [183]. Novel pharmacological agents aimed at down-regulating FABP4 include Sitagliptin, a dipeptidyl peptidase-4 (DPP-4) inhibitor which increases glucagon-like peptide 1 (GLP-1), has recently been demonstrated to reduce FABP4 in both T2M subjects and the 3T3-L1 adipocyte cell model [184]. While trials involving Sitagliptin in children are not currently available, trials involving DPP-4 inhibitors and GLP-1 receptor agonists in normal and obese children with T2D demonstrate positive effects on glycemic control [185].

Pediatric studies examining total body fat, VAT and SAT depots demonstrate each increase according to age, however, with puberty different trends in accumulation are evident and dependent on gender, maturational status and ethnicity [186]. While the accumulation of SAT is proposed to defend against T2D risk and potentially ectopic fat accumulation in adolescents, association between abdominal obesity and insulin resistance indexes are strong, highlighting the impact of abdominal obesity on the progression to metabolic syndrome in adolescents [187, 188]. In addition to a different metabolic activity and unique adipokine profile, SAT and VAT also differ in their responses to environmental stimuli, proliferation capacity, apoptotic and autophagic rates and adipocyte size [78]. On this basis, proteomic studies have been applied to understand the global differences between SAT and VAT depots. While most of these studies are animal in origin, a limited number have compared the two key adult human AT depots [189, 190], their relationship to epicardial depots [191] and the importance of the SVF in each [192]. As far as we were able to tell, there are no proteomic analyses in either children or adults for other AT depots such as dSAT, despite their emerging importance [85, 193].

The first comprehensive proteomic study comparing intact SAT and VAT biopsies from exclusively obese subjects (BMI>30kg/m^2) was performed by Perez *et al.* [189], where using 2D-DIGE and MALDI-TOF/TOF they identified 43 proteins related to glucose/lipid metabolism, lipid transport, protein synthesis and transport, stress response and inflammation differentially expressed between the two depots [189]. Their results highlighted the VAT overexpression of heat shock proteins (HSPs), specifically HSP90, HSP70 and HSP27 [189], chaperones regulating nascent protein folding in the endoplasmic reticulum, mitochondria and cytosol [194]. In particular, HSP90 has been shown using *in vitro* cell models to be an important player in endoplasmic reticulum stress through the regulation of endoplasmic reticulum stress sensors, IRE1α and protein kinase RNA-like endoplasmic reticulum kinase (PERK), being a critical modulator in the switch between apoptosis and autophagy in an environmental and cell-specific manner [195, 196]. Baring this in mind, environmental stressors which can cause the endoplasmic reticulum lumen to block with incorrectly folded proteins, is considered an important feature of pediatric obesity. In fact, HSP90 has been shown to chaperone peroxisome proliferator-activated receptor γ (PPARγ), regulating the differentiation and survival of 3T3-L1 adipocytes *in vitro* [197]. Moreover, HSP70, prior to the described proteomic study, was previously linked at a genetic level to obesity [198], while recently, plasma HSP70 levels were correlated to insulin resistance in the African American population [199]. Lastly HSP27, shown to participate in protective mechanisms to toxicity, has been proposed as a novel biomarker for vascular inflammation [200]. With HSPs identified as central modulators in cellular stress, it has been postulated that their modulation in AT and other relevant tissues could be a good therapeutic approach to obesity, in particular obesity-associated insulin resistance [201], a key feature of pediatric obesity. Radiciol and Geldanamycin derivatives which bind to HSP90, have been shown to inhibit differentiation and adipogenesis in 3T3-L1 cells, and in the case of the Geldanamycin derivatives, mice fed a high fat diet (HFD), highlighting HSP90 as a potent target for drug development in the control of obesity and its related metabolic complications [202, 203]. For the moment, HSP90 is a central therapeutic target for eradicating malignant cancers and overcoming chemotherapy resistance in adults and children, however, new developments with organelle specific HSP90 inhibitors, may have a functional relevance for obesity and its comorbidities in the future [204].

In a more in depth study, Isener *et al.* [190], with 2DE and MALDI-TOF/TOF examined the proteome profile in SAT and VAT intact biopsies, looking at the differences between lean and morbidly obese subjects matched for age and gender. This study identified 17 proteins differentially regulated as a function of obesity and/or AT depot, with the proteins identified involved in lipolysis (carboxylesterase-1), transcription (zinc finger protein 324A, ubiquitin carboxyl-terminal hydrolase) and enzymatic reactions (α1-antitrypsin). Amongst the proteins identified, 14-3-3γ and zinc finger protein 324A, demonstrated a three-way interaction between depots, the presence of obesity and gender, with 14-3-3γ elevated in obesity with the lowest expression in VAT of lean subjects [190]. The identification of 14-3-3γ is interesting in that the 14-3-3 isoforms are involved in a plethora of physiological processes and bind several hundred partner proteins, regulating intracellular signaling pathways and the intracellular localization of their target proteins [reviewed by 205]. The 14-3-3γ isoform, prior to this proteomic study, had been shown to be involved in the insulin-regulated glucose transport 4 (GLUT4) trafficking in 3T3-L1 adipocytes [206], as well as being shown by proteomics to be upregulated in BAT of obesity prone rats [207]. Of the 14-3-3 isoforms, 14-3-3γ has the highest expression in AT after the brain [205], it interacts with cytoskeletal actin filaments and contributes to the regulation apoptosis [208] and autophagy [209]. It also been found to be associated with the membranes of lysosomes, golgi and mitochondria, where in mitochondria it has been demonstrated to be key to mitochondrial quality control of proteins [210]. Due to their widespread biological functions, 14-3-3 isoforms have been recognized as potential candidates for pharmacological interventions. Despite this, however, their involvement in a range of physiological processes requires interventions which are target and tissue specific, with approaches in recent years focusing small molecules which inhibit and stabilize specific 14-3-3 protein-protein interactions [211]. While there are a few examples of small molecules which can interact and have a pharmacological function, including PRLX24905 which reduces the interaction between HSP20 and 14-3-3γ, in this case used for relaxing smooth muscle airways [212], their potential in obesity, and more specifically pediatric obesity awaits development.

While proteomics has unveiled important differences between SAT and VAT depots with respect to obesity, more tailored approaches looking at links between AT dysfunction and the emergence of obesity-associated co-morbidities such as T2D, which are highly relevant for children and their long term outcomes, have attempted to identify candidate molecules [213 - 216]. As described, obese children with IGT have an increased VAT depot with respect to those with a normal glucose homeostasis [94], with differences in the VAT biochemical and metabolic properties potentially explaining the association between children with IGT and those metabolically normal [217]. Three proteomic studies examining overweight [214], lean [215] and morbid obese [216] VAT biopsies or matched SAT/VAT biopsies from adults, have investigated the molecular processes leading to an early pathogenesis in diabetes using classic 2D or 2D-DIGE combined with MALDI-TOF/TOF, LC-MS/MS or linear trap quadrupole XL (LTQ XL). Common identified proteins between these studies is limited, most likely explained by the different patient populations studied and the locations in which biopsies were taken, considering regional differences within depots themselves (upper thigh SAT versus abdominal SAT), which leaves the extrapolation to children problematic. Annexin A1 and FABP4 are two of the few proteins repeatedly appearing in these studies. The potential of FABP4 for pediatric obesity we have already discussed. While differentially regulated between the different proteomic studies, Annexin A1 (ANXA1) is repeatedly highlighted in IGT/pre-diabetes in a majority of the studies described, including the first proteomic studies in VAT studying PCOS subjects [169], who characteristically are insulin resistant and go on to develop T2D. Annexin A1 is an endogenous glucocorticoid regulated protein [218] with a wide range of functions focused on the regulation of systemic anti-inflammatory processes [219 - 221]. To highlight its importance, a number of studies have suggested that ANXA1 dysregulation is central to the development of inflammatory diseases [221 - 223] with an increased adiposity documented in ANXA1-deficient mice [223]. While a link to obesity has been described with plasma ANXA1 inversely correlated to BMI, C-reactive protein (CRP) and leptin in adult males [224], early *in vivo* and *in vitro* studies have demonstrated that ANXA1 is able to modulate the secretion and signaling of insulin [225, 226], suggesting ANXA1 may be co-involved in the development of insulin resistance and the progression to T2D. Recently urine ANXA1 has been proposed as an index for glomerular injury in patients [227] with the prevalence of glomerular hyper filtration increasing with increasing stages of prediabetes and prehypertension [228], suggesting that it could be a could predictive marker of prediabetes in children and adolescents. With respect to a therapeutic feasibility, in elegant studies using mice AT explants and a 60% HFD obese mouse model, lipoxins (LXA) have been investigated as an approach to resolve the AT inflammatory response [229, 230]. Lipoxins are endogenously produced eicosanoids with anti-inflammatory, pro-resolution and antifibrotic bioactions, with LXA4 the most predominant [231]. In addition to attenuating obesity-induced chronic kidney disease including glomerular hyper filtration, administration of LXA4 was able to decrease obesity-induced adipose inflammation, attenuating tumor necrosis factor- α (TNF-α) and increasing Annexin-A1, amongst other inflammatory markers [230]. While results are promising, the use of LXA4 for treating obesity co-morbidities in both children and adults, as well as other inflammation-fueled disorders, is in its infancy, with studies in human AT and obese subjects necessary.

Proteomic studies of WAT are able to consider the global, time-resolved changes in this heterogenous tissue that are evident in this highly plastic organ. From the publication of the first proteome study of WAT more than a decade ago [164] and the continual advancement in proteomic technologies, numerous target proteins related to AT pathologies have been highlighted, as described herein. While this data can be extrapolated to a certain degree, it remains that direct studies in children and adolescents are lacking.

WAT Secretome

The AT secretome is the "signature" to understanding the molecular events of body weight regulation and the link to the obesity-associated co-morbidities in both children and adults. Adipose tissue, comprised of adipocytes and the SVF, releases proteins into the extracellular fluid, as either intact or cleaved peptides. Several of these AT-derived proteins can end up in circulation thus reflecting an individual's response to genetic/environmental conditions. These proteins have the potential to serve as potential serum/plasma biomarkers.

Despite being considered more reflective of the physiological state due to the paracrine interactions within this heterogeneous tissue and the final endocrine effects, very few proteomic AT secretome studies have been performed and none of these are in children due to the difficulties in tissue handling, contamination by serum proteins and damaged cells, the highly reactive nature of AT biopsies, as well as the ethical issues previously described. The first characterization of human AT biopsy secretomes was done in adult VAT, due to its importance in the development of metabolic syndrome and T2D [232]. In this study they optimized the best protocol to elucidate true proteins secreted by AT devoid of contamination and identified by SELDI-TOF MS 70 VAT-specific secreted proteins including adiponectin, endothelial plasminogen activator inhibitor (PAI-1), retinol binding protein (RBP), interleukin-6 (IL6), adipsin, gelsolin and SPARC. While this study was exclusively descriptive, the first comparative study of AT secretomes used the isotope-labeled amino acid incorporation rates (CILAIR), a modification of the SILAC method, to investigate VAT from 1 subject treated with and without 60nM insulin [233]. They identified 24 up-regulated and 4 down-regulated proteins with Search Tool for the Retrieval of Interacting Genes/Proteins (STRING) highlighting two major clusters; endoplasmic reticulum stress response (peptidyl-prolyl cis-trans isomerase B [PP1B], endoplasmin, calreticulin, protein-disulfide isomerase A1 and A3, HSP5A) and extracellular matrix remodeling (tenascin, metalloproteinase inhibitor 1 [TIMP1], CHI3L1). They hypothesize that these cluster changes are the result of the chronic administration of insulin and tissue rearrangements to accommodate the accumulation triglycerides. Interestingly, they also identified the IGF carrier proteins, IGF-binding protein-4 (IGFBP-4) and -6 (IGFBP-6), as significantly upregulated with insulin treatments. While 98% of IGF-1 is bound to one of six IGFBPs, some of these binding proteins have also been shown to have important independent biological functions [234, 235]. While there are no pediatric obesity associated studies currently present within the literature, in animal models the brain over expression of IGFBP-6 has been found to have a significant impact on the regulation of energy homeostasis in mice fed a HFD for 3 months, with mice developing obesity and a mild insulin resistance [236]. Similarly for IGFBP-4 a negative regulator of IGF-1, in mouse AT organ cultures, IGF-1/IGFBP-4 signaling was implicated in AT expansion in response to HFD [237]. With respect to human studies, an interesting observation in a plasma proteomic study of >300 postmenopausal women with coronary heart disease and >300 stroke cases, demonstrated that IGFBP-4 is a validated stroke risk marker

[238]. IGFBP-4 has also been demonstrated to have independent functions inhibiting angiogenesis and glioblastoma tumor growth *in vitro* [239]. Despite these important studies and potential relevance of IGFBPs, whether IGFBP-4 can be exploited with respect to cardiovascular markers in obese children, awaits the clarification of the function of VAT-produced IGFBP-4 and -6 in pediatric obesity.

Animal AT secretome studies offer an alternative to the problems of studying human AT, particularly from children and healthy lean subjects. On this basis lean versus obese rat epididymal AT following treatment with thiazolidinediones analyzed by 2DE LC-MS/MS and ^{18}O-proteolytic labeling, demonstrated obese AT secretomes contain more inflammatory and ECM proteins which could be inhibited with thiazolidinediones, emphasizing the clinical relevance of these anti-diabetic agents [240]. As described, the use of thiazolinediones in children and adolescents is not recommended. In another rat AT secretome study, AT-specific depot differences (SAT, VAT, gluteal) were compared using 2DE-MALDI-TOF/TOF approaches [241]. Overall a higher secretion of adipokines/gm of AT was demonstrated for VAT with a total of 45 proteins differentially expressed between these 3 tissues selected for identification. Amongst these, thrombospondin-1, angiotensinogen, FABPs and galectin-1 were elevated in VAT. On the contrary vitamin D binding protein (VDBP) was more elevated in SAT. This research reinforces numerous previous studies which have demonstrated that it is important to consider the anatomical distribution of AT in both children and adults. For the moment computed tomography (CT) and magnetic resonance imaging (MRI) are considered the most valid methods to measure intra-abdominal fat distribution [242, 243], however, each have important limitations (radiation and cost) for their use in children. Ultrasound overcomes these limitations and is considered a promising technique which capable of measuring intra-abdominal adiposity in children, however, for the moment it requires further validation [244].

BAT

In contrast to WAT, BAT is extensively vascularized with a high concentration of mitochondria which through the activation of uncoupling protein 1 (UCP1), uncouples the oxidation of fatty acids from ATP synthesis to dissipate heat as energy. While found only in mammals and originally thought to be found exclusively in newborn children as opposed to children and adults, this thermogenic organ which protects the body from low temperatures, has also been found in adult humans in cold environments [245]. Further, it has been demonstrated that a daily 2-hour cold exposure at 17°C for 6 weeks causes a parallel increase in BAT activity and energy expenditure and a concomitant decrease in body fat mass [246]. These and numerous other important studies have prompted investigations into the potential role of BAT in fighting against obesity and its associated co-morbidities. Interestingly in children, it has very recently been demonstrated that brown-like/beige adipocytes are present well beyond infancy in SAT depots, specifically lean as opposed to obese children [104], highlighting that BAT may have important "browning agents" that can increase energy expenditure and reduce the body fat mass. As a result, proteomics in BAT using exclusively animal models have evaluated the physiological processes this tissue goes through in response to cold exposure as well as in obese phenotypes, with a particular focus on mitochondria and the mitochondrial proteome between WAT and BAT [207, 247 - 250]. At the proteome level, Navet *et al.*, 2007 [247] demonstrated a 10-fold increase in respiratory function, 8-fold in β-oxidation, 8-fold for ATP-synthase with UCP1 increasing 20-fold in the rat BAT mitochondrial proteome following 20 day cold-exposure. Controlling UCP1 has been proposed as a potent strategy to treat morbid obesity, as UCP1 ablation has been shown to induce obesity in mice kept at thermoneutrality [251]. While a temperature-based therapy for obese children and adolescents is unrealistic, pharmacological targets to increase UCP1 expression in WAT are being investigated at the molecular level. Recently, Moisan *et al.* [252], using human *in vitro* adipocyte cell models, identified two inhibitors, Tofacitinib and R406, that increase UCP1 expression and mitochondrial activity. Interestingly, these pharmacological agents achieve these results through the inhibition of the Janus Kinase (JAK)-Signal Transducer and Activator of Transcription (STAT) pathway, a key second messenger pathway that connects environmental stimuli to the transcriptional machinery [252]. These results while promising for the "browning" of WAT are in the early stages of development. Studies in WAT from rats treated with the insulin sensitizing agent Rosiglitazone, have also demonstrated that this drug is able to increase adipogenesis, mitochondrial mass, fatty acid oxidation, electron transport as well as inducing a 20-fold increase in UCP1, suggesting that rosiglitazone has the potential to activate BAT characteristics in WAT [253]. Rosiglitazone, a member of the thiazolidinediones, are a class of controversial therapeutical agents for T2D, with rosiglitazone withdrawn in 2007 due to an association with an increased risk of heart attack and stroke in adults [254]. While restrictions have been reduced, the use of rosiglitazone in children and adolescents is not recommended with Treatment Options for T2D in Adolescents and Youth (TODAY) study being the first multiethnic, multicenter randomized trial which compared 3 treatment approaches in obese youth with new-onset T2D (n=699; ages 10-17 years). These treatments included monotherapy with Metformin, Metformin with Rosiglitazone, and Metformin with an intensive lifestyle intervention with Metformin plus Rosiglitazone treatment causing a modest increase in adiposity, but demonstrating the best overall glycemic control [255]. Whether these positive responses are associated to the "browning" of WAT in children remains to be elaborated.

Similar results were obtained with another proteomic study of mouse BAT and WAT mitochondria using, on this occasion, a quantitative approach with SILAC-labelled cells combined to MS [248]. In addition to the aforementioned results, this group demonstrated functional differences between the two mitochondrial populations with BAT mitochondria having metabolic characteristics similar to muscle, while WAT demonstrated protective proteome profile with anabolic functions. Amongst the specific BAT mitochondrial proteins identified was pyruvate dehydrogenase lipoamide kinase isozyme 4 (PDK4), a central regulator of glucose metabolism in the process of glyceroneogenesis [248]. For the browning of WAT to enhance the expenditure of excess stored energy, these proteins offer potential therapeutic targets. Bearing this in mind, resveratrol a naturally occurring poly-phenolic substance from plants, particularly the skin of red grapes has been found to display anti-inflammatory, vasoprotective and insulin-sensitizing effects in obese adults [256], although the overall benefits are questioned [257]. While most studies have focused on the muscle, Beaudoin *et al.* [258], examined its effects on WAT depots and demonstrated that reversatrol is able to induce the mitochondrial biogenesis in WAT with the induction of PDK4 and the activation of the process of glyceroneogenesis with a concomitant increase in adiponectin secretion [258]. While reversatrol is gaining a new interest in the treatment of obesity and in particular T2D, we await the results of proposed controlled trials in children [259].

The most recent BAT proteome studies present in the literature have investigated BAT adipogenesis [249] and the BAT lipid drop proteome in response to cold treatment [250], aiming at understanding the interaction between BAT mitochondria and lipid drops. The studies have highlighted further proteins which could be of therapeutic benefit in obesity including cofilin-1, a regulator of actin filament non-equilibrium assembly or disassembly [260], which inhibits BAT adipogenesis and represses, amongst other proteins, UCP1 expression. A further identified protein is perilipin 2, one of 3 isoforms regulated and phosphorylated by protein kinase A (PKA) and acts as a coating for lipid droplets protecting them from lipases such as hormone sensitive lipase (HSL), enzymes essential for lipolysis. Polymorphisms in the human perilipin gene have been associated with variance in body-weight regulation, with a Pro251 mutation associating with a lower insulin secretion and increased insulin-sensitivity [261, 262]. Up until this point in time, the therapeutic potential for cofilin-1 is focused on the invasive machinery of cancer using small molecule inhibitors BMS-5 and Cucurbitacin I to curtail tumor progression [263]. Alternatively, for perilipin 2 it has been shown that the perilipins are differentially expressed in hepatocyte steatosis and are expressed *de novo* and have been proposed as a differential marker for the differential diagnosis of chronic vs. acute steatosis [264]. This application is also relevant for the pediatric obese population, being that an association between NAFLD and cardiovascular disease among children is increasingly being recognized [265].

Stromal-Vascular Fraction (SVF)

The SVF, which includes preadipocytes, fibroblasts, endothelial cells, multipotent stem cells and immune cells such as macrophages, neutrophils, lymphocytes and T-cells outnumber the adipocytes with 4-6 x 10^6 cells/gm of AT versus 1-2 x 10^6 adipocytes in both healthy and obese subjects [96]. With respect to AT depots, the number of SVF cells is higher in VAT as opposed to SAT, with 10% of the VAT SVF endothelial cells and comprised of a larger accumulation of lymphocytes, including B, alphabetaT, gammadeltaT, NK and NKT, due to the presence of lymph nodes. Alternatively, the preadipocyte cell population is reported to be higher in SAT than VAT [266, 267]. While adipocytes contribute to the release of adipokines such as leptin and adiponectin, the SVF is the major contributor of inflammatory cytokines, such as TNFα and IL6 and IL-1 [268], which are key to the inflammatory state associated to obesity and its associated co-morbidities, in particular insulin resistance and T2D [269]. On the basis of clear role for the SVF in obesity and the technological development of efficient cell separation methodologies for AT [217], a few proteomic studies have profiled the SVF and compared its protein profile between SAT and VAT [194], or with respect to the accompanying adipocytes in abdominal and arm AT depots [270]. The comparison between adipocytes and the SVF in both studies described herein, each independently demonstrated that adipocytes and SVF share at least 60% of their proteome, including proteins involved acid/base balance, free radical oxidation, lipid binding and intermediate filament proteins [192, 270]. Amongst these proteins was carbonic anhydrase 1, found to be expressed at higher levels in the SVF [192, 270]. The carbonic anhydrases are a family of metalloenzymes that catalyze the rapid interconversion of CO_2 and water to bicarbonate and protons and vice versa [271]. This simple reaction is involved in a plethora of biological processes including maintaining the acid-base balance in blood and tissues, helping to transport CO_2 out of tissues, electrolyte balance, respiration, bone remodeling as well as metabolic processes such as glucogenesis, ureagenesis and lipogenesis [272]. Interest in the carbonic anhydrases as an obesity therapy has evolved following the identification that treatment with topirimate, an anticonvulsant drug, had a dramatic effect on weight reduction [273]. These results were further demonstrated in both lean and obese Zucker rats that topirimate was able to reduce fat and energy gains through reducing energetic efficiency [274]. With respect to pediatric obesity, the first assessment of topirimate has been recently performed in a small cohort of adolescents (n=28; mean age 15.2 ± 2.5 years, mean baseline BMI 46.2 ± 10.3 kg/m2) over a 6 month period, where a positive effect on weight loss was observed [275]. Despite these positive results, the potential for topirimate and zonisamide, another carbonic anhydrase target with weight loss effects [276], as therapeutic agents for pediatric obesity must wait for long term randomized controlled clinical trials.

Using 2DE-combined MALDI-TOF-MS with verification, Peinado *et al.* [192], identified 24 proteins differentially expressed between the SAT and VAT SVF of lean subjects amongst which was a higher expression of omentin in the VAT SVF. Omentin, discovered in 2005, is a new member of the adipocytokine family which control insulin sensitivity, inflammatory activity, neuroendocrine activity, cardiovascular function, food and water intake, fertility, and bone metabolism with omentin playing a role in the "positive metabolism" as an anti-inflammatory factor [277]. Lower circulating omentin levels contribute to the pathogenesis of insulin resistance, T2D and CVD in overweight and obese adults [278, 279] suggesting that an upregulation of this adipocytokine could be of a significant benefit to these phenotypes. With respect to children, studies to date are limited and those described in the literature are conflicting. It has been observed in a small cohort of obese subjects (n=49) that low omentin-1 levels are related to clinical and metabolic parameters in obese children [280], while in another examining a more extreme obese phenotype, higher levels were demonstrated [281]. While more comprehensive clinical studies in obese children are required, research has moved forward examining the potential therapeutic applications of omentin. *In vitro* and *in vivo* studies have recently demonstrated that omentin has hypotensive effects and in addition is able to attenuate the pathological process of myocardial hypertrophy via the activation of AMP-activated protein kinase (AMPK) in the heart, suggesting that it may represent a target molecule for the treatment of cardiac hypertrophy [282, 283]. Despite promising results, whether omentin is clinically useful for pediatric obesity and the prognostic outcome for these children, particularly with respect to CVD, needs to be further investigated.

PROTEOMIC STUDIES IN ADIPOCYTES: STEM CELLS AND CELL LINES

The accumulation of AT is dependent on the proliferation of preadipocytes, their differentiation into and the hypertrophy of existing adipocytes. Early studies defined obese phenotypes in terms of AT cellularity, introducing the terms "hyperplastic" and "hypertrophic" obesity [284]. Hyperplasia, an increase in cell number and hypertrophy an increase in cell size, are two growth mechanisms for AT. The hyperplastic growth of AT occurs in the early stages of AT development with a genetic foundation [97, 98], with hypertrophy occurring prior to hyperplasia to meet the need of for additional fat storage [97, 98]. Adipocyte number while an important determinant of fat mass, remains constant in adulthood with adipocyte cell numbers increasing and being set during childhood and adolescence with a 10% turnover annually for all adult ages and BMI [97]. Even with extreme weight loss, fat cell numbers remain constant, confirming that the differences observed in fat cell number between lean and obese subjects, is set during childhood [97]. Therefore the key to the accumulation of AT and obesity is preadipocyte differentiation and adipocyte hypertrophy. To elucidate the molecular mechanisms of differentiation and hypertrophy in relation to obesity and its associated co-morbidities, proteomic approaches have been applied to the murine 3T3-L1 cell line and adipose-derived stem cells.

Adipogenesis: Adipo-proteomics

Blocking adipocyte differentiation is considered a key anti-obesity strategy, as such understanding the molecular mechanisms of adipogenesis are essential for the development of novel therapies.

Murine 3T3-L1 Preadipocytes

Murine cell models, in particular 3T3-L1 preadipocytes, form the basis of a majority of studies examining adipogenesis, as they differentiate within 5-7 days when given a differentiation medium containing insulin, glucocorticoids and a source of cyclic-adenosine monophosphate (cAMP) [285]. As early as 1979 the changes in mouse 3T3-L1 cells with adipogenesis were investigated using 2DE, where 30 cytoplasmic, 9 non-histone chromosome associated and 24 membrane proteins were significantly altered, with actin identified and a decrease in actin observed with differentiation [163]. With subsequent "adipo-proteome" studies, it has been demonstrated that actin and the remodeling of the cytoskeletal network, is an essential for adipocyte differentiation, insulin signaling and the GLUT4, independent of the experimental conditions [286 - 290]. In contrast to Sidhu [163], the study by Welsh *et al.* [286], used a more complex differentiation cocktail including the PPARγ agonist, ciglitazone, which could activate its own specific subset of proteins. Amongst the proteins identified in this study was an increased expression of adiponectin and Eps15 homology domain-containing protein 1 (EDH1), amongst others. Adiponectin, an adipokine, has been well studied since this identification and is well recognized for its "positive" metabolic function, having insulin-sensitizing effects [291], central regulation of food intake and body weight [292], cardioprotective [293], anti-inflammatory and anti-oxidant properties [294], demonstrating that it has a clear clinical relevance with respect to pediatric obesity and its associated complications. Circulating concentrations of adiponectin are known to be significantly decreased with the development of childhood obesity and with altered glycemic control, with the high molecular weight form more strictly involved in insulin resistance [94, 295]. Due to the complex nature of the adiponectin multimers in circulation, studies regarding the direct administration of adiponectin to resolve the complications of obesity are limited, where therapeutic approaches have focused more on alternative therapies which aim to upregulate the synthesis and secretion of adiponectin. We have previously demonstrated using a 2DE approach that adiponectin levels a significantly decreased in vitamin D deficient pediatric obese subjects and that the administration of vitamin D is able to upregulate the synthesis and secretion of adiponectin in 3T3-L1 adipocytes [296] suggesting that vitamin D administration could have a long term benefit for pediatric obese subjects. Another study involving traditional oriental medicine, *Allium fistulosum* and *Viola mandshurica*, considered to be effective in promoting blood circulation, have been shown in a HFD-mouse model to increase the expression of adiponectin in epididymal WAT [297] suggesting natural products to treat obesity are of potential benefit, particularly with respect to childhood obesity.

In addition to adiponectin, Welsh *et al.* [286], identified 4 isoforms of Eps15 (EDH1) differentially regulated with 3T3-L1 differentiation, with these changes said to be post-translational events [286]. This protein is interesting in that regulates both clathrin-dependent and –independent endocytosis of proteins from the endosomal recycling compartment [298]. In addition, it has also been shown to be a candidate gene involved in Bardet Biedl syndrome, a heterogeneous autosomal dominant disorder associated to developmental abnormalities and obesity [299], with another proteomic based study demonstrating that EHD1 is reduced in normal and obesity-resistant rats suggesting that it may play a suppressive role in obesity development [207]. With respect to a therapeutical application, in early studies EDH1 was shown to down-regulate the insulin-like growth factor-1 (IGF-1) signaling pathway through a direct association with the IGF-I receptor (IGF-1R) [300], however, to our knowledge this aspect has not been further developed with respect to obesity-associated therapies.

The following proteomic studies by Choi *et al.* [287], and Rahman *et al.* [289], employed classic 2DE-combined MS methodologies to evaluate 3T3-L1 adipogenesis. Rahman *et al.* [289], identified phosphororibosyl pyrophosphate synthetase-associated protein (PRPS), a previously unidentified protein which was significantly downregulated with adipogenesis. It is known that PRPS is a central enzyme in the metabolism of nitrogenous compounds, used for both *de novo* nucleotide synthesis and the salvage pathway [301], with a demonstration of its involvement in DNA synthesis [302]. They propose its involvement in normal cellular proliferation, yet beyond this study there have been no further developments of PRPS as a therapeutic or diagnostic marker. Alternatively, Choi *et al.* [287], followed the classic 2DE with 2DE of 35S metabolic labelled products, where they confirmed the involvement of adiponectin and identified that a 20kDa α2 macroglobulin fragment is significantly downregulated with adipogenesis, and not as a result of *de novo* synthesis. The depletion of these fragments using an anti-α2 macroglobulin polyclonal antibody, demonstrated that adipogenesis was enhanced, suggesting that these fragments serve to inhibit adipogenesis [287]. Despite this interesting finding, there appears to be no further development to decipher the mechanism/s of these fragments and their potential application with respect to obesity and therapeutical targets. One abstract has shown that retinoic acid regulates α2 macroglobulin in bovine intramuscular adipogenesis [303]. For now these results reinforce the importance of the proteolytic processes in adipogenesis [304].

With technological advances in proteomic methodologies including iTRAQ-coupled 2D LC-MS/MS a high-throughput proteomic technology, the group of Ye *et al.* [290], was able to increase the list of key adipogenic proteins. Amongst the 24 new proteins they identified was pyruvate carboxylase (PCX) and voltage-dependent anion-selective channel protein 2 (VDAC2), both significantly upregulated with adipogenesis. Importantly, they were able to show that silencing both PCX and VDAC2 using siRNA technology could significantly inhibit adipocyte differentiation [290]. Pyruvate carboxylase is a regulatory metabolic enzyme that provides acetyl-coA and NADPH for the *de novo* biosynthesis of fatty acids and is regulated by glucagon, glucocorticoids, insulin and PPARγ [305]. Alternatively, the VDACS are a class of porin ion channels located on the outer mitochondrial membrane, constituting a major pathway for metabolic exchange across the mitochondria [306]. The VDACs have been proposed to be involved in ligand activated non-apoptotic cell death [307] and as such have been proposed to key to the viability of pre-adipocytes during adipogenesis. The potential of this protein awaits further development. With respect to PCX, a dramatic increase in PCX expression (40-fold) has been observed in the first 2 days of 3T3-L1 differentiation, which drops off progressively over the following days [308]. This group has also shown that if they block the autophagic pathway with either asparagine or 3-methyladenine within the first 2 days of the differentiation protocol, the peak expression of PCX is ablated suggesting autophagy is a key regulator of PCX and adipogenesis [308]. Autophagy, the orderly degradation and recycling of cellular components, is a central "cell fate" process in most tissues and organs and with respect to AT could be a key anti-obesity strategy. Bearing this in mind, recent studies in mesenchymal stem cells have demonstrated that Notch signaling via the activation of autophagy and PTEN-PI3K/Akt/mTOR pathway is able to induce adipogenic differentiation, highlighting the Notch signaling as a potential therapeutic target for future investigations [309].

Adipocyte-Derived Stem Cells (ASCs)

While murine 3T3-L1 cells have provided the most extensive information with respect to adipogenesis and the complications of obesity, its species-related differences to humans must also be considered. Bearing this in mind, the SVF contains lineage-committed preadipocytes and ASCs, with the difference between the two being that preadipocytes have a limited lifespan, while ASCs have a renewal capacity [310]. The AT is one of the richest sources of stem cells with >500 times more stem cells in 1 gram of AT than in 1 gram of aspirated bone marrow. General proteomic studies in ASCs are limited, however, one using ASC *in vitro* model of adipogenesis identified >40 proteins differentially expressed with differentiation, confirming the involvement of cytoskeletal proteins, metabolic, proteins involved in redox protein degradation and HSPs observed in 3T3-L1 cells and more importantly WAT tissue [311]. The therapeutical potential of the HSPs were discussed earlier.

In a second study, Lee *et al.* [312], using classic 2DE-MS methods, identified 32 proteins including syntaxin-3, oxysterol-binding protein (OSBP)-related protein 3, PPARγ and glycophorin. Syntaxins (STXs), a family (16 members) of **membrane** integrated **Q-SNAREproteins** participating in **exocytosis** [313], have been found to be involved in the complex orchestra of proteins involved in insulin-responsive GLUT4 trafficking [314]. More recently, an increased STX8 expression in VAT was shown to be associated to the presence of T2D in obese patients through a potential GLUT4 mechanism, highlighting that the family of syntaxins may offer a novel target for obesity and its associated co-morbidities [315]. For now, STX4 has been shown to increase pancreatic insulin release in human subjects in the presence or absence of T2D, suggesting there could be a therapeutic potential for this family of proteins [316]. Alternatively, the OSBP-related proteins (ORPs), are members of the OSBP-family which is comprised of sterol and phosphoinositide binding proteins which are conserved in eukaryotes, emphasizing a central regulatory role. The ORPs have been implicated as lipid sensor transporters that regulate a broad range of cellular functions from lipid metabolism and transport to membrane trafficking and cell signaling [317]. Most ORPs are capable of associating with ER membranes, where ORP3 has been shown to control cell adhesion [318]. To our knowledge, no further investigations of this protein with respect to obesity have been done, despite what appears to be an important role.

Adipocyte Secretome

It is the adipocytes which secrete an exclusive class of proteins known as adipokines. These include amongst others leptin, adiponectin, PAI-1, resistin, vaspin and a range of pro-inflammatory cytokines which act as endocrine-like factors to modulate physiological functions systemically. The first adipocyte secretome study compared epididymal, inguinal and omental derived cells treated with insulin using 2D-LC-MS/MS and ^{18}O proteolytic labelling [319]. In this study they identified 53 novel adipokines including RBP4 and clusterin, and they demonstrated that the chronic administration of insulin regulates PAI-1, osteonectin, complement factor B, complement component 4 and serine protease inhibitor 2c [319]. At the same time as this investigation, RBP4, a transport protein for retinol (Vitamin A) exploded into the arena. It was observed that this adipokine could act on muscle and liver in a retinol-dependent or –independent way regulating insulin sensitivity, thus conferring a link between obesity and insulin resistance [320]. Despite these promising results, RBP4 has sparked controversial debates due to numerous confounding factors including gender, genetic background and age, which influence its association to obesity and insulin resistance [321, 322]. Despite this, the majority of clinical studies in children and adolescents support a role for RBP4, which appears to have a role in the early development of insulin resistance and aspects of metabolic syndrome in the pediatric population [323, 324]. Longitudinal studies are required to investigate the prognostic value in obese children and adolescents. Recently, the thiazolinedione pioglitazone has been shown to inhibit scrum RPB4 by suppressing rat AT RBP4 expression, suggesting that inhibiting RBP4 expression in adipocytes may provide a mechanism by which pioglitazone improves insulin sensitivity in insulin-resistant subjects [325].

The first secretome studies of human, as opposed to rat, adipocytes used 2-DE MALDI-TOF methodologies where they identified Pigment epithelium-derived factor (PEDF), dipeptidyl peptidase 4 (DPP4) and heme oxygenase 1 (HO-1) as novel adipokines [326 - 328]. Famulla et al. [326], went on to confirm that PEDF is inversely regulated by insulin and hypoxia and is able to induce insulin resistance in adipocytes and human skeletal muscle cells, leading to inflammatory signaling. PEDF is recognized as anti-angiogenic, immunomodulatory, and neurotrophic serine protease inhibitor protein, however, the diverse actions seen by Famulla et al. [326], suggest that PEDF is a key adipokine, which could have an important role in diabetes and obesity-related disorders. Plasma PEDF levels have been shown to be elevated in overweight adolescents with a positive association with insulin resistance, highlighting that PEDF may play a role in the development of cardiometabolic dysfunction in adolescents [329]. With respect to DPP4, an antigenic enzyme involved in immune regulation, signal transduction and apoptosis, confirmation studies demonstrated that this adipokine has higher expression adipocytes than preadipocytes and that VAT explant cultures from obese individuals secrete higher levels of DPP4 [327]. Obese children with a substantial weight loss as opposed to those without, had significantly reduced DPP-4 levels and insulin concentrations, while insulin sensitivity indexes at fasting were significantly increased [330]. In their conformational studies, Lamers *et al.* [327], demonstrated that DPP4 administration to AT, skeletal as well as smooth muscle explants, impeded insulin signaling, suggesting that DPP4 could be a key link between obesity and metabolic syndrome [327]. In fact, DPP4 has been shown to be responsible for the degradation of incretins such as GLP-1 [331, 332]. As described previously, GLP-1 is responsible for amplifying the glucose response to insulin and as a result, DPP4 inhibitors such as vildagliptin (Novartis), sitagliptin (Merck Sharp & Dohme) and saxagliptin (Britstol-Meyers Squibb) have been developed to enhance GLP-1 activity [333]. Finally, adipocyte produced HO-1 was demonstrated to be significantly higher from adipocytes of obese subjects with respect to normal controls [328]. The HO system is part of an intricate network involved in mitigating the deleterious effects of oxidative stress in obesity and CVD [reviewed by 334]. The HO-1 enzyme is the exclusive enzyme which degrades the pro-oxidant heme to generate antioxidant products carbon monoxide and bilirubin, which have anti-inflammatory properties. In contrast, suppression of HO-1 is associated with hypertension, atherosclerosis and stroke, as such HO-1 has become a novel target in the development of potential therapeutic strategies [reviewed by 334].

Post-Translational Modifications (PTMs)

It is important to recognize that it may not only be the type of protein and its concentrations which determine its impact with respect to cell activity and the physiological state. It is now becoming more evident that more often than not it is the PTMs of proteins which determine the final outcome, thus offer important therapeutical targets. For example, protein kinases which regulate cell growth, differentiation, immune function and energy homeostasis, do so via phosphorylation [335]. As described, proteomic technologies have the possibility to collectively investigate the pattern of PTMs at one and the same time, thus enabling researchers to decipher the signaling cascades and protein modifications relevant to pediatric obesity.

Despite these important modifications there are very few reports regarding PTMs with respect to AT in a normal and obese state, with most studies in the literature focusing on adipogenesis and the role of phosphorylation, acetylation and succination [336 - 342], with one group evaluating BAT following insulin stimulation via the SILAC method [343]. The group of Schmelze *et al.* [336], profiled 3T3-L1 adipocytes following insulin treatments over time, where they identified 122 phosphorylation sites on 89 proteins. Their method involved an immune purification step using anti-tyrosine antibodies, purification by immobilized metal affinity chromatography (IMAC). Amongst the phosphorylated proteins identified, they identified novel proteins involved in

GLUT4 translocation, including Munc18c, APS and Gab1 which were activated 10-fold within 5min of insulin stimulation. The groups of Kim *et al.*, and Jung *et al.* [337, 338, 340], also examined the phosphoproteome in 3T3-L1 human mesenchymal stem cells, however, they evaluated the activated cascades during adipogenesis. They identified phosphorylated PTP-RQ, LAR and RPTPµ as positive or negative regulators of adipogenesis and confirmed these findings with functional investigations [337, 338, 340]. Despite these important findings, there have been no further demonstrations of these proteins as potential therapeutic targets in pediatric obesity, even though they could be potentially sites of AT dysregulation providing a link between obesity to insulin resistance.

With respect to other PTMs identified by proteomics, protein acetylation has also been identified during adipogenesis [340, 341]. Acetylation refers to the process of introducing an acetyl group into proteins, namely the substitution of an acetyl group for an active hydrogen atom, with deacetylation the removal. There is now a renewed interest in reversible acetylation and its ability to link energy status to adaptive cellular and organismal homeostasis [344]. In differentiating 3T3-L1 cells, a proteomic approach identified acetylated malate dehydrogenase 1 (MDH1), with the group going on to demonstrate that this acetylation was essential for MDH1 enzymatic activity and increasing intracellular NADPH levels [340]. They also identified in an independent study that MDH2 acetylation depended on the cells energy status and that this in turn could influence adipogenesis [340, 345]. Other groups have also demonstrated the importance of succination during 3T3-L1 differentiation [342] and protein carbonylation [345]. Protein carbonylation has been discussed for FABP4. Succination, on the other hand, is a chemical modification of cysteines in proteins by the Krebs cycle intermediate, fumarate, yielding S-(2-succino) cysteine (2SC). It is known that many proteins including enzymes, adipokines, cytoskeletal proteins and endoplasmic reticulum chaperones which have functional cysteine residues are succinylated [reviewed by 346]. In fact the succination of adipocyte proteins increases due to nutrient excess derived mitochondrial stress, suggesting that succination is a mechanistic link between mitochondrial dysfunction, oxidative and endoplasmic reticulum stress, and cellular progression toward apoptosis [347]. For the moment the significance of these findings and the potential applications with respect to pediatric obesity need to be further investigated.

PROTEOMIC PROFILING: TISSUES AND CIRCULATION

Parental obesity is a key amongst the known risk factors for pediatric obesity. Currently emphasis is being given to prenatal events, including maternal nutrition and lifestyle [10, 348, 349]. It was the Dutch famine in the Winter of 1944, which highlighted the importance of maternal nutrition and fetal programming, with children born in that period demonstrating a decreased fetal growth and decreased glucose tolerance in adulthood [350]. Fetal programming is the fetal adaptive responses to the intrauterine environment which may alter gene expression and permanently change the structure/function of one or more organs, influencing an individual's neurodevelopment and metabolic programming and susceptibility to chronic disorders [350, 351]. Despite the emergence of fetal programming in the early 1990s, related genes, proteins and pathways which determine an individual's susceptibility remain to be clearly defined. Proteomic investigations related to fetal programming are only now emerging, with the most relevant studies utilizing rodent model systems focusing on the influence of maternal nutrition and pre-existing maternal obesity in the liver, placenta and brain proteomes [352 - 356].

Circulating proteomic profiles provide essential information for biomarker discoveries; in particular profiles which are related to the developmental stages of obesity and the progressive steps associated co-morbidities, such as insulin resistance and T2D, which are of particular relevance for pediatric obesity. In addition to providing targets for innovative therapies and building protein reference maps for personalized care, proteomic profiles should help to improve our understanding of these pathologies and provide prognostic outcomes for obese children. Proteomic tissue based studies provide mechanistic data and biomarkers. They exclude, however, the collective influence of important peripheral tissues. Circulating biomarkers in serum/plasma and urine collectively define the physiological state. As such proteomic profiling in these fluids in pediatric obesity with respect to normal subjects, or according to different clinical parameters or during lifestyle intervention or treatment/s in a time related study, offer a global insight into these pathologies.

Fetal Programming: Tissue-Specific Biomarkers

Due to the significant and broad range effects that a maternal diet/lifestyle can have on the fetal environment, proteomics offers a global approach to understanding the maternal effect on offspring. These studies are restricted to rodent models with one of the earliest proteomic studies by Novak *et al.* [352], examining the effect of a maternal diet containing high versus low unsaturated fatty acids (UFAs) on 3-day old rodent pup livers through gestation and lactation. Of the 800 resolved proteins, 3-fold changes were observed in 11 proteins, with MALDI-TOF MS identifying proteins associated to gluconeogenic and lipolytic pathways which regulate the liver accretion of long chain n-3 fatty acids, thought to be essential for the sequence of liver differentiation in preparation for extra-uterine life. Proteomic studies have also been used to assess maternal food restriction, where the group of You *et al.* [356], investigated one-carbon metabolism in the livers of newborn rodent pups during gestation. One-carbon metabolism has been shown to be essential for placental function and fetal growth, with an impaired function increasing homocysteine levels. This study was able to demonstrate that male pups have an increased susceptibility to diseases in adult life through maternal food restriction and fetal programming. Proteomic investigations have also focused on other key tissues including the placenta [353] and brains [354, 355]. In these tissues, a large array of proteins associated to cellular growth, apoptosis, oxidative stress and inflammation were identified. Of these, Lee *et al.* [354], confirmed the expression pattern of ubiquitin carboxy-terminal hydrolase L1 (UCHL1) and secernin 1 (SCRN1), proposing these two proteins as fetal-programming-related obesity markers. While clear biomarkers still remain to be defined, proteomic studies have collectively highlighted that maternal nutrition/lifestyle does regulates fetal metabolic pathways and the adaption to birth.

Circulating Biomarkers

Human plasma is one of the most central and accessible body fluids for biomarker discovery, particularly with respect to the ethical issues associated to pediatric population. Despite this, however, there are very few proteomic evaluations, most likely due to the complexity of plasma and serum proteomes and the fact that 95% of serum proteins are albumin and immunoglobulins, thus masking the less abundant cytokines, hormones and enzymes, amongst other proteins. While it is logical to think an immunodepletion will resolve this issue, a large number of proteins interact with albumin and as such its removal introduces a bias. One of the first plasma proteomic studies examining childhood obesity, evaluated 10 age matched obese, 10 overweight and 10 lean pre-pubertal boys, in all aspects healthy, to see if obesity could alter the plasma proteome [357]. This investigation targeted 9 relevant proteins by classic 2DE combined with MALDI-TOF MS, where fibrinogen β (FIBB) was found to have a significantly higher expression in obese boys, while complement factor B was highest in overweight and obese with respect to lean boys. Additionally, ApoA-I was lower in overweight and obese boys while ApoA-IV was higher, with respect to lean boys. The dysregulation of the apolipoprotein profile they confirmed by clinical laboratory evaluations with plasma ApoA-1 shown to decline prior to HDL-cholesterol in this small cohort of pediatric subjects. The relevance of ApoA-1 with respects to pediatric obesity has been described, with ApoA-1 and ApoB concentrations in childhood predictive of carotid intima-media and brachial flow-mediated dilation in adulthood [358]. The other interesting findings in this study were the differential levels of FIBB which suggest that obese pre-pubertal children may be predisposed to atherosclerotic cardiovascular disease. It is well recognized that FIBB is a key protein the coagulation and acute phase response, with levels reflecting an inflammatory state and shown to be associated CVD. In fact, FIBB is considered a key cardiovascular risk factor in adults [359]. This proteomic study has highlighted the importance of FIBB levels in obese children and has further introduced the concept of screening ApoA-1 levels in obese children for disease prognoses.

In addition to comparing lean and obese phenotypes, proteomic plasma approaches have also been used as a strategy to differentiate pediatric obese phenotypes and study diagnostic approaches and lifestyle/therapeutic interventions. With evidence accumulating to suggest that there is a potential link between obesity and vitamin D deficiency amongst global pediatric populations [360], our group as described, examined the plasma proteome by 2DE in 42 pediatric obese children divided according to their vitamin D levels, with vitamin D deficient children having calcidiol < 15ng/ml (n=18) and normal calcidiol levels >30ng/ml (n=24). In this study we identified and confirmed with functional studies that adiponectin is a key link between obesity and vitamin D status with beneficial results observed with cholecalciferol administration to the vitamin D deficient children [296]. Alternatively, Martos-Moreno *et al.* [361], evaluated the ability of serum proteomic profiles to detect metabolic changes compared to standardized clinical assays, with the goal being to find novel biomarkers for metabolic impairment in obese children (n=22) compared to lean controls (n=21). They identified isoforms of ApoA-1 and haptoglobin, Apo-J/clusterin, VDBP and transthyretin were all downregulated in obese children. In the case of ApoA-1 and clusterin, these results were enhanced by the presence of insulin resistance, while ApoA-1 and transthyretin were upregulated with weight loss. Apo- J/clusterin is an abundant plasma chaperone protein involved in the clearance of cellular debris and apoptosis [362]. The fasting plasma levels of clusterin have been shown to correlate with the parameters of adiposity and systemic inflammation in healthy adults, suggesting that circulating clusterin level may be a surrogate marker for obesity-associated systemic inflammation [363]. Circulating clusterin levels in pediatric obese in addition to its prognostic value with respect to pediatric obesity and the step to insulin resistance, await further investigations. An interesting observation was the enhancement of haptoglobin isoforms with insulin resistance and that weight-loss could regulate its levels. Haptoglobin functions as a "suicide" protein binding free hemoglobin to allow degradative enzymes to gain access to it, while at the same time preventing loss of iron through the kidneys and protecting them from damage by hemoglobin [364]. Martos-Moreno *et al.* [361], identified that haptoglobin levels correlate with IL6 and visfatin and propose that haptoglobin is a good potential biomarker which relates specifically to metabolic complications in children.

In the majority of cases, as discussed above, weight gain is attributable to lifestyle-related and social factors, although a genetic contribution to body weight regulation is also recognized. Moreover, the contribution of life-style factors and environment on obesity comorbidities is largely unexplored, in particular in children and adolescents. The WHO found that some countries have managed to contain the obesity epidemic "through a whole-of-government approach" which helped to maintain its levels stable. This approach includes promoting vegetable and fruit consumption in schools, employing good surveillance and promoting physical activity. Lifestyle intervention, in terms of low caloric restriction, empowerment of a healthy nutrition, and promotion of physical exercise are the first steps in the management of obesity beyond its prevention and this is truer in children. It has been recently shown in a large cohort of obese youths that a BMI-SDS reduction of 0.25 or greater significantly improved hypertension, hypertriglyceridemia, and low HDL-cholesterol, whereas a BMI-SDS greater than 0.5 doubled the effect but without an improvement on fasting glucose and LDL-cholesterol [365]. Moreover, age at intervention seems to be another crucial factor with more weight loss in those younger than 10 years [366]. These data suggest that the interaction between obesity and cardiovascular comorbidities is complex and that some processes are irreversible. However, lifestyle intervention is difficult and often unsuccessful in the long term and most children who are obese will stay obese in adulthood [367]. The difficulty of an obese child or adolescent to reduce weight might be attributable also to genetic background and/or adaptive changes in basal metabolic rate, hunger and satiety hormones that occur with weight loss. With respect to this background proteomics, in particular in the plasma, could be useful to identify biomarkers of "success" or "not" to lifestyle interventions, risk of long-term relapse, and healing or the development of comorbidities. The search of biomarkers of success in weight management to precociously stratify patients at higher risk by other approaches is a real challenge. Some candidate proteins or adipokines have been explored [368], however to date; proteomic studies in children have still to be published. On the other hand, some recent proteomic reports are present in the adult obesity lifestyle management. In studies on fat biopsies after weight loss or high intensity intermitting training, several authors identified changes in the same proteins. In particular, fructose-bisphosphate aldolase C and tubulin beta 5 are candidate protein responsive to caloric restriction, in association to proteins indicating a reduced intracellular scaffolding of GLUT4 (ALDOC, TUBB5, annexin 2), an increased uptake of fatty acids (FABP4), an improved inflammatory profile of the adipose tissue (ApoA1, AOP1) and a change in fat droplet organization (vimentin). Annexin 2 and FABP4 are also modulated by the exercise training [369 - 372]. Furthermore, some data on plasma proteomics have been published. Obesity-associated (complement C3), and diet-associated proteins (apolipoproteins, especially apolipoprotein A-IV) were also identified in the plasma of type 2 diabetes patients after a very low caloric diet (450/Kcal/day) in addiction to an exercise program [373]. Apolipoprotein A-IV has been identified also after weight loss due to Roux-en-Y gastric bypass surgery [374]. Interestingly, other proteins identified to be higher in obese patients than in normal-weight subjects, after surgery showed a biphasic pattern of variation, decreasing after 3 months before rising back to baseline values after 6 months with a kinetic parallel to changes in calorie and carbohydrate intake [375]. All these preliminary data suggest that circulating proteomic is useful in the studying and management of obesity with respect to different type of diets and exercise programs and the research should be more addressed to children in which growth and pubertal dynamics have an intriguing role.

Urine Biomarkers

Recent epidemiological data highlight that childhood obesity is associated with an increased risk of renal injury [376]. As the onset of obesity-associated renal disease is asymptomatic, the searches for early diagnostic markers are essential for prevention and therapeutic approaches. Of the urine proteins found in normal physiological conditions, 70% are derived from kidney and urinary tract, with the remainder transported from the blood and filtered by the kidney. As such, urine contains not only markers of kidney disease but also markers relative to the cause of kidney disease, such as obesity. In contrast to plasma and serum, urine does not contain the highly abundant plasma proteins such as albumin which can mask other proteins, its collection is non-invasive and large quantities can be obtained. While normalization is required in consideration of fluid intake, physical activity, diet and so forth, urine proteomics offers obesity-associated renal disease potential diagnostic and prognostic markers. Despite this potential, to our knowledge there are no pediatric obesity-associated urine proteomic studies present within the literature with current studies in children focusing on idiopathic nephrotic syndrome [377], T2D nephropathy [378] and posterior urethral valves [379], amongst others with a specific focus on rare diseases/syndromes.

OUTLOOKS

The pediatric obesity prevalence rates in certain countries have slowed in recent years due to national prevention programs reinforcing the importance of diet and exercise. Despite these positive trends the results to date have not resolved this global problem and emphasize an urgent need for additional strategies. Current lifestyle and pharmacological approaches for children are limited and are useful only once obesity is diagnosed. While a small number of drugs have shown beneficial effects over the short term with the primary endpoint being a reduction in BMI, each pharmacological agent still requires long-term studies to assess safety and efficacy with orlistat the only FDA-approved drug for the treatment of pediatric obesity at this point in time [380].

In addressing how to treat and prevent pediatric obesity, one needs to consider the cause. Adipose tissue with a central role in body weight homeostasis, inflammation and insulin resistance, is a highly orchestrated tissue involving receptor and second messenger pathways with steps and passes that influence hyperplasia, hypertrophy, adipocyte differentiation, turnover, lipolysis, FFA metabolism, lipogenesis and the secretome profile. It is AT dysfunction which is the major contributor to the pathogenesis of obesity-related insulin resistance and MetS. These conditions are characterized by an abnormal secretion of adipokines, inflammatory cytokines as well as a dysregulation in glucose and lipid homeostasis and mitochondrial dysfunction. While significant efforts have been made in the last 50 years via extensive clinical investigations, animal models, tissue and cell line studies to understand AT dysregulation, these investigations have been only able to understand a small number of aspects without taking into consideration the global time resolved changes. "Proteomics", first coined in 1995 is a large-scale characterization of the entire protein profile of a cell line, tissue, fluid or organism not only from the perspective of expression but also PTMs. With the development of various quantitative and qualitative proteomic methodologies in the last decade, valuable information has been obtained in the changes/activities of key AT proteins in both WAT and BAT, with a long list of adipokines/cytokines, signaling, PTMs and mitochondrial proteins contributors to AT dysregulation. Moreover another player should be considered, the gut microbiota. It is an environmental factor which influences whole-body metabolism by affecting energy balance but also inflammation and gut barrier function, integrates peripheral and central food intake regulatory signals and thereby increases body weight. Gut microbiota maintains a relatively constant abundance, with an altered bacterial density among the phyla associated with complex diseases such as obesity, type 2 diabetes and cancer [381 - 383]. Studies on microbiota are increasing because it has emerged as an important field of research in order to achieve better health. Several efforts have been put in pediatric research, considering gut microbiota as an element strictly linked to lifestyle interventions, in particular on nutrition, as well as treatments, antibiotics among the others. It appears as a field of prevention and/or treatment in which probiotics and prebiotics could restore an imbalance in homeostasis without being classified as pharmacological treatments. In the present review we have addressed the recent advances in the proteomic characterization of pediatric obesity, in particular proteins that potentially play relevant roles and those which may offer targets for novel therapies, considering either/or pharmacological or natural approaches. With the future offering the rapid development of high-throughput methodologies, technological advances in MS, as well as the completion of the international human proteome sequencing program (http://www.thehpp.org/ human HUPO) in the next few years, the generation of reference maps applicable to pediatric obesity will become available making drug discoveries, combination therapies, trials, and nutritional/environmental influences easier to evaluate. Furthermore, proteomics of gut microbiota is in its infancy and the scenario of dynamic interactions among proteins of bacteria and of the host could offer further prospective.

CONFLICT OF INTEREST

The authors confirm that they have no conflict of interest to declare for this publication.

ACKNOWLEDGEMENTS

The authors would like to acknowledge Drs. Giulia Genoni, Roberta Ricotti and Stefania Moia for their technical assistance.

ABBREVIATIONS

2DE	Two-dimensional electrophoresis	EDH1	Eps15 homology domain-containing protein 1
2D-DIGE	2D-difference gel electrophoresis	ELISA	Enzyme-Linked Immuno Sorbent Assay
3-AR	3-adrenergic receptor	ENCODE	Encyclopedia of DNA Elements
AgRP	Agouti-related protein	ESI	electron spray ionization
AMPK	AMP-activated protein kinase	FABP4	fatty acid binding protein 4
ANXA1	Annexin A1	FFA	free-fatty acids
ApoA1	proapolipoprotein A-1	FIBB	fibrinogen β (FIBB)
AT	adipose tissue	FTO	fat mass and obesity-associated gene
BMI	body mass index	GLP	glucagon like peptide
BAT	brown/beige adipose tissue	GLUT4	glucose transport-4
cAMP	cyclic-adenosine monophosphate	GWAS	genome-wide association study
CHAPS	3-[3-cholamidopropyl) dimethylammonio]-1-propanesulfonate	HDL	high density lipoprotein
CID	collision induced dissociation	HED	hydroxyethyl disulphide
CNS	central nervous system	HFD	high fat diet
CNV	copy number variation	HO-1	heme oxygenase 1
CRP	C-reactive protein	HSL	hormone sensitive lipase
CVD	cardiovascular disease	HSP	heat shock protein
DPP-4	dipeptidyl peptidase-4	ICAT	isotope-coded affinity tags
dSAT	deep superficial adipose tissue	IEF	isoelectric focusing
DTT	dithiothrietol	IGF-1	insulin-like growth factor-1
ECD	electron capture dissociation	IGF-1R	IGF-1 receptor

IGFBP	IGF-binding proteins	POMC	pro-opiomelanocortin
IGT	impaired glucose tolerance	PPARγ	peroxisome proliferator-activated receptor γ
IPG	immobilized pH gradient		
iTRAQ	isobaric tags for relative and absolute quantification	PRPS	phosphororibosyl pyrophosphate synthetase-associated protein
JAK	Janus Kinase	PTMs	post-translational modifications
LC	liquid chromatography	PYY	peptide YY
LXN	lipoxins	RBP	retinol binding protein
MALDI	matrix-assisted laser desorption ionization	ROS	reactive oxygen species
		SAT	superficial adipose tissue
MS	mass spectrometry	SDS	sodium dodecyl sulphate
MW	molecular weight	SDS-PAGE	SDS-Polyacrylamide Gel Electrophoresis
NAFLD	non-alcoholic fatty liver disease		
NEPHGE	non-equilibrium pH gel electrophoresis	SILAC	stable-isotope labeling by amino acids in cell culture
		sSAT	superficial-SAT
NGS	next generation sequencing	STAT	Signal Transducer and Activator of Transcription
NPY	neuropeptide Y		
OW	overweight	SVF	stromal vascular fraction
PAI-1	plasminogen activator inhibitor	STXs	Syntaxins
PCOS	polycystic ovary syndrome	T2D	type 2 diabetes mellitus
PDK4	pyruvate dehydrogenase lipoamide kinase isozyme 4	TNFα	tumor necrosis factor α
		UCP1	uncoupling protein 1
PERK	protein kinase RNA-like endoplasmic reticulum kinase	VAT	visceral adipose tissue
		VDBP	vitamin D binding protein
PEDF	Pigment epithelium-derived factor PKA: protein kinase A	WAT	white adipose tissue
		WHO	World Health Organization
pI	isoelectric point		
PMF	peptide map fingerprinting	WIB	western immunoblot

REFERENCES

[1] Ogden CL, Carroll MD, Flegal KM. Prevalence of obesity in the United States. JAMA 2014; 312(2): 189-90.
[http://dx.doi.org/10.1001/jama.2014.6228] [PMID: 25005661]

[2] Peeters A, Bonneux L, Barendregt J, Nusselder W. Methods of estimating years of life lost due to obesity. JAMA 2003; 289(22): 2941-2.
[http://dx.doi.org/10.1001/jama.289.22.2941-a] [PMID: 12799399]

[3] Hotamisligil GS, Erbay E. Nutrient sensing and inflammation in metabolic diseases. Nat Rev Immunol 2008; 8(12): 923-34.
[http://dx.doi.org/10.1038/nri2449] [PMID: 19029988]

[4] Alley DE, Chang VW. The changing relationship of obesity and disability, 19882004. JAMA 2007; 298(17): 2020-7.
[http://dx.doi.org/10.1001/jama.298.17.2020] [PMID: 17986695]

[5] Levy-Marchal C, Arslanian S, Cutfield W, *et al.* Insulin resistance in children: consensus, perspective, and future directions. J Clin Endocrinol Metab 2010; 95(12): 5189-98.
[http://dx.doi.org/10.1210/jc.2010-1047] [PMID: 20829185]

[6] Liang Y, Hou D, Zhao X, *et al.* Childhood obesity affects adult metabolic syndrome and diabetes. Endocrine 2015; 50(1): 87-92.
[http://dx.doi.org/10.1007/s12020-015-0560-7] [PMID: 25754912]

[7] Serdula MK, Ivery D, Coates RJ, Freedman DS, Williamson DF, Byers T. Do obese children become obese adults? A review of the literature. Prev Med 1993; 22(2): 167-77.
[http://dx.doi.org/10.1006/pmed.1993.1014] [PMID: 8483856]

[8] Druet C, Stettler N, Sharp S, *et al.* Prediction of childhood obesity by infancy weight gain: an individual-level meta-analysis. Paediatr Perinat Epidemiol 2012; 26(1): 19-26.
[http://dx.doi.org/10.1111/j.1365-3016.2011.01213.x] [PMID: 22150704]

[9] Sandholt CH, Hansen T, Pedersen O. Beyond the fourth wave of genome-wide obesity association studies. Nutr Diabetes 2012; 2: e37.
[http://dx.doi.org/10.1038/nutd.2012.9] [PMID: 23168490]

[10] Brown CL, Halvorson EE, Cohen GM, Lazorick S, Skelton JA. Addressing childhood obesity: opportunities for prevention. Pediatr Clin North Am 2015; 62(5): 1241-61.
[http://dx.doi.org/10.1016/j.pcl.2015.05.013] [PMID: 26318950]

[11] Bouchard C, Tremblay A, Després JP, *et al.* The response to long-term overfeeding in identical twins. N Engl J Med 1990; 322(21): 1477-82.
[http://dx.doi.org/10.1056/NEJM199005243222101] [PMID: 2336074]

[12] Speakman JR. A nonadaptive scenario explaining the genetic predisposition to obesity: the predation release hypothesis. Cell Metab 2007; 6(1): 5-12.
[http://dx.doi.org/10.1016/j.cmet.2007.06.004] [PMID: 17618852]

[13] van der Klaauw AA, Farooqi IS. The hunger genes: pathways to obesity. Cell 2015; 161(1): 119-32.
[http://dx.doi.org/10.1016/j.cell.2015.03.008] [PMID: 25815990]

[14] Haslam DW, James WP. Obesity. Lancet 2005; 366(9492): 1197-209.
[http://dx.doi.org/10.1016/S0140-6736(05)67483-1] [PMID: 16198769]

[15] Xia Q, Grant SF. The genetics of human obesity. Ann N Y Acad Sci 2013; 1281: 178-90.
[http://dx.doi.org/10.1111/nyas.12020] [PMID: 23360386]

[16] Montague CT, Farooqi IS, Whitehead JP, *et al.* Congenital leptin deficiency is associated with severe early-onset obesity in humans. Nature 1997; 387(6636): 903-8.
[http://dx.doi.org/10.1038/43185] [PMID: 9202122]

[17] Strobel A, Issad T, Camoin L, Ozata M, Strosberg AD. A leptin missense mutation associated with hypogonadism and morbid obesity. Nat Genet 1998; 18(3): 213-5.
[http://dx.doi.org/10.1038/ng0398-213] [PMID: 9500540]

[18] Clément K, Vaisse C, Lahlou N, *et al.* A mutation in the human leptin receptor gene causes obesity and pituitary dysfunction. Nature 1998; 392(6674): 398-401.
[http://dx.doi.org/10.1038/32911] [PMID: 9537324]

[19] Farooqi IS, Wangensteen T, Collins S, *et al.* Clinical and molecular genetic spectrum of congenital deficiency of the leptin receptor. N Engl J Med 2007; 356(3): 237-47.
[http://dx.doi.org/10.1056/NEJMoa063988] [PMID: 17229951]

[20] Wabitsch M, Funcke JB, von Schnurbein J, *et al.* Severe early-onset obesity due to bioinactive leptin caused by a p.N103K mutation in the leptin gene. J Clin Endocrinol Metab 2015; 100(9): 3227-30.
[http://dx.doi.org/10.1210/jc.2015-2263] [PMID: 26186301]

[21] Moitra J, Mason MM, Olive M, *et al.* Life without white fat: a transgenic mouse. Genes Dev 1998; 12(20): 3168-81.

[http://dx.doi.org/10.1101/gad.12.20.3168] [PMID: 9784492]

[22] Antuna-Puente B, Feve B, Fellahi S, Bastard JP. Adipokines: the missing link between insulin resistance and obesity. Diabetes Metab 2008; 34(1): 2-11.
[http://dx.doi.org/10.1016/j.diabet.2007.09.004] [PMID: 18093861]

[23] Halaas JL, Gajiwala KS, Maffei M, et al. Weight-reducing effects of the plasma protein encoded by the obese gene. Science 1995; 269(5223): 543-6.
[http://dx.doi.org/10.1126/science.7624777] [PMID: 7624777]

[24] Fruebis J, Tsao TS, Javorschi S, et al. Proteolytic cleavage product of 30-kDa adipocyte complement-related protein increases fatty acid oxidation in muscle and causes weight loss in mice. Proc Natl Acad Sci USA 2001; 98(4): 2005-10.
[http://dx.doi.org/10.1073/pnas.98.4.2005] [PMID: 11172066]

[25] Wilkins MR, Pasquali C, Appel RD, et al. From proteins to proteomes: large scale protein identification by two-dimensional electrophoresis and amino acid analysis. Biotechnology (N Y) 1996; 14(1): 61-5.
[http://dx.doi.org/10.1038/nbt0196-61] [PMID: 9636313]

[26] Tyers M, Mann M. From genomics to proteomics. Nature 2003; 422(6928): 193-7.
[http://dx.doi.org/10.1038/nature01510] [PMID: 12634792]

[27] Cravatt BF, Simon GM, Yates JR III. The biological impact of mass-spectrometry-based proteomics. Nature 2007; 450(7172): 991-1000.
[http://dx.doi.org/10.1038/nature06525] [PMID: 18075578]

[28] Yang W, Steen H, Freeman MR. Proteomic approaches to the analysis of multiprotein signaling complexes. Proteomics 2008; 8(4): 832-51.
[http://dx.doi.org/10.1002/pmic.200700650] [PMID: 18297654]

[29] Ghosh D, Poisson LM. Omics data and levels of evidence for biomarker discovery. Genomics 2009; 93(1): 13-6.
[http://dx.doi.org/10.1016/j.ygeno.2008.07.006] [PMID: 18723089]

[30] Mallick P, Kuster B. Proteomics: a pragmatic perspective. Nat Biotechnol 2010; 28(7): 695-709.
[http://dx.doi.org/10.1038/nbt.1658] [PMID: 20622844]

[31] Sperrin M, Marshall AD, Higgins V, Buchan IE, Renehan AG. Slowing down of adult body mass index trend increases in England: a latent class analysis of cross-sectional surveys (19922010). Int J Obes 2014; 38(6): 818-24.
[http://dx.doi.org/10.1038/ijo.2013.161] [PMID: 23995474]

[32] Maggio AB, Martin XE, Saunders Gasser C, et al. Medical and non-medical complications among children and adolescents with excessive body weight. BMC Pediatr 2014; 14: 232.
[http://dx.doi.org/10.1186/1471-2431-14-232] [PMID: 25220473]

[33] Neovius MG, Linné YM, Barkeling BS, Rossner SO. Sensitivity and specificity of classification systems for fatness in adolescents. Am J Clin Nutr 2004; 80(3): 597-603.
[PMID: 15321798]

[34] Wang Y, Lobstein T. Worldwide trends in childhood overweight and obesity. Int J Pediatr Obes 2006; 1(1): 11-25.
[http://dx.doi.org/10.1080/17477160600586747] [PMID: 17902211]

[35] Farooqi IS, O'Rahilly S. Monogenic obesity in humans. Annu Rev Med 2005; 56: 443-58.
[http://dx.doi.org/10.1146/annurev.med.56.062904.144924] [PMID: 15660521]

[36] Ozanne SE, Hales CN. Lifespan: catch-up growth and obesity in male mice. Nature 2004; 427(6973): 411-2.
[http://dx.doi.org/10.1038/427411b] [PMID: 14749819]

[37] Nicholas LM, Morrison JL, Rattanatray L, Zhang S, Ozanne SE, McMillen IC. The early origins of obesity and insulin resistance: timing, programming and mechanisms. Int J Obes 2015.
[http://dx.doi.org/10.1038/ijo.2015.178] [PMID: 26367335]

[38] Škledar MT, Milošević M. Breastfeeding and time of complementary food introduction as predictors of obesity in children. Cent Eur J Public Health 2015; 23(1): 26-31.
[http://dx.doi.org/10.21101/cejph.a3956] [PMID: 26036095]

[39] Braithwaite I, Stewart AW, Hancox RJ, Beasley R, Murphy R, Mitchell EA. Fast-food consumption and body mass index in children and adolescents: an international cross-sectional study. BMJ Open 2014; 4(12): e005813.
[http://dx.doi.org/10.1136/bmjopen-2014-005813] [PMID: 25488096]

[40] Cantoral A, Téllez-Rojo MM, Ettinger AS, Hu H, Hernández-Ávila M, Peterson K. Early introduction and cumulative consumption of sugar-sweetened beverages during the pre-school period and risk of obesity at 8 14 years of age. Pediatr Obes 2015.
[http://dx.doi.org/10.1111/ijpo.12023] [PMID: 25891908]

[41] Miller AL, Lumeng JC, LeBourgeois MK. Sleep patterns and obesity in childhood. Curr Opin Endocrinol Diabetes Obes 2015; 22(1): 41-7.
[http://dx.doi.org/10.1097/MED.0000000000000125] [PMID: 25517022]

[42] Takizawa R, Danese A, Maughan B, Arseneault L. Bullying victimization in childhood predicts inflammation and obesity at mid-life: a five-decade birth cohort study. Psychol Med 2015; 45(13): 2705-15.
[http://dx.doi.org/10.1017/S0033291715000653] [PMID: 25988703]

[43] Tanaka C, Reilly JJ, Huang WY. Longitudinal changes in objectively measured sedentary behaviour and their relationship with adiposity in children and adolescents: systematic review and evidence appraisal. Obes Rev 2014; 15(10): 791-803.
[http://dx.doi.org/10.1111/obr.12195] [PMID: 24899125]

[44] Bourguignon JP, Parent AS. Early homeostatic disturbances of human growth and maturation by endocrine disrupters. Curr Opin Pediatr 2010; 22(4): 470-7.
[http://dx.doi.org/10.1097/MOP.0b013e32833a6eef] [PMID: 20489638]

[45] Atkinson RL, Lee I, Shin HJ, He J. Human adenovirus-36 antibody status is associated with obesity in children. Int J Pediatr Obes 2010; 5(2): 157-60.
[http://dx.doi.org/10.3109/17477160903111789] [PMID: 19593728]

[46] Genoni G, Prodam F, Marolda A, et al. Obesity and infection: two sides of one coin. Eur J Pediatr 2014; 173(1): 25-32.
[http://dx.doi.org/10.1007/s00431-013-2178-1] [PMID: 24146165]

[47] Waalen J. The genetics of human obesity. Transl Res 2014; 164(4): 293-301.
[http://dx.doi.org/10.1016/j.trsl.2014.05.010] [PMID: 24929207]

[48] Albuquerque D, Stice E, Rodríguez-López R, Manco L, Nóbrega C. Current review of genetics of human obesity: from molecular mechanisms to an evolutionary perspective. Mol Genet Genomics 2015; 290(4): 1191-221.
[http://dx.doi.org/10.1007/s00438-015-1015-9] [PMID: 25749980]

[49] Mutch DM, Clément K. Genetics of human obesity. Best Pract Res Clin Endocrinol Metab 2006; 20(4): 647-64.
[http://dx.doi.org/10.1016/j.beem.2006.09.006] [PMID: 17161337]

[50] Finucane MM, Stevens GA, Cowan MJ, et al. Global Burden of Metabolic Risk Factors of Chronic Diseases Collaborating Group (Body Mass Index). National, regional, and global trends in body-mass index since 1980: systematic analysis of health examination surveys and epidemiological studies with 960 country-years and 9·1 million participants. Lancet 2011; 377(9765): 557-67.
[http://dx.doi.org/10.1016/S0140-6736(10)62037-5] [PMID: 21295846]

[51] Paciorek CJ, Stevens GA, Finucane MM, Ezzati M. Childrens height and weight in rural and urban populations in low-income and middle-income countries: a systematic analysis of population-representative data. Lancet Glob Health 2013; 1(5): e300-9.
[http://dx.doi.org/10.1016/S2214-109X(13)70109-8] [PMID: 25104494]

[52] Allison DB, Kaprio J, Korkeila M, Koskenvuo M, Neale MC, Hayakawa K. The heritability of body mass index among an international sample of monozygotic twins reared apart. Int J Obes Relat Metab Disord 1996; 20(6): 501-6.
[PMID: 8782724]

[53] Maes HH, Neale MC, Eaves LJ. Genetic and environmental factors in relative body weight and human adiposity. Behav Genet 1997; 27(4): 325-51.
[http://dx.doi.org/10.1023/A:1025635913927] [PMID: 9519560]

[54] Stunkard AJ, Harris JR, Pedersen NL, McClearn GE. The body-mass index of twins who have been reared apart. N Engl J Med 1990; 322(21): 1483-7.
[http://dx.doi.org/10.1056/NEJM199005243222102] [PMID: 2336075]

[55] Naidoo N, Pawitan Y, Soong R, Cooper DN, Ku CS. Human genetics and genomics a decade after the release of the draft sequence of the human genome. Hum Genomics 2011; 5(6): 577-622.
[http://dx.doi.org/10.1186/1479-7364-5-6-577] [PMID: 22155605]

[56] Lu Y, Loos RJ. Obesity genomics: assessing the transferability of susceptibility loci across diverse populations. Genome Med 2013; 5(6): 55.
[http://dx.doi.org/10.1186/gm459] [PMID: 23806069]

[57] Zhang D, Li Z, Wang H, et al. Interactions between obesity-related copy number variants and dietary behaviors in childhood obesity. Nutrients 2015; 7(4): 3054-66.
[http://dx.doi.org/10.3390/nu7043054] [PMID: 25912042]

[58] Apalasamy YD, Mohamed Z. Obesity and genomics: role of technology in unraveling the complex genetic architecture of obesity. Hum Genet 2015; 134(4): 361-74.
[http://dx.doi.org/10.1007/s00439-015-1533-x] [PMID: 25687726]

[59] Bray GA, York DA. Hypothalamic and genetic obesity in experimental animals: an autonomic and endocrine hypothesis. Physiol Rev 1979; 59(3): 719-809.
[PMID: 379887]

[60] Jéquier E. Leptin signaling, adiposity, and energy balance. Ann N Y Acad Sci 2002; 967: 379-88.
[http://dx.doi.org/10.1111/j.1749-6632.2002.tb04293.x] [PMID: 12079865]

[61] Cole TJ. Conditional reference charts to assess weight gain in British infants. Arch Dis Child 1995; 73(1): 8-16.
[http://dx.doi.org/10.1136/adc.73.1.8] [PMID: 7639558]

[62] Reynolds CM, Gray C, Li M, Segovia SA, Vickers MH. Early life nutrition and energy balance disorders in offspring in later life. Nutrients 2015; 7(9): 8090-111.
[http://dx.doi.org/10.3390/nu7095384] [PMID: 26402696]

[63] Hetherington AW, Ranson SW. Hypothalamic lesions and adiposity in the rat. Anat Rec 1940; 78: 149-72.
[http://dx.doi.org/10.1002/ar.1090780203]

[64] Wilson JL, Enriori PJ. A talk between fat tissue, gut, pancreas and brain to control body weight. Mol Cell Endocrinol 2015; 418 Pt 2: 108-19.
[http://dx.doi.org/10.1016/j.mce.2015.08.022] [PMID: 26316427]

[65] Yi CX, Tschöp MH. Brain-gut-adipose-tissue communication pathways at a glance. Dis Model Mech 2012; 5(5): 583-7.
[http://dx.doi.org/10.1242/dmm.009902] [PMID: 22915019]

[66] Näslund E, Hellström PM. Appetite signaling: from gut peptides and enteric nerves to brain. Physiol Behav 2007; 92(1-2): 256-62.
[http://dx.doi.org/10.1016/j.physbeh.2007.05.017] [PMID: 17582445]

[67] Williams KW, Margatho LO, Lee CE, *et al*. Segregation of acute leptin and insulin effects in distinct populations of arcuate proopiomelanocortin neurons. J Neurosci 2010; 30(7): 2472-9.
[http://dx.doi.org/10.1523/JNEUROSCI.3118-09.2010] [PMID: 20164331]

[68] Berthoud HR. The neurobiology of food intake in an obesogenic environment. Proc Nutr Soc 2012; 71(4): 478-87.
[http://dx.doi.org/10.1017/S0029665112000602] [PMID: 22800810]

[69] Fernandez-Twinn DS, Ozanne SE. Early life nutrition and metabolic programming. Ann N Y Acad Sci 2010; 1212: 78-96.
[http://dx.doi.org/10.1111/j.1749-6632.2010.05798.x] [PMID: 21070247]

[70] Ross MG, Desai M. Developmental programming of offspring obesity, adipogenesis, and appetite. Clin Obstet Gynecol 2013; 56(3): 529-36.
[http://dx.doi.org/10.1097/GRF.0b013e318299c39d] [PMID: 23751877]

[71] Vickers MH. Developmental programming and transgenerational transmission of obesity. Ann Nutr Metab 2014; 64 (Suppl. 1): 26-34.
[http://dx.doi.org/10.1159/000360506] [PMID: 25059803]

[72] Gali Ramamoorthy T, Begum G, Harno E, White A. Developmental programming of hypothalamic neuronal circuits: impact on energy balance control. Front Neurosci 2015; 9: 126.
[http://dx.doi.org/10.3389/fnins.2015.00126] [PMID: 25954145]

[73] Waterland RA. Epigenetic mechanisms affecting regulation of energy balance: many questions, few answers. Annu Rev Nutr 2014; 34: 337-55.
[http://dx.doi.org/10.1146/annurev-nutr-071813-105315] [PMID: 24850387]

[74] Allard C, Desgagné V, Patenaude J, *et al*. Mendelian randomization supports causality between maternal hyperglycemia and epigenetic regulation of leptin gene in newborns. Epigenetics 2015; 10(4): 342-51.
[http://dx.doi.org/10.1080/15592294.2015.1029700] [PMID: 25800063]

[75] Godfrey KM, Sheppard A, Gluckman PD, *et al*. Epigenetic gene promoter methylation at birth is associated with childs later adiposity. Diabetes 2011; 60(5): 1528-34.
[http://dx.doi.org/10.2337/db10-0979] [PMID: 21471513]

[76] Lawlor DA, Relton C, Sattar N, Nelson SM. Maternal adiposity a determinant of perinatal and offspring outcomes? Nat Rev Endocrinol 2012; 8(11): 679-88.
[http://dx.doi.org/10.1038/nrendo.2012.176] [PMID: 23007319]

[77] Wajchenberg BL. Subcutaneous and visceral adipose tissue: their relation to the metabolic syndrome. Endocr Rev 2000; 21(6): 697-738.
[http://dx.doi.org/10.1210/edrv.21.6.0415] [PMID: 11133069]

[78] Walker GE, Marzullo P, Ricotti R, Bona G, Prodam F. The pathophysiology of abdominal adipose tissue depots in health and disease. Horm Mol Biol Clin Investig 2014; 19(1): 57-74.
[http://dx.doi.org/10.1515/hmbci-2014-0023] [PMID: 25390016]

[79] Harms M, Seale P. Brown and beige fat: development, function and therapeutic potential. Nat Med 2013; 19(10): 1252-63.
[http://dx.doi.org/10.1038/nm.3361] [PMID: 24100998]

[80] Giordano A, Smorlesi A, Frontini A, Barbatelli G, Cinti S. White, brown and pink adipocytes: the extraordinary plasticity of the adipose organ. Eur J Endocrinol 2014; 170(5): R159-71.
[http://dx.doi.org/10.1530/EJE-13-0945] [PMID: 24468979]

[81] Mraz M, Haluzik M. The role of adipose tissue immune cells in obesity and low-grade inflammation. J Endocrinol 2014; 222(3): R113-27.
[http://dx.doi.org/10.1530/JOE-14-0283] [PMID: 25006217]

[82] Grant RW, Dixit VD. Adipose tissue as an immunological organ. Obesity (Silver Spring) 2015; 23(3): 512-8.
[http://dx.doi.org/10.1002/oby.21003] [PMID: 25612251]

[83] Sinha R, Fisch G, Teague B, et al. Prevalence of impaired glucose tolerance among children and adolescents with marked obesity. N Engl J Med 2002; 346(11): 802-10.
[http://dx.doi.org/10.1056/NEJMoa012578] [PMID: 11893791]

[84] Vague J. The degree of masculine differentiation of obesities: a factor determining predisposition to diabetes, atherosclerosis, gout, and uric calculous disease. Am J Clin Nutr 1956; 4(1): 20-34.
[PMID: 13282851]

[85] Walker GE, Verti B, Marzullo P, Savia G, Mencarelli M, Zurleni F, et al. Deep sub-cutaneous adipose tissue (dSAT): A metabolically distinct abdominal adipose depot. Obesity (Silver Spring) 2007; 15: 1933-43.
[http://dx.doi.org/10.1038/oby.2007.231] [PMID: 17712110]

[86] Britton KA, Fox CS. Ectopic fat depots and cardiovascular disease. Circulation 2011; 124(24): e837-41.
[http://dx.doi.org/10.1161/CIRCULATIONAHA.111.077602] [PMID: 22156000]

[87] Smith SR, Lovejoy JC, Greenway F, et al. Contributions of total body fat, abdominal subcutaneous adipose tissue compartments, and visceral adipose tissue to the metabolic complications of obesity. Metabolism 2001; 50(4): 425-35.
[http://dx.doi.org/10.1053/meta.2001.21693] [PMID: 11288037]

[88] Shen W, Punyanitya M, Silva AM, et al. Sexual dimorphism of adipose tissue distribution across the lifespan: a cross-sectional whole-body magnetic resonance imaging study. Nutr Metab (Lond) 2009; 6: 17.
[http://dx.doi.org/10.1186/1743-7075-6-17] [PMID: 19371437]

[89] Hocking S, Samocha-Bonet D, Milner KL, Greenfield JR, Chisholm DJ. Adiposity and insulin resistance in humans: the role of the different tissue and cellular lipid depots. Endocr Rev 2013; 34(4): 463-500.
[http://dx.doi.org/10.1210/er.2012-1041] [PMID: 23550081]

[90] Golan R, Shelef I, Rudich A, et al. Abdominal superficial subcutaneous fat: a putative distinct protective fat subdepot in type 2 diabetes. Diabetes Care 2012; 35(3): 640-7.
[http://dx.doi.org/10.2337/dc11-1583] [PMID: 22344612]

[91] Virtue S, Vidal-Puig A. Its not how fat you are, its what you do with it that counts. PLoS Biol 2008; 6(9): e237.
[http://dx.doi.org/10.1371/journal.pbio.0060237] [PMID: 18816166]

[92] Gray SL, Vidal-Puig AJ. Adipose tissue expandability in the maintenance of metabolic homeostasis. Nutr Rev 2007; 65(6 Pt 2): S7-S12.
[http://dx.doi.org/10.1301/nr.2007.jun.S7-S12] [PMID: 17605308]

[93] Desai M, Beall M, Ross MG. Developmental origins of obesity: programmed adipogenesis. Curr Diab Rep 2013; 13(1): 27-33.
[http://dx.doi.org/10.1007/s11892-012-0344-x] [PMID: 23188593]

[94] Weiss R, Dufour S, Taksali SE, et al. Prediabetes in obese youth: a syndrome of impaired glucose tolerance, severe insulin resistance, and altered myocellular and abdominal fat partitioning. Lancet 2003; 362(9388): 951-7.
[http://dx.doi.org/10.1016/S0140-6736(03)14364-4] [PMID: 14511928]

[95] Larson-Meyer DE, Newcomer BR, Ravussin E, *et al.* Intrahepatic and intramyocellular lipids are determinants of insulin resistance in prepubertal children. Diabetologia 2011; 54(4): 869-75.
[http://dx.doi.org/10.1007/s00125-010-2022-3] [PMID: 21181394]

[96] Cinti S. The adipose organ. Milano: Editrice Kurtis s..r.l 1999.

[97] Spalding KL, Arner E, Westermark PO, *et al.* Dynamics of fat cell turnover in humans. Nature 2008; 453(7196): 783-7.
[http://dx.doi.org/10.1038/nature06902] [PMID: 18454136]

[98] Jo J, Gavrilova O, Pack S, *et al.* Hypertrophy and/or hyperplasia: dynamics of adipose tissue growth. PLOS Comput Biol 2009; 5(3): e1000324.
[http://dx.doi.org/10.1371/journal.pcbi.1000324] [PMID: 19325873]

[99] Faust IM, Johnson PR, Stern JS, Hirsch J. Diet-induced adipocyte number increase in adult rats: a new model of obesity. Am J Physiol 1978; 235(3): E279-86.
[PMID: 696822]

[100] Plum L, Rother E, Münzberg H, *et al.* Enhanced leptin-stimulated Pi3k activation in the CNS promotes white adipose tissue transdifferentiation. Cell Metab 2007; 6(6): 431-45.
[http://dx.doi.org/10.1016/j.cmet.2007.10.012] [PMID: 18054313]

[101] Barbatelli G, Murano I, Madsen L, *et al.* The emergence of cold-induced brown adipocytes in mouse white fat depots is determined predominantly by white to brown adipocyte transdifferentiation. Am J Physiol Endocrinol Metab 2010; 298(6): E1244-53.
[http://dx.doi.org/10.1152/ajpendo.00600.2009] [PMID: 20354155]

[102] Himms-Hagen J, Cui J, Danforth E Jr, *et al.* Effect of CL-316,243, a thermogenic beta 3-agonist, on energy balance and brown and white adipose tissues in rats. Am J Physiol 1994; 266: R1371-82.
[PMID: 7910436]

[103] Bi S, Li L. Browning of white adipose tissue: role of hypothalamic signaling. Ann N Y Acad Sci 2013; 1302: 30-4.
[http://dx.doi.org/10.1111/nyas.12258] [PMID: 23980536]

[104] Rockstroh D, Landgraf K, Wagner IV, *et al.* Direct evidence of brown adipocytes in different fat depots in children. PLoS One 2015; 10(2): e0117841.
[http://dx.doi.org/10.1371/journal.pone.0117841] [PMID: 25706927]

[105] Kopecký J, Hodný Z, Rossmeisl M, Syrový I, Kozak LP. Reduction of dietary obesity in aP2-Ucp transgenic mice: physiology and adipose tissue distribution. Am J Physiol 1996; 270(5 Pt 1): E768-75.
[PMID: 8967464]

[106] Collins S, Daniel KW, Petro AE, Surwit RS. Strain-specific response to beta 3-adrenergic receptor agonist treatment of diet-induced obesity in mice. Endocrinology 1997; 138(1): 405-13.
[PMID: 8977430]

[107] Ghorbani M, Claus TH, Himms-Hagen J. Hypertrophy of brown adipocytes in brown and white adipose tissues and reversal of diet-induced obesity in rats treated with a beta3-adrenoceptor agonist. Biochem Pharmacol 1997; 54(1): 121-31.
[http://dx.doi.org/10.1016/S0006-2952(97)00162-7] [PMID: 9296358]

[108] Ninomiya Y, Davies TJ, Gardner RL. Experimental analysis of the transdifferentiation of visceral to parietal endoderm in the mouse. Dev Dyn 2005; 233(3): 837-46.
[http://dx.doi.org/10.1002/dvdy.20405] [PMID: 15880460]

[109] Cypess AM, Kahn CR. Brown fat as a therapy for obesity and diabetes. Curr Opin Endocrinol Diabetes Obes 2010; 17(2): 143-9.
[http://dx.doi.org/10.1097/MED.0b013e328337a81f] [PMID: 20160646]

[110] An integrated encyclopedia of DNA elements in the human genome. Nature 2012; 489(7414): 57-74.
[http://dx.doi.org/10.1038/nature11247] [PMID: 22955616]

[111] Lu CT, Huang KY, Su MG, *et al.* DbPTM 3.0: an informative resource for investigating substrate site specificity and functional association of protein post-translational modifications. Nucleic Acids Res 2013; 41(Database issue): D295-305.
[http://dx.doi.org/10.1093/nar/gks1229] [PMID: 23193290]

[112] Wittmann-Liebold B, Graack HR, Pohl T. Two-dimensional gel electrophoresis as tool for proteomics studies in combination with protein identification by mass spectrometry. Proteomics 2006; 6(17): 4688-703.
[http://dx.doi.org/10.1002/pmic.200500874] [PMID: 16933336]

[113] Rogowska-Wrzesinska A, Le Bihan MC, Thaysen-Andersen M, Roepstorff P. 2D gels still have a niche in proteomics. J Proteomics 2013; 88: 4-13.
[http://dx.doi.org/10.1016/j.jprot.2013.01.010] [PMID: 23353020]

[114] Oliveira BM, Coorssen JR, Martins-de-Souza D. 2DE: the phoenix of proteomics. J Proteomics 2014; 104: 140-50.
[http://dx.doi.org/10.1016/j.jprot.2014.03.035] [PMID: 24704856]

[115] Chen G, Pramanik BN. Application of LC/MS to proteomics studies: current status and future prospects. Drug Discov Today 2009; 14(9-10): 465-71.
[http://dx.doi.org/10.1016/j.drudis.2009.02.007] [PMID: 19429505]

[116] Holčapek M, Jirásko R, Lísa M. Recent developments in liquid chromatography-mass spectrometry and related techniques. J Chromatogr A 2012; 1259: 3-15.
[http://dx.doi.org/10.1016/j.chroma.2012.08.072] [PMID: 22959775]

[117] Gallien S, Duriez E, Demeure K, Domon B. Selectivity of LC-MS/MS analysis: implication for proteomics experiments. J Proteomics 2013; 81: 148-58.
[http://dx.doi.org/10.1016/j.jprot.2012.11.005] [PMID: 23159602]

[118] Lueking A, Cahill DJ, Müllner S. Protein biochips: A new and versatile platform technology for molecular medicine. Drug Discov Today 2005; 10(11): 789-94.
[http://dx.doi.org/10.1016/S1359-6446(05)03449-5] [PMID: 15922937]

[119] Gahoi N, Ray S, Srivastava S. Array-based proteomic approaches to study signal transduction pathways: prospects, merits and challenges. Proteomics 2015; 15(2-3): 218-31.
[http://dx.doi.org/10.1002/pmic.201400261] [PMID: 25266292]

[120] Dunn MJ, Corbett JM. Two-dimensional polyacrylamide gel electrophoresis. Methods Enzymol 1996; 271: 177-203.
[http://dx.doi.org/10.1016/S0076-6879(96)71010-8] [PMID: 8782554]

[121] Görg A, Weiss W, Dunn MJ. Current two-dimensional electrophoresis technology for proteomics. Proteomics 2004; 4(12): 3665-85.
[http://dx.doi.org/10.1002/pmic.200401031] [PMID: 15543535]

[122] Carrette O, Burkhard PR, Sanchez JC, Hochstrasser DF. State-of-the-art two-dimensional gel electrophoresis: a key tool of proteomics research. Nat Protoc 2006; 1(2): 812-23.
[http://dx.doi.org/10.1038/nprot.2006.104] [PMID: 17406312]

[123] Vercauteren FG, Arckens L, Quirion R. Applications and current challenges of proteomic approaches, focusing on two-dimensional electrophoresis. Amino Acids 2007; 33(3): 405-14.
[http://dx.doi.org/10.1007/s00726-006-0460-5] [PMID: 17136510]

[124] Issaq H, Veenstra T. Two-dimensional polyacrylamide gel electrophoresis (2D-PAGE): advances and perspectives. Biotechniques 2008; 44(5): 697-698, 700.
[http://dx.doi.org/10.2144/000112823] [PMID: 18474047]

[125] Slibinskas R, Ražanskas R, Zinkevičiūtė R, Čiplys E. Comparison of first dimension IPG and NEPHGE techniques in two-dimensional gel electrophoresis experiment with cytosolic unfolded protein response in Saccharomyces cerevisiae. Proteome Sci 2013; 11(1): 36.
[http://dx.doi.org/10.1186/1477-5956-11-36] [PMID: 23889826]

[126] Neuhoff V, Arold N, Taube D, Ehrhardt W. Improved staining of proteins in polyacrylamide gels including isoelectric focusing gels with clear background at nanogram sensitivity using Coomassie Brilliant Blue G-250 and R-250. Electrophoresis 1988; 9(6): 255-62.
[http://dx.doi.org/10.1002/elps.1150090603] [PMID: 2466658]

[127] Chevallet M, Luche S, Rabilloud T. Silver staining of proteins in polyacrylamide gels. Nat Protoc 2006; 1(4): 1852-8.
[http://dx.doi.org/10.1038/nprot.2006.288] [PMID: 17487168]

[128] Patton WF. A thousand points of light: the application of fluorescence detection technologies to two-dimensional gel electrophoresis and proteomics. Electrophoresis 2000; 21(6): 1123-44.
[http://dx.doi.org/10.1002/(SICI)1522-2683(20000401)21:6<1123::AID-ELPS1123>3.0.CO;2-E] [PMID: 10786886]

[129] Tannu NS, Hemby SE. Two-dimensional fluorescence difference gel electrophoresis for comparative proteomics profiling. Nat Protoc 2006; 1(4): 1732-42.
[http://dx.doi.org/10.1038/nprot.2006.256] [PMID: 17487156]

[130] Panchaud A, Affolter M, Moreillon P, Kussmann M. Experimental and computational approaches to quantitative proteomics: status quo and outlook. J Proteomics 2008; 71(1): 19-33.
[http://dx.doi.org/10.1016/j.jprot.2007.12.001] [PMID: 18541471]

[131] Fenn JB, Mann M, Meng CK, Wong SF, Whitehouse CM. Electrospray ionization for mass spectrometry of large biomolecules. Science 1989; 246(4926): 64-71.
[http://dx.doi.org/10.1126/science.2675315] [PMID: 2675315]

[132] Hillenkamp F, Karas M. Mass spectrometry of peptides and proteins by matrix-assisted ultraviolet laser desorption/ionization. Methods Enzymol 1990; 193: 280-95.
[http://dx.doi.org/10.1016/0076-6879(90)93420-P] [PMID: 1963669]

[133] James P, Quadroni M, Carafoli E, Gonnet G. Protein identification by mass profile fingerprinting. Biochem Biophys Res Commun 1993; 195(1): 58-64.
[http://dx.doi.org/10.1006/bbrc.1993.2009] [PMID: 8363627]

[134] Mann M, Højrup P, Roepstorff P. Use of mass spectrometric molecular weight information to identify proteins in sequence databases. Biol Mass Spectrom 1993; 22(6): 338-45.
[http://dx.doi.org/10.1002/bms.1200220605] [PMID: 8329463]

[135] Pappin DJ, Hojrup P, Bleasby AJ. Rapid identification of proteins by peptide-mass fingerprinting. Curr Biol 1993; 3(6): 327-32.
[http://dx.doi.org/10.1016/0960-9822(93)90195-T] [PMID: 15335725]

[136] Henzel WJ, Billeci TM, Stults JT, Wong SC, Grimley C, Watanabe C. Identifying proteins from two-dimensional gels by molecular mass searching of peptide fragments in protein sequence databases. Proc Natl Acad Sci USA 1993; 90(11): 5011-5.
[http://dx.doi.org/10.1073/pnas.90.11.5011] [PMID: 8506346]

[137] Mann M, Wilm M. Error-tolerant identification of peptides in sequence databases by peptide sequence tags. Anal Chem 1994; 66(24): 4390-9.
[http://dx.doi.org/10.1021/ac00096a002] [PMID: 7847635]

[138] McDonald WH, Yates JR III. Shotgun proteomics and biomarker discovery. Dis Markers 2002; 18(2): 99-105.
[http://dx.doi.org/10.1155/2002/505397] [PMID: 12364816]

[139] Righetti PG, Castagna A, Herbert B, Candiano G. How to bring the unseen proteome to the limelight via electrophoretic pre-fractionation techniques. Biosci Rep 2005; 25(1-2): 3-17.
[http://dx.doi.org/10.1007/s10540-005-2844-2] [PMID: 16222416]

[140] Hu Q, Noll RJ, Li H, Makarov A, Hardman M, Graham Cooks R. The Orbitrap: a new mass spectrometer. J Mass Spectrom 2005; 40(4): 430-43.
[http://dx.doi.org/10.1002/jms.856] [PMID: 15838939]

[141] Schwartz JC, Senko MW, Syka JE. A two-dimensional quadrupole ion trap mass spectrometer. J Am Soc Mass Spectrom 2002; 13(6): 659-69.
[http://dx.doi.org/10.1016/S1044-0305(02)00384-7] [PMID: 12056566]

[142] Bogdanov B, Smith RD. Proteomics by FTICR mass spectrometry: top down and bottom up. Mass Spectrom Rev 2005; 24(2): 168-200.
[http://dx.doi.org/10.1002/mas.20015] [PMID: 15389855]

[143] Mann M. Functional and quantitative proteomics using SILAC. Nat Rev Mol Cell Biol 2006; 7(12): 952-8.
[http://dx.doi.org/10.1038/nrm2067] [PMID: 17139335]

[144] Chahrour O, Cobice D, Malone J. Stable isotope labelling methods in mass spectrometry-based quantitative proteomics. J Pharm Biomed Anal 2015; 113: 2-20.
[http://dx.doi.org/10.1016/j.jpba.2015.04.013] [PMID: 25956803]

[145] Gygi SP, Rist B, Gerber SA, Turecek F, Gelb MH, Aebersold R. Quantitative analysis of complex protein mixtures using isotope-coded affinity tags. Nat Biotechnol 1999; 17(10): 994-9.
[http://dx.doi.org/10.1038/13690] [PMID: 10504701]

[146] Aggarwal K, Choe LH, Lee KH. Shotgun proteomics using the iTRAQ isobaric tags. Brief Funct Genomics Proteomics 2006; 5(2): 112-20.
[http://dx.doi.org/10.1093/bfgp/ell018] [PMID: 16772272]

[147] Ge Y, Lawhorn BG, ElNaggar M, et al. Top down characterization of larger proteins (45 kDa) by electron capture dissociation mass spectrometry. J Am Chem Soc 2002; 124(4): 672-8.
[http://dx.doi.org/10.1021/ja011335z] [PMID: 11804498]

[148] Ntai I, Kim K, Fellers RT, et al. Applying label-free quantitation to top down proteomics. Anal Chem 2014; 86(10): 4961-8.
[http://dx.doi.org/10.1021/ac500395k] [PMID: 24807621]

[149] Moradian A, Kalli A, Sweredoski MJ, Hess S. The top-down, middle-down, and bottom-up mass spectrometry approaches for characterization of histone variants and their post-translational modifications. Proteomics 2014; 14(4-5): 489-97.
[http://dx.doi.org/10.1002/pmic.201300256] [PMID: 24339419]

[150] Hennrich ML, Gavin AC. Quantitative mass spectrometry of posttranslational modifications: keys to confidence. Sci Signal 2015; 8(371): re5.
[http://dx.doi.org/10.1126/scisignal.aaa6466] [PMID: 25852188]

[151] Butte A. The use and analysis of microarray data. Nat Rev Drug Discov 2002; 1(12): 951-60.
[http://dx.doi.org/10.1038/nrd961] [PMID: 12461517]

[152] Haddon RC, Lamola AA. The molecular electronic device and the biochip computer: present status. Proc Natl Acad Sci USA 1985; 82(7): 1874-8.
[http://dx.doi.org/10.1073/pnas.82.7.1874] [PMID: 3856865]

[153] Xiao Z, Adam BL, Cazares LH, et al. Quantitation of serum prostate-specific membrane antigen by a novel protein biochip immunoassay discriminates benign from malignant prostate disease. Cancer Res 2001; 61(16): 6029-33.
[PMID: 11507047]

[154] Wang CC. Protein array-based multiplexed cytokine assays. Methods Mol Biol 2007; 385: 177-92.
[http://dx.doi.org/10.1007/978-1-59745-426-1_13] [PMID: 18365712]

[155] Kuang Z, Wilson JJ, Luo S, Zhu SW, Huang RP. Deciphering asthma biomarkers with protein profiling technology. Int J Inflam 2015; 2015: 630637.
[http://dx.doi.org/10.1155/2015/630637]

[156] Tampoia M, Zucano A, Villalta D, Antico A, Bizzaro N. Anti-skin specific autoantibodies detected by a new immunofluorescence multiplex biochip method in patients with autoimmune bullous diseases.

Dermatology 2012; 225(1): 37-44.
[http://dx.doi.org/10.1159/000339776] [PMID: 22907099]

[157] Stich N, van Steen G, Schalkhammer T. Design and peptide-based validation of phage display antibodies for proteomic biochips. Comb Chem High Throughput Screen 2003; 6(1): 67-78.
[http://dx.doi.org/10.2174/1386207033329841] [PMID: 12570753]

[158] Guijarro C, Fuchs K, Bohrn U, Stütz E, Wölfl S. Simultaneous detection of multiple bioactive pollutants using a multiparametric biochip for water quality monitoring. Biosens Bioelectron 2015; 72: 71-9.
[http://dx.doi.org/10.1016/j.bios.2015.04.092] [PMID: 25957833]

[159] Brunner C, Hoffmann K, Thiele T, Schedler U, Jehle H, Resch-Genger U. Novel calibration tools and validation concepts for microarray-based platforms used in molecular diagnostics and food safety control. Anal Bioanal Chem 2015; 407(11): 3181-91.
[http://dx.doi.org/10.1007/s00216-014-8450-z] [PMID: 25616702]

[160] Chan SM, Ermann J, Su L, Fathman CG, Utz PJ. Protein microarrays for multiplex analysis of signal transduction pathways. Nat Med 2004; 10(12): 1390-6.
[http://dx.doi.org/10.1038/nm1139] [PMID: 15558056]

[161] Boellner S, Becker KF. Recent progress in protein profiling of clinical tissues for next-generation molecular diagnostics. Expert Rev Mol Diagn 2015; 15(10): 1277-92.
[http://dx.doi.org/10.1586/14737159.2015.1070098] [PMID: 26211480]

[162] Creighton CJ, Huang S. Reverse phase protein arrays in signaling pathways: a data integration perspective. Drug Des Devel Ther 2015; 9: 3519-27.
[PMID: 26185419]

[163] Sidhu RS. Two-dimensional electrophoretic analyses of proteins synthesized during differentiation of 3T3-L1 preadipocytes. J Biol Chem 1979; 254(21): 11111-8.
[PMID: 500628]

[164] Lanne B, Potthast F, Höglund A, et al. Thiourea enhances mapping of the proteome from murine white adipose tissue. Proteomics 2001; 1(7): 819-28.
[http://dx.doi.org/10.1002/1615-9861(200107)1:7<819::AID-PROT819>3.0.CO;2-V] [PMID: 11503206]

[165] Sanchez JC, Chiappe D, Converset V, et al. The mouse SWISS-2D PAGE database: a tool for proteomics study of diabetes and obesity. Proteomics 2001; 1(1): 136-63.
[http://dx.doi.org/10.1002/1615-9861(200101)1:1<136::AID-PROT136>3.0.CO;2-1] [PMID: 11680894]

[166] Frizzell N, Rajesh M, Jepson MJ, et al. Succination of thiol groups in adipose tissue proteins in diabetes: succination inhibits polymerization and secretion of adiponectin. J Biol Chem 2009; 284(38): 25772-81.
[http://dx.doi.org/10.1074/jbc.M109.019257] [PMID: 19592500]

[167] Parray HA, Yun JW. Proteomic identification of target proteins of thiodigalactoside in white adipose tissue from diet-induced obese rats. Int J Mol Sci 2015; 16(7): 14441-63.
[http://dx.doi.org/10.3390/ijms160714441] [PMID: 26121299]

[168] Cortón M, Villuendas G, Botella JI, San Millán JL, Escobar-Morreale HF, Peral B. Improved resolution of the human adipose tissue proteome at alkaline and wide range pH by the addition of hydroxyethyl disulfide. Proteomics 2004; 4(2): 438-41.
[http://dx.doi.org/10.1002/pmic.200300644] [PMID: 14760714]

[169] Cortón M, Botella-Carretero JI, López JA, et al. Proteomic analysis of human omental adipose tissue in the polycystic ovary syndrome using two-dimensional difference gel electrophoresis and mass spectrometry. Hum Reprod 2008; 23(3): 651-61.
[http://dx.doi.org/10.1093/humrep/dem380] [PMID: 18156650]

[170] Jowsey IR, Smith SA, Hayes JD. Expression of the murine glutathione S-transferase alpha3 (GSTA3) subunit is markedly induced during adipocyte differentiation: activation of the GSTA3 gene promoter by the pro-adipogenic eicosanoid 15-deoxy-Delta12,14-prostaglandin J2. Biochem Biophys Res Commun 2003; 312(4): 1226-35.
[http://dx.doi.org/10.1016/j.bbrc.2003.11.068] [PMID: 14652005]

[171] Mooradian AD, Haas MJ, Wong NC. The effect of select nutrients on serum high-density lipoprotein cholesterol and apolipoprotein A-I levels. Endocr Rev 2006; 27(1): 2-16.
[http://dx.doi.org/10.1210/er.2005-0013] [PMID: 16243964]

[172] Christensen SB, Black MH, Smith N, et al. Prevalence of polycystic ovary syndrome in adolescents. Fertil Steril 2013; 100(2): 470-7.
[http://dx.doi.org/10.1016/j.fertnstert.2013.04.001] [PMID: 23756098]

[173] Yin Q, Chen X, Li L, Zhou R, Huang J, Yang D. Apolipoprotein B/apolipoprotein A1 ratio is a good predictive marker of metabolic syndrome and pre-metabolic syndrome in Chinese adolescent women with polycystic ovary syndrome. J Obstet Gynaecol Res 2013; 39(1): 203-9.
[http://dx.doi.org/10.1111/j.1447-0756.2012.01907.x] [PMID: 22672648]

[174] Stoekenbroek RM, Stroes ES, Hovingh GK. ApoA-I mimetics. Handbook Exp Pharmacol 2015; 224: 631-48.
[http://dx.doi.org/10.1007/978-3-319-09665-0_21] [PMID: 25523005]

[175] Xie X, Yi Z, Bowen B, et al. Characterization of the human adipocyte proteome and reproducibility of protein abundance by one-dimensional gel electrophoresis and HPLC-ESI-MS/MS. J Proteome Res 2010; 9(9): 4521-34.
[http://dx.doi.org/10.1021/pr100268f] [PMID: 20812759]

[176] De Pauw A, Tejerina S, Raes M, Keijer J, Arnould T. Mitochondrial (dys)function in adipocyte (de)differentiation and systemic metabolic alterations. Am J Pathol 2009; 175(3): 927-39.
[http://dx.doi.org/10.2353/ajpath.2009.081155] [PMID: 19700756]

[177] Frohnert BI, Sinaiko AR, Serrot FJ, et al. Increased adipose protein carbonylation in human obesity. Obesity (Silver Spring) 2011; 19(9): 1735-41.
[http://dx.doi.org/10.1038/oby.2011.115] [PMID: 21593812]

[178] Furuhashi M, Tuncman G, Görgün CZ, et al. Treatment of diabetes and atherosclerosis by inhibiting fatty-acid-binding protein aP2. Nature 2007; 447(7147): 959-65.
[http://dx.doi.org/10.1038/nature05844] [PMID: 17554340]

[179] Furuhashi M, Fucho R, Görgün CZ, Tuncman G, Cao H, Hotamisligil GS. Adipocyte/macrophage fatty acid-binding proteins contribute to metabolic deterioration through actions in both macrophages and adipocytes in mice. J Clin Invest 2008; 118(7): 2640-50.
[PMID: 18551191]

[180] Siahanidou T, Margeli A, Davradou M, et al. Circulating adipocyte fatty acid binding protein levels in healthy preterm infants: Positive correlation with weight gain and total-cholesterol levels. Early Hum Dev 2010; 86(4): 197-201.
[http://dx.doi.org/10.1016/j.earlhumdev.2010.02.008] [PMID: 20231079]

[181] Choi KM, Yannakoulia M, Park MS, et al. Serum adipocyte fatty acid-binding protein, retinol-binding protein 4, and adiponectin concentrations in relation to the development of the metabolic syndrome in Korean boys: a 3-y prospective cohort study. Am J Clin Nutr 2011; 93(1): 19-26.
[http://dx.doi.org/10.3945/ajcn.2010.29667] [PMID: 21106915]

[182] Hotamisligil GS, Johnson RS, Distel RJ, Ellis R, Papaioannou VE, Spiegelman BM. Uncoupling of obesity from insulin resistance through a targeted mutation in aP2, the adipocyte fatty acid binding protein. Science 1996; 274(5291): 1377-9.
[http://dx.doi.org/10.1126/science.274.5291.1377] [PMID: 8910278]

[183] Wu LE, Samocha-Bonet D, Whitworth PT, *et al.* Identification of fatty acid binding protein 4 as an adipokine that regulates insulin secretion during obesity. Mol Metab 2014; 3(4): 465-73.
[http://dx.doi.org/10.1016/j.molmet.2014.02.005] [PMID: 24944906]

[184] Furuhashi M, Hiramitsu S, Mita T, Fuseya T, Ishimura S, Omori A, *et al.* Reduction of serum concentration of FABP4 by sitagliptin, a dipeptidyl peptidase-4 inhibitor, in patients with type 2 diabetes mellitus. J Lipid Res. 2015; pii: jlr.M059469.

[185] Urakami T, Kuwabara R, Habu M, *et al.* Pharmacologic treatment strategies in children with type 2 diabetes mellitus. Clin Pediatr Endocrinol 2013; 22(1): 1-8.
[http://dx.doi.org/10.1297/cpe.22.1] [PMID: 23966754]

[186] Staiano AE, Katzmarzyk PT. Ethnic and sex differences in body fat and visceral and subcutaneous adiposity in children and adolescents. Int J Obes 2012; 36(10): 1261-9.
[http://dx.doi.org/10.1038/ijo.2012.95] [PMID: 22710928]

[187] Gyllenhammer LE, Alderete TL, Toledo-Corral CM, Weigensberg M, Goran MI. Saturation of subcutaneous adipose tissue expansion and accumulation of ectopic fat associated with metabolic dysfunction during late and post-pubertal growth. Int J Obes 2016; 40(4): 601-6.
[http://dx.doi.org/10.1038/ijo.2015.207] [PMID: 26443340]

[188] He F, Rodriguez-Colon S, Fernandez-Mendoza J, *et al.* Abdominal obesity and metabolic syndrome burden in adolescents--Penn State Children Cohort study. J Clin Densitom 2015; 18(1): 30-6.
[http://dx.doi.org/10.1016/j.jocd.2014.07.009] [PMID: 25220887]

[189] Pérez-Pérez R, Ortega-Delgado FJ, García-Santos E, *et al.* Differential proteomics of omental and subcutaneous adipose tissue reflects their unalike biochemical and metabolic properties. J Proteome Res 2009; 8(4): 1682-93.
[http://dx.doi.org/10.1021/pr800942k] [PMID: 19714809]

[190] Insenser M, Montes-Nieto R, Vilarrasa N, *et al.* A nontargeted proteomic approach to the study of visceral and subcutaneous adipose tissue in human obesity. Mol Cell Endocrinol 2012; 363(1-2): 10-9.
[http://dx.doi.org/10.1016/j.mce.2012.07.001] [PMID: 22796336]

[191] Salgado-Somoza A, Teijeira-Fernández E, Fernández AL, González-Juanatey JR, Eiras S. Proteomic analysis of epicardial and subcutaneous adipose tissue reveals differences in proteins involved in oxidative stress. Am J Physiol Heart Circ Physiol 2010; 299(1): H202-9.
[http://dx.doi.org/10.1152/ajpheart.00120.2010] [PMID: 20435850]

[192] Peinado JR, Jimenez-Gomez Y, Pulido MR, *et al.* The stromal-vascular fraction of adipose tissue contributes to major differences between subcutaneous and visceral fat depots. Proteomics 2010; 10(18): 3356-66.
[http://dx.doi.org/10.1002/pmic.201000350] [PMID: 20706982]

[193] Walker GE, Marzullo P, Verti B, *et al.* Subcutaneous abdominal adipose tissue subcompartments: potential role in rosiglitazone effects. Obesity (Silver Spring) 2008; 16(9): 1983-91.
[http://dx.doi.org/10.1038/oby.2008.326] [PMID: 19186324]

[194] Young JC, Agashe VR, Siegers K, Hartl FU. Pathways of chaperone-mediated protein folding in the cytosol. Nat Rev Mol Cell Biol 2004; 5(10): 781-91.
[http://dx.doi.org/10.1038/nrm1492] [PMID: 15459659]

[195] Marcu MG, Doyle M, Bertolotti A, Ron D, Hendershot L, Neckers L. Heat shock protein 90 modulates the unfolded protein response by stabilizing IRE1alpha. Mol Cell Biol 2002; 22(24): 8506-13.
[http://dx.doi.org/10.1128/MCB.22.24.8506-8513.2002] [PMID: 12446770]

[196] Jiang Q, Wang Y, Li T, *et al.* Heat shock protein 90-mediated inactivation of nuclear factor-κB switches autophagy to apoptosis through becn1 transcriptional inhibition in selenite-induced NB4 cells. Mol Biol Cell 2011; 22(8): 1167-80.
[http://dx.doi.org/10.1091/mbc.E10-10-0860] [PMID: 21346199]

[197] Nguyen MT, Csermely P, Sőti C. Hsp90 chaperones PPARγ and regulates differentiation and survival of 3T3-L1 adipocytes. Cell Death Differ 2013; 20(12): 1654-63.
[http://dx.doi.org/10.1038/cdd.2013.129] [PMID: 24096869]

[198] Chouchane L, Danguir J, Beji C, *et al.* Genetic variation in the stress protein hsp702 gene is highly associated with obesity. Int J Obes Relat Metab Disord 2001; 25(4): 462-6.
[http://dx.doi.org/10.1038/sj.ijo.0801545] [PMID: 11319647]

[199] Islam A, Hait SH, Andrews-Shigaki B, Carus S, Deuster PA. Plasma HSP70 levels correlate with health risk factors and insulin resistance in African American subjects. Exp Clin Endocrinol Diabetes 2014; 122(8): 496-501.
[http://dx.doi.org/10.1055/s-0034-1374636] [PMID: 24841720]

[200] Rayner K, Chen YX, Siebert T, OBrien ER. Heat shock protein 27: clue to understanding estrogen-mediated atheroprotection? Trends Cardiovasc Med 2010; 20(2): 54-8.
[http://dx.doi.org/10.1016/j.tcm.2010.03.008] [PMID: 20656216]

[201] Henstridge DC, Whitham M, Febbraio MA. Chaperoning to the metabolic party: The emerging therapeutic role of heat-shock proteins in obesity and type 2 diabetes. Mol Metab 2014; 3(8): 781-93.
[http://dx.doi.org/10.1016/j.molmet.2014.08.003] [PMID: 25379403]

[202] He Y, Li Y, Zhang S, *et al.* Radicicol, a heat shock protein 90 inhibitor, inhibits differentiation and adipogenesis in 3T3-L1 preadipocytes. Biochem Biophys Res Commun 2013; 436(2): 169-74.
[http://dx.doi.org/10.1016/j.bbrc.2013.05.068] [PMID: 23727383]

[203] Desarzens S, Liao WH, Mammi C, Caprio M, Faresse N. Hsp90 blockers inhibit adipocyte differentiation and fat mass accumulation. PLoS One 2014; 9(4): e94127.
[http://dx.doi.org/10.1371/journal.pone.0094127] [PMID: 24705830]

[204] Seo YH. Organelle-specific Hsp90 inhibitors. Arch Pharm Res 2015; 38(9): 1582-90.
[http://dx.doi.org/10.1007/s12272-015-0636-1] [PMID: 26195286]

[205] Aghazadeh Y, Papadopoulos V. The role of the 1433 protein family in health, disease, and drug development. Drug Discov Today 2016; 21(2): 278-87.
[http://dx.doi.org/10.1016/j.drudis.2015.09.012] [PMID: 26456530]

[206] Ramm G, Larance M, Guilhaus M, James DE. A role for 1433 in insulin-stimulated GLUT4 translocation through its interaction with the RabGAP AS160. J Biol Chem 2006; 281(39): 29174-80.
[http://dx.doi.org/10.1074/jbc.M603274200] [PMID: 16880201]

[207] Joo JI, Oh TS, Kim DH, *et al.* Differential expression of adipose tissue proteins between obesity-susceptible and -resistant rats fed a high-fat diet. Proteomics 2011; 11(8): 1429-48.
[http://dx.doi.org/10.1002/pmic.201000515] [PMID: 21365757]

[208] Chen XQ, Yu AC. The association of 1433gamma and actin plays a role in cell division and apoptosis in astrocytes. Biochem Biophys Res Commun 2002; 296(3): 657-63.
[http://dx.doi.org/10.1016/S0006-291X(02)00895-1] [PMID: 12176032]

[209] Lee JH, Lu H. 1433Gamma inhibition of MDMX-mediated p21 turnover independent of p53. J Biol Chem 2011; 286(7): 5136-42.
[http://dx.doi.org/10.1074/jbc.M110.190470] [PMID: 21148311]

[210] Miyamoto T, Kitamura N, Ono M, *et al.* Identification of 1433γ as a Mieap-interacting protein and its role in mitochondrial quality control. Sci Rep 2012; 2: 379.
[http://dx.doi.org/10.1038/srep00379] [PMID: 22532927]

[211] Ottmann C. Small-molecule modulators of 1433 protein-protein interactions. Bioorg Med Chem 2013; 21(14): 4058-62.
[http://dx.doi.org/10.1016/j.bmc.2012.11.028] [PMID: 23266179]

[212] An SS, Askovich PS, Zarembinski TI, *et al.* A novel small molecule target in human airway smooth muscle for potential treatment of obstructive lung diseases: a staged high-throughput biophysical

screening. Respir Res 2011; 12: 8.
[http://dx.doi.org/10.1186/1465-9921-12-8] [PMID: 21232113]

[213] Boden G, Duan X, Homko C, et al. Increase in endoplasmic reticulum stress-related proteins and genes in adipose tissue of obese, insulin-resistant individuals. Diabetes 2008; 57(9): 2438-44.
[http://dx.doi.org/10.2337/db08-0604] [PMID: 18567819]

[214] Murri M, Insenser M, Bernal-Lopez MR, Perez-Martinez P, Escobar-Morreale HF, Tinahones FJ. Proteomic analysis of visceral adipose tissue in pre-obese patients with type 2 diabetes. Mol Cell Endocrinol 2013; 376(1-2): 99-106.
[http://dx.doi.org/10.1016/j.mce.2013.06.010] [PMID: 23791845]

[215] Kim SJ, Chae S, Kim H, et al. A protein profile of visceral adipose tissues linked to early pathogenesis of type 2 diabetes mellitus. Mol Cell Proteomics 2014; 13(3): 811-22.
[http://dx.doi.org/10.1074/mcp.M113.035501] [PMID: 24403596]

[216] Fang L, Kojima K, Zhou L, Crossman DK, Mobley JA, Grams J. Analysis of the human proteome in subcutaneous and visceral fat depots in diabetic and non-diabetic patients with morbid obesity. J Proteomics Bioinform 2015; 8(6): 133-41.
[PMID: 26472921]

[217] Fain JN, Madan AK, Hiler ML, Cheema P, Bahouth SW. Comparison of the release of adipokines by adipose tissue, adipose tissue matrix, and adipocytes from visceral and subcutaneous abdominal adipose tissues of obese humans. Endocrinology 2004; 145(5): 2273-82.
[http://dx.doi.org/10.1210/en.2003-1336] [PMID: 14726444]

[218] Goulding NJ, Godolphin JL, Sharland PR, et al. Anti-inflammatory lipocortin 1 production by peripheral blood leucocytes in response to hydrocortisone. Lancet 1990; 335(8703): 1416-8.
[http://dx.doi.org/10.1016/0140-6736(90)91445-G] [PMID: 1972208]

[219] DAcquisto F, Perretti M, Flower RJ. Annexin-A1: a pivotal regulator of the innate and adaptive immune systems. Br J Pharmacol 2008; 155(2): 152-69.
[http://dx.doi.org/10.1038/bjp.2008.252] [PMID: 18641677]

[220] Pupjalis D, Goetsch J, Kottas DJ, Gerke V, Rescher U. Annexin A1 released from apoptotic cells acts through formyl peptide receptors to dampen inflammatory monocyte activation via JAK/STAT/SOCS signalling. EMBO Mol Med 2011; 3(2): 102-14.
[http://dx.doi.org/10.1002/emmm.201000113] [PMID: 21254404]

[221] Dalli J, Rosignoli G, Hayhoe RP, Edelman A, Perretti M. CFTR inhibition provokes an inflammatory response associated with an imbalance of the annexin A1 pathway. Am J Pathol 2010; 177(1): 176-86.
[http://dx.doi.org/10.2353/ajpath.2010.091149] [PMID: 20489160]

[222] Yang YH, Song W, Deane JA, et al. Deficiency of annexin A1 in CD4+ T cells exacerbates T cell-dependent inflammation. J Immunol 2013; 190(3): 997-1007.
[http://dx.doi.org/10.4049/jimmunol.1202236] [PMID: 23267026]

[223] Akasheh RT, Pini M, Pang J, Fantuzzi G. Increased adiposity in annexin A1-deficient mice. PLoS One 2013; 8(12): e82608.
[http://dx.doi.org/10.1371/journal.pone.0082608] [PMID: 24312665]

[224] Kosicka A, Cunliffe AD, Mackenzie R, et al. Attenuation of plasma annexin A1 in human obesity. FASEB J 2013; 27(1): 368-78.
[http://dx.doi.org/10.1096/fj.12-213728] [PMID: 23038751]

[225] Hong SH, Won JH, Yoo SA, Auh CK, Park YM. Effect of annexin I on insulin secretion through surface binding sites in rat pancreatic islets. FEBS Lett 2002; 532(1-2): 17-20.
[http://dx.doi.org/10.1016/S0014-5793(02)03613-X] [PMID: 12459455]

[226] Won JH, Kang NN, Auh CK, Park YM. The surface receptor is involved in annexin I-stimulated insulin secretion in MIN6N8a cells. Biochem Biophys Res Commun 2003; 307(2): 389-94.
[http://dx.doi.org/10.1016/S0006-291X(03)01197-5] [PMID: 12859969]

[227] Ka SM, Tsai PY, Chao TK, *et al.* Urine annexin A1 as an index for glomerular injury in patients Dis Markers. 2014; 2014: 854163.
[http://dx.doi.org/10.1155/2014/854163]

[228] Okada R, Yasuda Y, Tsushita K, Wakai K, Hamajima N, Matsuo S. Glomerular hyperfiltration in prediabetes and prehypertension. Nephrol Dial Transplant 2012; 27(5): 1821-5.
[http://dx.doi.org/10.1093/ndt/gfr651] [PMID: 22140135]

[229] Börgeson E, McGillicuddy FC, Harford KA, *et al.* Lipoxin A4 attenuates adipose inflammation. FASEB J 2012; 26(10): 4287-94.
[http://dx.doi.org/10.1096/fj.12-208249] [PMID: 22700871]

[230] Börgeson E, Johnson AM, Lee YS, *et al.* Lipoxin A4 attenuates obesity-induced adipose inflammation and associated liver and kidney disease. Cell Metab 2015; 22(1): 125-37.
[http://dx.doi.org/10.1016/j.cmet.2015.05.003] [PMID: 26052006]

[231] Serhan CN, Chiang N, Van Dyke TE. Resolving inflammation: dual anti-inflammatory and pro-resolution lipid mediators. Nat Rev Immunol 2008; 8(5): 349-61.
[http://dx.doi.org/10.1038/nri2294] [PMID: 18437155]

[232] Alvarez-Llamas G, Szalowska E, de Vries MP, *et al.* Characterization of the human visceral adipose tissue secretome. Mol Cell Proteomics 2007; 6(4): 589-600.
[http://dx.doi.org/10.1074/mcp.M600265-MCP200] [PMID: 17255083]

[233] Roelofsen H, Dijkstra M, Weening D, de Vries MP, Hoek A, Vonk RJ. Comparison of isotope-labeled amino acid incorporation rates (CILAIR) provides a quantitative method to study tissue secretomes. Mol Cell Proteomics 2009; 8(2): 316-24.
[http://dx.doi.org/10.1074/mcp.M800254-MCP200] [PMID: 18840871]

[234] Hwa V, Oh Y, Rosenfeld RG. The insulin-like growth factor-binding protein (IGFBP) superfamily. Endocr Rev 1999; 20(6): 761-87.
[PMID: 10605625]

[235] Walker GE, Kim H, Yang Y. Oh Y IGF-independent effects of the IGFBP superfamily Insulin-like growth factors. Georgetown, TX: Kluwer Academic/Plenum Publishers 2003; pp. 262-80.

[236] Bienvenu G, Seurin D, Le Bouc Y, Even P, Babajko S, Magnan C. Dysregulation of energy homeostasis in mice overexpressing insulin-like growth factor-binding protein 6 in the brain. Diabetologia 2005; 48(6): 1189-97.
[http://dx.doi.org/10.1007/s00125-005-1767-6] [PMID: 15889232]

[237] Gealekman O, Gurav K, Chouinard M, *et al.* Control of adipose tissue expandability in response to high fat diet by the insulin-like growth factor-binding protein-4. J Biol Chem 2014; 289(26): 18327-38.
[http://dx.doi.org/10.1074/jbc.M113.545798] [PMID: 24778188]

[238] Prentice RL, Zhao S, Johnson M, *et al.* Proteomic risk markers for coronary heart disease and stroke: validation and mediation of randomized trial hormone therapy effects on these diseases. Genome Med 2013; 5(12): 112.
[http://dx.doi.org/10.1186/gm517] [PMID: 24373343]

[239] Moreno MJ, Ball M, Andrade MF, McDermid A, Stanimirovic DB. Insulin-like growth factor binding protein-4 (IGFBP-4) is a novel anti-angiogenic and anti-tumorigenic mediator secreted by dibutyryl cyclic AMP (dB-cAMP)-differentiated glioblastoma cells. Glia 2006; 53(8): 845-57.
[http://dx.doi.org/10.1002/glia.20345] [PMID: 16586492]

[240] Chen X, Hunt D, Cushman SW, Hess S. Proteomic characterization of thiazolidinedione regulation of obese adipose secretome in Zucker obese rats. Proteomics Clin Appl 2009; 3(9): 1099-111.
[http://dx.doi.org/10.1002/prca.200900026] [PMID: 21137009]

[241] Roca-Rivada A, Alonso J, Al-Massadi O, *et al.* Secretome analysis of rat adipose tissues shows location-specific roles for each depot type. J Proteomics 2011; 74(7): 1068-79.

[http://dx.doi.org/10.1016/j.jprot.2011.03.010] [PMID: 21439414]

[242] Yoshizumi T, Nakamura T, Yamane M, *et al.* Abdominal fat: standardized technique for measurement at CT. Radiology 1999; 211(1): 283-6.
[http://dx.doi.org/10.1148/radiology.211.1.r99ap15283] [PMID: 10189485]

[243] Siegel MJ, Hildebolt CF, Bae KT, Hong C, White NH. Total and intraabdominal fat distribution in preadolescents and adolescents: measurement with MR imaging. Radiology 2007; 242(3): 846-56.
[http://dx.doi.org/10.1148/radiol.2423060111] [PMID: 17244720]

[244] Horan M, Gibney E, Molloy E, McAuliffe F. Methodologies to assess paediatric adiposity. Ir J Med Sci 2015; 184(1): 53-68.
[http://dx.doi.org/10.1007/s11845-014-1124-1] [PMID: 24791970]

[245] van Marken Lichtenbelt WD, Vanhommerig JW, Smulders NM, *et al.* Cold-activated brown adipose tissue in healthy men. N Engl J Med 2009; 360(15): 1500-8.
[http://dx.doi.org/10.1056/NEJMoa0808718] [PMID: 19357405]

[246] Yoneshiro T, Aita S, Matsushita M, *et al.* Recruited brown adipose tissue as an antiobesity agent in humans. J Clin Invest 2013; 123(8): 3404-8.
[http://dx.doi.org/10.1172/JCI67803] [PMID: 23867622]

[247] Navet R, Mathy G, Douette P, *et al.* Mitoproteome plasticity of rat brown adipocytes in response to cold acclimation. J Proteome Res 2007; 6(1): 25-33.
[http://dx.doi.org/10.1021/pr060064u] [PMID: 17203945]

[248] Forner F, Kumar C, Luber CA, Fromme T, Klingenspor M, Mann M. Proteome differences between brown and white fat mitochondria reveal specialized metabolic functions. Cell Metab 2009; 10(4): 324-35.
[http://dx.doi.org/10.1016/j.cmet.2009.08.014] [PMID: 19808025]

[249] Kamal AH, Kim WK, Cho K, *et al.* Investigation of adipocyte proteome during the differentiation of brown preadipocytes. J Proteomics 2013; 94: 327-36.
[http://dx.doi.org/10.1016/j.jprot.2013.10.005] [PMID: 24129212]

[250] Yu J, Zhang S, Cui L, *et al.* Lipid droplet remodeling and interaction with mitochondria in mouse brown adipose tissue during cold treatment. Biochim Biophys Acta 2015; 1853(5): 918-28.
[http://dx.doi.org/10.1016/j.bbamcr.2015.01.020] [PMID: 25655664]

[251] Feldmann HM, Golozoubova V, Cannon B, Nedergaard J. UCP1 ablation induces obesity and abolishes diet-induced thermogenesis in mice exempt from thermal stress by living at thermoneutrality. Cell Metab 2009; 9(2): 203-9.
[http://dx.doi.org/10.1016/j.cmet.2008.12.014] [PMID: 19187776]

[252] Moisan A, Lee YK, Zhang JD, *et al.* White-to-brown metabolic conversion of human adipocytes by JAK inhibition. Nat Cell Biol 2015; 17(1): 57-67.
[http://dx.doi.org/10.1038/ncb3075] [PMID: 25487280]

[253] Wilson-Fritch L, Nicoloro S, Chouinard M, *et al.* Mitochondrial remodeling in adipose tissue associated with obesity and treatment with rosiglitazone. J Clin Invest 2004; 114(9): 1281-9.
[http://dx.doi.org/10.1172/JCI21752] [PMID: 15520860]

[254] Nissen SE, Wolski K. Effect of rosiglitazone on the risk of myocardial infarction and death from cardiovascular causes. N Engl J Med 2007; 356(24): 2457-71.
[http://dx.doi.org/10.1056/NEJMoa072761] [PMID: 17517853]

[255] Narasimhan S, Weinstock RS. Youth-onset type 2 diabetes mellitus: lessons learned from the TODAY study. Mayo Clin Proc 2014; 89(6): 806-16.
[http://dx.doi.org/10.1016/j.mayocp.2014.01.009] [PMID: 24702733]

[256] Timmers S, Konings E, Bilet L, *et al.* Calorie restriction-like effects of 30 days of resveratrol supplementation on energy metabolism and metabolic profile in obese humans. Cell Metab 2011; 14(5): 612-22.

[http://dx.doi.org/10.1016/j.cmet.2011.10.002] [PMID: 22055504]

[257] Carpene C, Gomez-Zorita S, Deleruyelle S, Carpene MA. Novel strategies for preventing diabetes and obesity complications with natural polyphenols. Curr Med Chem 2015; 22(1): 150-64.
[http://dx.doi.org/10.2174/0929867321666140815124052] [PMID: 25139462]

[258] Beaudoin MS, Snook LA, Arkell AM, Simpson JA, Holloway GP, Wright DC. Resveratrol supplementation improves white adipose tissue function in a depot-specific manner in Zucker diabetic fatty rats. Am J Physiol Regul Integr Comp Physiol 2013; 305(5): R542-51.
[http://dx.doi.org/10.1152/ajpregu.00200.2013] [PMID: 23824959]

[259] Wicklow B, Wittmeier K, T Jong GW, et al. Proposed trial: safety and efficacy of resveratrol for the treatment of non-alcoholic fatty liver disease (NAFLD) and associated insulin resistance in adolescents who are overweight or obese adolescents - rationale and protocol. Biochem Cell Biol 2015; 93(5): 522-30.
[http://dx.doi.org/10.1139/bcb-2014-0136] [PMID: 26305052]

[260] Van Troys M, Huyck L, Leyman S, Dhaese S, Vandekerkhove J, Ampe C. Ins and outs of ADF/cofilin activity and regulation. Eur J Cell Biol 2008; 87(8-9): 649-67.
[http://dx.doi.org/10.1016/j.ejcb.2008.04.001] [PMID: 18499298]

[261] Soenen S, Mariman EC, Vogels N, et al. Relationship between perilipin gene polymorphisms and body weight and body composition during weight loss and weight maintenance. Physiol Behav 2009; 96(4-5): 723-8.
[http://dx.doi.org/10.1016/j.physbeh.2009.01.011] [PMID: 19385027]

[262] Sentinelli F, Capoccia D, Incani M, Bertoccini L, Severino A, Pani MG, et al. The Perilipin 2 (PLIN2) gene Ser251Pro missense mutation is associated with reduced insulin secretion and increased insulin sensitivity in Italian obese subjects. Diabetes Metab Res Rev 2015.
[http://dx.doi.org/10.1002/dmrr.2751] [PMID: 26443937]

[263] Park JB, Agnihotri S, Golbourn B, et al. Transcriptional profiling of GBM invasion genes identifies effective inhibitors of the LIM kinase-Cofilin pathway. Oncotarget 2014; 5(19): 9382-95.
[http://dx.doi.org/10.18632/oncotarget.2412] [PMID: 25237832]

[264] Pawella LM, Hashani M, Eiteneuer E, et al. Perilipin discerns chronic from acute hepatocellular steatosis. J Hepatol 2014; 60(3): 633-42.
[http://dx.doi.org/10.1016/j.jhep.2013.11.007] [PMID: 24269473]

[265] AlKhater SA. Paediatric non-alcoholic fatty liver disease: an overview. Obes Rev 2015; 16(5): 393-405.
[http://dx.doi.org/10.1111/obr.12271] [PMID: 25753407]

[266] Van Harmelen V, Röhrig K, Hauner H. Comparison of proliferation and differentiation capacity of human adipocyte precursor cells from the omental and subcutaneous adipose tissue depot of obese subjects. Metabolism 2004; 53(5): 632-7.
[http://dx.doi.org/10.1016/j.metabol.2003.11.012] [PMID: 15131769]

[267] Lee MJ, Wu Y, Fried SK. Adipose tissue heterogeneity: implication of depot differences in adipose tissue for obesity complications. Mol Aspects Med 2013; 34(1): 1-11.
[http://dx.doi.org/10.1016/j.mam.2012.10.001] [PMID: 23068073]

[268] Zeyda M, Farmer D, Todoric J, et al. Human adipose tissue macrophages are of an anti-inflammatory phenotype but capable of excessive pro-inflammatory mediator production. Int J Obes 2007; 31(9): 1420-8.
[http://dx.doi.org/10.1038/sj.ijo.0803632] [PMID: 17593905]

[269] Shoelson SE, Lee J, Goldfine AB. Inflammation and insulin resistance. J Clin Invest 2006; 116(7): 1793-801.
[http://dx.doi.org/10.1172/JCI29069] [PMID: 16823477]

[270] Kheterpal I, Ku G, Coleman L, *et al.* Proteome of human subcutaneous adipose tissue stromal vascular fraction cells versus mature adipocytes based on DIGE. J Proteome Res 2011; 10(4): 1519-27.
[http://dx.doi.org/10.1021/pr100887r] [PMID: 21261302]

[271] Badger MR, Price GD. The role of carbonic anhydrase in photosynthesis. Annu Rev Plant Physiol Plant Mol Biol 1994; 45: 369-92.
[http://dx.doi.org/10.1146/annurev.pp.45.060194.002101]

[272] Supuran CT. Carbonic anhydrases: novel therapeutic applications for inhibitors and activators. Nat Rev Drug Discov 2008; 7(2): 168-81.
[http://dx.doi.org/10.1038/nrd2467] [PMID: 18167490]

[273] Gordon A, Price LH. Mood stabilization and weight loss with topiramate. Am J Psychiatry 1999; 156(6): 968-9.
[http://dx.doi.org/10.1176/ajp.156.6.968a] [PMID: 10360144]

[274] Picard F, Deshaies Y, Lalonde J, Samson P, Richard D. Topiramate reduces energy and fat gains in lean (Fa/?) and obese (fa/fa) Zucker rats. Obes Res 2000; 8(9): 656-63.
[http://dx.doi.org/10.1038/oby.2000.84] [PMID: 11225714]

[275] Fox CK, Marlatt KL, Rudser KD, Kelly AS. Topiramate for weight reduction in adolescents with severe obesity. Clin Pediatr (Phila) 2015; 54(1): 19-24.
[http://dx.doi.org/10.1177/0009922814542481] [PMID: 25027265]

[276] Zareba G. Zonisamide: review of its use in epilepsy therapy. Drugs Today (Barc) 2005; 41(9): 589-97.
[http://dx.doi.org/10.1358/dot.2005.41.9.921095] [PMID: 16341290]

[277] Jaikanth C, Gurumurthy P, Cherian KM, Indhumathi T. Emergence of omentin as a pleiotropic adipocytokine. Exp Clin Endocrinol Diabetes 2013; 121(7): 377-83.
[http://dx.doi.org/10.1055/s-0033-1345123] [PMID: 23839538]

[278] Pan HY, Guo L, Li Q. Changes of serum omentin-1 levels in normal subjects and in patients with impaired glucose regulation and with newly diagnosed and untreated type 2 diabetes. Diabetes Res Clin Pract 2010; 88(1): 29-33.
[http://dx.doi.org/10.1016/j.diabres.2010.01.013] [PMID: 20129687]

[279] Shibata R, Ouchi N, Kikuchi R, *et al.* Circulating omentin is associated with coronary artery disease in men. Atherosclerosis 2011; 219(2): 811-4.
[http://dx.doi.org/10.1016/j.atherosclerosis.2011.08.017] [PMID: 21925659]

[280] Catli G, Anik A, Abaci A, Kume T, Bober E. Low omentin-1 levels are related with clinical and metabolic parameters in obese children. Exp Clin Endocrinol Diabetes 2013; 121(10): 595-600.
[http://dx.doi.org/10.1055/s-0033-1355338] [PMID: 24085389]

[281] Prats-Puig A, Bassols J, Bargalló E, *et al.* Toward an early marker of metabolic dysfunction: omentin-1 in prepubertal children. Obesity (Silver Spring) 2011; 19(9): 1905-7.
[http://dx.doi.org/10.1038/oby.2011.198] [PMID: 21720428]

[282] Brunetti L, Leone S, Orlando G, *et al.* Hypotensive effects of omentin-1 related to increased adiponectin and decreased interleukin-6 in intra-thoracic pericardial adipose tissue. Pharmacol Rep 2014; 66(6): 991-5.
[http://dx.doi.org/10.1016/j.pharep.2014.06.014] [PMID: 25443726]

[283] Matsuo K, Shibata R, Ohashi K, *et al.* Omentin functions to attenuate cardiac hypertrophic response. J Mol Cell Cardiol 2015; 79: 195-202.
[http://dx.doi.org/10.1016/j.yjmcc.2014.11.019] [PMID: 25479337]

[284] Salans LB, Cushman SW, Weismann RE. Studies of human adipose tissue. Adipose cell size and number in nonobese and obese patients. J Clin Invest 1973; 52(4): 929-41.
[http://dx.doi.org/10.1172/JCI107258] [PMID: 4693656]

[285] Student AK, Hsu RY, Lane MD. Induction of fatty acid synthetase synthesis in differentiating 3T3-L1 preadipocytes. J Biol Chem 1980; 255(10): 4745-50.
[PMID: 7372608]

[286] Welsh GI, Griffiths MR, Webster KJ, Page MJ, Tavaré JM. Proteome analysis of adipogenesis. Proteomics 2004; 4(4): 1042-51.
[http://dx.doi.org/10.1002/pmic.200300675] [PMID: 15048985]

[287] Choi KL, Wang Y, Tse CA, Lam KS, Cooper GJ, Xu A. Proteomic analysis of adipocyte differentiation: Evidence that alpha2 macroglobulin is involved in the adipose conversion of 3T3 L1 preadipocytes. Proteomics 2004; 4(6): 1840-8.
[http://dx.doi.org/10.1002/pmic.200300697] [PMID: 15174150]

[288] Renes J, Bouwman F, Noben JP, Evelo C, Robben J, Mariman E. Protein profiling of 3T3-L1 adipocyte differentiation and (tumor necrosis factor alpha-mediated) starvation. Cell Mol Life Sci 2005; 62(4): 492-503.
[http://dx.doi.org/10.1007/s00018-004-4498-9] [PMID: 15719175]

[289] Rahman A, Kumar SG, Kim SW, et al. Proteomic analysis for inhibitory effect of chitosan oligosaccharides on 3T3-L1 adipocyte differentiation. Proteomics 2008; 8(3): 569-81.
[http://dx.doi.org/10.1002/pmic.200700888] [PMID: 18175373]

[290] Ye F, Zhang H, Yang YX, et al. Comparative proteome analysis of 3T3-L1 adipocyte differentiation using iTRAQ-coupled 2D LC-MS/MS. J Cell Biochem 2011; 112(10): 3002-14.
[http://dx.doi.org/10.1002/jcb.23223] [PMID: 21678470]

[291] Shetty S, Kusminski CM, Scherer PE. Adiponectin in health and disease: evaluation of adiponectin-targeted drug development strategies. Trends Pharmacol Sci 2009; 30(5): 234-9.
[http://dx.doi.org/10.1016/j.tips.2009.02.004] [PMID: 19359049]

[292] Qi Y, Takahashi N, Hileman SM, et al. Adiponectin acts in the brain to decrease body weight. Nat Med 2004; 10(5): 524-9.
[http://dx.doi.org/10.1038/nm1029] [PMID: 15077108]

[293] Shibata R, Sato K, Pimentel DR, et al. Adiponectin protects against myocardial ischemia-reperfusion injury through AMPK- and COX-2-dependent mechanisms. Nat Med 2005; 11(10): 1096-103.
[http://dx.doi.org/10.1038/nm1295] [PMID: 16155579]

[294] Sun X, Zemel MB. Calcium and 1,25-dihydroxyvitamin D3 regulation of adipokine expression. Obesity (Silver Spring) 2007; 15(2): 340-8.
[http://dx.doi.org/10.1038/oby.2007.540] [PMID: 17299106]

[295] Araki S, Dobashi K, Kubo K, Asayama K, Shirahata A. High molecular weight, rather than total, adiponectin levels better reflect metabolic abnormalities associated with childhood obesity. J Clin Endocrinol Metab 2006; 91(12): 5113-6.
[http://dx.doi.org/10.1210/jc.2006-1051] [PMID: 16984991]

[296] Walker GE, Ricotti R, Roccio M, et al. Pediatric obesity and vitamin D deficiency: a proteomic approach identifies multimeric adiponectin as a key link between these conditions. PLoS One 2014; 9(1): e83685.
[http://dx.doi.org/10.1371/journal.pone.0083685] [PMID: 24404137]

[297] Sung YY, Kim SH, Yoo BW, Kim HK. The nutritional composition and anti-obesity effects of an herbal mixed extract containing Allium fistulosum and Viola mandshurica in high-fat-diet-induced obese mice. BMC Complement Altern Med 2015; 15(1): 370.
[http://dx.doi.org/10.1186/s12906-015-0875-1] [PMID: 26474757]

[298] Reineke JB, Xie S, Naslavsky N, Caplan S. Qualitative and quantitative analysis of endocytic recycling. Methods Cell Biol 2015; 130: 139-55.
[http://dx.doi.org/10.1016/bs.mcb.2015.04.002] [PMID: 26360033]

[299] Haider NB, Searby C, Galperin E, *et al.* Evaluation and molecular characterization of EHD1, a candidate gene for Bardet-Biedl syndrome 1 (BBS1). Gene 1999; 240(1): 227-32.
[http://dx.doi.org/10.1016/S0378-1119(99)00395-9] [PMID: 10564830]

[300] Rotem-Yehudar R, Galperin E, Horowitz M. Association of insulin-like growth factor 1 receptor with EHD1 and SNAP29. J Biol Chem 2001; 276(35): 33054-60.
[http://dx.doi.org/10.1074/jbc.M009913200] [PMID: 11423532]

[301] Hovi T, Allison AC, Raivio K, Vaheri A. Purine metabolism and control of cell proliferation. Ciba Found Symp 1977; 48(48): 225-48.
[PMID: 204461]

[302] Kaida A, Ariumi Y, Baba K, Matsubae M, Takao T, Shimotohno K. Identification of a novel p300-specific-associating protein, PRS1 (phosphoribosylpyrophosphate synthetase subunit 1). Biochem J 2005; 391(Pt 2): 239-47.
[http://dx.doi.org/10.1042/BJ20041308] [PMID: 15943588]

[303] Taniguchi D, Hasegawa A, Harigaya T, Mizoguchi Y. Retinoic acids alter alpha-2-macroglobulin and ceruloplasmin bovine intramuscular adipogenesis. SUN-665; The Endocrine Society's 95th Annual Meeting and Expo, June 15-18.

[304] Christiaens V, Scroyen I, Lijnen HR. Role of proteolysis in development of murine adipose tissue. Thromb Haemost 2008; 99(2): 290-4.
[PMID: 18278177]

[305] Jitrapakdee S, St Maurice M, Rayment I, Cleland WW, Wallace JC, Attwood PV. Structure, mechanism and regulation of pyruvate carboxylase. Biochem J 2008; 413(3): 369-87.
[http://dx.doi.org/10.1042/BJ20080709] [PMID: 18613815]

[306] Hoogenboom BW, Suda K, Engel A, Fotiadis D. The supramolecular assemblies of voltage-dependent anion channels in the native membrane. J Mol Biol 2007; 370(2): 246-55.
[http://dx.doi.org/10.1016/j.jmb.2007.04.073] [PMID: 17524423]

[307] Yagoda N, von Rechenberg M, Zaganjor E, *et al.* RAS-RAF-MEK-dependent oxidative cell death involving voltage-dependent anion channels. Nature 2007; 447(7146): 864-8.
[http://dx.doi.org/10.1038/nature05859] [PMID: 17568748]

[308] Skop V, Cahova M, Dankova H, *et al.* Autophagy inhibition in early but not in later stages prevents 3T3-L1 differentiation: Effect on mitochondrial remodeling. Differentiation 2014; 87(5): 220-9.
[http://dx.doi.org/10.1016/j.diff.2014.06.002] [PMID: 25041706]

[309] Song BQ, Chi Y, Li X, *et al.* Inhibition of notch signaling promotes the adipogenic differentiation of mesenchymal stem cells through autophagy activation and PTEN-PI3K/AKT/mTOR pathway. Cell Physiol Biochem 2015; 36(5): 1991-2002.
[http://dx.doi.org/10.1159/000430167] [PMID: 26202359]

[310] Casteilla L, Dani C. Adipose tissue-derived cells: from physiology to regenerative medicine. Diabetes Metab 2006; 32(5 Pt 1): 393-401.
[http://dx.doi.org/10.1016/S1262-3636(07)70297-5] [PMID: 17110894]

[311] DeLany JP, Floyd ZE, Zvonic S, *et al.* Proteomic analysis of primary cultures of human adipose-derived stem cells: modulation by Adipogenesis. Mol Cell Proteomics 2005; 4(6): 731-40.
[http://dx.doi.org/10.1074/mcp.M400198-MCP200] [PMID: 15753122]

[312] Lee HK, Lee BH, Park SA, Kim CW. The proteomic analysis of an adipocyte differentiated from human mesenchymal stem cells using two-dimensional gel electrophoresis. Proteomics 2006; 6(4): 1223-9.
[http://dx.doi.org/10.1002/pmic.200500385] [PMID: 16421933]

[313] Bennett MK, García-Arrarás JE, Elferink LA, *et al.* The syntaxin family of vesicular transport receptors. Cell 1993; 74(5): 863-73.
[http://dx.doi.org/10.1016/0092-8674(93)90466-4] [PMID: 7690687]

[314] Hatakeyama H, Kanzaki M. Molecular basis of insulin-responsive GLUT4 trafficking systems revealed by single molecule imaging. Traffic 2011; 12(12): 1805-20.
[http://dx.doi.org/10.1111/j.1600-0854.2011.01279.x] [PMID: 21910807]

[315] Lancha A, López-Garrido S, Rodríguez A, et al. Expression of syntaxin 8 in visceral adipose tissue is increased in obese patients with type 2 diabetes and related to markers of insulin resistance and inflammation. Arch Med Res 2015; 46(1): 47-53.
[http://dx.doi.org/10.1016/j.arcmed.2014.12.003] [PMID: 25523146]

[316] Oh E, Stull ND, Mirmira RG, Thurmond DC. Syntaxin 4 up-regulation increases efficiency of insulin release in pancreatic islets from humans with and without type 2 diabetes mellitus. J Clin Endocrinol Metab 2014; 99(5): E866-70.
[http://dx.doi.org/10.1210/jc.2013-2221] [PMID: 24552216]

[317] Olkkonen VM, Li S. Oxysterol-binding proteins: sterol and phosphoinositide sensors coordinating transport, signaling and metabolism. Prog Lipid Res 2013; 52(4): 529-38.
[http://dx.doi.org/10.1016/j.plipres.2013.06.004] [PMID: 23830809]

[318] Lehto M, Mäyränpää MI, Pellinen T, et al. The R-Ras interaction partner ORP3 regulates cell adhesion. J Cell Sci 2008; 121(Pt 5): 695-705.
[http://dx.doi.org/10.1242/jcs.016964] [PMID: 18270267]

[319] Chen X, Cushman SW, Pannell LK, Hess S. Quantitative proteomic analysis of the secretory proteins from rat adipose cells using a 2D liquid chromatography-MS/MS approach. J Proteome Res 2005; 4(2): 570-7.
[http://dx.doi.org/10.1021/pr049772a] [PMID: 15822936]

[320] Yang Q, Graham TE, Mody N, et al. Serum retinol binding protein 4 contributes to insulin resistance in obesity and type 2 diabetes. Nature 2005; 436(7049): 356-62.
[http://dx.doi.org/10.1038/nature03711] [PMID: 16034410]

[321] Graham TE, Yang Q, Blüher M, et al. Retinol-binding protein 4 and insulin resistance in lean, obese, and diabetic subjects. N Engl J Med 2006; 354(24): 2552-63.
[http://dx.doi.org/10.1056/NEJMoa054862] [PMID: 16775236]

[322] Janke J, Engeli S, Boschmann M, et al. Retinol-binding protein 4 in human obesity. Diabetes 2006; 55(10): 2805-10.
[http://dx.doi.org/10.2337/db06-0616] [PMID: 17003346]

[323] Aeberli I, Biebinger R, Lehmann R, Lallemand D, Spinas GA, Zimmermann MB. Serum retinol-binding protein 4 concentration and its ratio to serum retinol are associated with obesity and metabolic syndrome components in children. J Clin Endocrinol Metab 2007; 92(11): 4359-65.
[http://dx.doi.org/10.1210/jc.2007-0468] [PMID: 17726085]

[324] Lee DC, Lee JW, Im JA. Association of serum retinol binding protein 4 and insulin resistance in apparently healthy adolescents. Metabolism 2007; 56(3): 327-31.
[http://dx.doi.org/10.1016/j.metabol.2006.10.011] [PMID: 17292720]

[325] Zhu C, Xiao Y, Liu X, et al. Pioglitazone lowers serum retinol binding protein 4 by suppressing its expression in adipose tissue of obese rats. Cell Physiol Biochem 2015; 35(2): 778-88.
[http://dx.doi.org/10.1159/000369737] [PMID: 25634757]

[326] Famulla S, Lamers D, Hartwig S, et al. Pigment epithelium-derived factor (PEDF) is one of the most abundant proteins secreted by human adipocytes and induces insulin resistance and inflammatory signaling in muscle and fat cells. Int J Obes 2011; 35(6): 762-72.
[http://dx.doi.org/10.1038/ijo.2010.212] [PMID: 20938440]

[327] Lamers D, Famulla S, Wronkowitz N, et al. Dipeptidyl peptidase 4 is a novel adipokine potentially linking obesity to the metabolic syndrome. Diabetes 2011; 60(7): 1917-25.
[http://dx.doi.org/10.2337/db10-1707] [PMID: 21593202]

[328] Lehr S, Hartwig S, Lamers D, *et al*. Identification and validation of novel adipokines released from primary human adipocytes. Mol Cell Proteomics 2012; 11(1): 010504.
[http://dx.doi.org/10.1074/mcp.M111.010504] [PMID: 21947364]

[329] Sunderland KL, Tryggestad JB, Wang JJ, *et al*. Pigment epithelium-derived factor (PEDF) varies with body composition and insulin resistance in healthy young people. J Clin Endocrinol Metab 2012; 97(11): E2114-8.
[http://dx.doi.org/10.1210/jc.2012-1894] [PMID: 22930782]

[330] Reinehr T, Roth CL, Enriori PJ, Masur K. Changes of dipeptidyl peptidase IV (DPP-IV) in obese children with weight loss: relationships to peptide YY, pancreatic peptide, and insulin sensitivity. J Pediatr Endocrinol Metab 2010; 23(1-2): 101-8.
[http://dx.doi.org/10.1515/JPEM.2010.23.1-2.101] [PMID: 20432813]

[331] Deacon CF, Nauck MA, Toft-Nielsen M, Pridal L, Willms B, Holst JJ. Both subcutaneously and intravenously administered glucagon-like peptide I are rapidly degraded from the NH2-terminus in type II diabetic patients and in healthy subjects. Diabetes 1995; 44(9): 1126-31.
[http://dx.doi.org/10.2337/diab.44.9.1126] [PMID: 7657039]

[332] Lambeir AM, Durinx C, Scharpé S, De Meester I. Dipeptidyl-peptidase IV from bench to bedside: an update on structural properties, functions, and clinical aspects of the enzyme DPP IV. Crit Rev Clin Lab Sci 2003; 40(3): 209-94.
[http://dx.doi.org/10.1080/713609354] [PMID: 12892317]

[333] Barnett A. DPP-4 inhibitors and their potential role in the management of type 2 diabetes. Int J Clin Pract 2006; 60(11): 1454-70.
[http://dx.doi.org/10.1111/j.1742-1241.2006.01178.x] [PMID: 17073841]

[334] Abraham NG, Junge JM, Drummond GS. Translational significance of heme oxygenase in obesity and metabolic syndrome. Trends Pharmacol Sci 2016; 37(1): 17-36.
[http://dx.doi.org/10.1016/j.tips.2015.09.003] [PMID: 26515032]

[335] Ubersax JA, Ferrell JE Jr. Mechanisms of specificity in protein phosphorylation. Nat Rev Mol Cell Biol 2007; 8(7): 530-41.
[http://dx.doi.org/10.1038/nrm2203] [PMID: 17585314]

[336] Schmelzle K, Kane S, Gridley S, Lienhard GE, White FM. Temporal dynamics of tyrosine phosphorylation in insulin signaling. Diabetes 2006; 55(8): 2171-9.
[http://dx.doi.org/10.2337/db06-0148] [PMID: 16873679]

[337] Kim WK, Jung H, Kim DH, *et al*. Regulation of adipogenic differentiation by LAR tyrosine phosphatase in human mesenchymal stem cells and 3T3-L1 preadipocytes. J Cell Sci 2009; 122(Pt 22): 4160-7.
[http://dx.doi.org/10.1242/jcs.053009] [PMID: 19910497]

[338] Jung H, Kim WK, Kim DH, *et al*. Involvement of PTP-RQ in differentiation during adipogenesis of human mesenchymal stem cells. Biochem Biophys Res Commun 2009; 383(2): 252-7.
[http://dx.doi.org/10.1016/j.bbrc.2009.04.001] [PMID: 19351528]

[339] Kim WK, Jung H, Kim EY, *et al*. RPTPμ tyrosine phosphatase promotes adipogenic differentiation via modulation of p120 catenin phosphorylation. Mol Biol Cell 2011; 22(24): 4883-91.
[http://dx.doi.org/10.1091/mbc.E11-03-0175] [PMID: 21998202]

[340] Kim EY, Han BS, Kim WK, Lee SC, Bae KH. Acceleration of adipogenic differentiation via acetylation of malate dehydrogenase 2. Biochem Biophys Res Commun 2013; 441(1): 77-82.
[http://dx.doi.org/10.1016/j.bbrc.2013.10.016] [PMID: 24134846]

[341] Xu Z, Ande SR, Mishra S. Temporal analysis of protein lysine acetylation during adipocyte differentiation. Adipocyte 2013; 2(1): 33-40.
[http://dx.doi.org/10.4161/adip.21916] [PMID: 23700550]

[342] Manuel AM, Frizzell N. Adipocyte protein modification by Krebs cycle intermediates and fumarate

ester-derived succination. Amino Acids 2013; 45(5): 1243-7.
[http://dx.doi.org/10.1007/s00726-013-1568-z] [PMID: 23892396]

[343] Krüger M, Kratchmarova I, Blagoev B, Tseng YH, Kahn CR, Mann M. Dissection of the insulin signaling pathway via quantitative phosphoproteomics. Proc Natl Acad Sci USA 2008; 105(7): 2451-6.
[http://dx.doi.org/10.1073/pnas.0711713105] [PMID: 18268350]

[344] Menzies KJ, Zhang H, Katsyuba E, Auwerx J. Protein acetylation in metabolism-metabolites and cofactors. Nat Rev Endocrinol 2015.
[http://dx.doi.org/10.1038/nrendo.2015.181] [PMID: 26503676]

[345] Grimsrud PA, Picklo MJ Sr, Griffin TJ, Bernlohr DA. Carbonylation of adipose proteins in obesity and insulin resistance: identification of adipocyte fatty acid-binding protein as a cellular target of 4-hydroxynonenal. Mol Cell Proteomics 2007; 6(4): 624-37.
[http://dx.doi.org/10.1074/mcp.M600120-MCP200] [PMID: 17205980]

[346] Merkley ED, Metz TO, Smith RD, Baynes JW, Frizzell N. The succinated proteome. Mass Spectrom Rev 2014; 33(2): 98-109.
[http://dx.doi.org/10.1002/mas.21382] [PMID: 24115015]

[347] Frizzell N, Thomas SA, Carson JA, Baynes JW. Mitochondrial stress causes increased succination of proteins in adipocytes in response to glucotoxicity. Biochem J 2012; 445(2): 247-54.
[http://dx.doi.org/10.1042/BJ20112142] [PMID: 22524437]

[348] Mennitti LV, Oliveira JL, Morais CA, et al. Type of fatty acids in maternal diets during pregnancy and/or lactation and metabolic consequences of the offspring. J Nutr Biochem 2015; 26(2): 99-111.
[http://dx.doi.org/10.1016/j.jnutbio.2014.10.001] [PMID: 25459884]

[349] Monzani A, Rapa A, Fuiano N, et al. Metabolic syndrome is strictly associated with parental obesity beginning from childhood. Clin Endocrinol (Oxf) 2014; 81(1): 45-51.
[http://dx.doi.org/10.1111/cen.12261] [PMID: 23746346]

[350] Ravelli AC, van der Meulen JH, Michels RP, et al. Glucose tolerance in adults after prenatal exposure to famine. Lancet 1998; 351(9097): 173-7.
[http://dx.doi.org/10.1016/S0140-6736(97)07244-9] [PMID: 9449872]

[351] Barker DJ. The effect of nutrition of the fetus and neonate on cardiovascular disease in adult life. Proc Nutr Soc 1992; 51(2): 135-44.
[http://dx.doi.org/10.1079/PNS19920023] [PMID: 1438321]

[352] Novak EM, Lee EK, Innis SM, Keller BO. Identification of novel protein targets regulated by maternal dietary fatty acid composition in neonatal rat liver. J Proteomics 2009; 73(1): 41-9.
[http://dx.doi.org/10.1016/j.jprot.2009.07.008] [PMID: 19651254]

[353] Oliva K, Barker G, Riley C, et al. The effect of pre-existing maternal obesity on the placental proteome: two-dimensional difference gel electrophoresis coupled with mass spectrometry. J Mol Endocrinol 2012; 48(2): 139-49.
[http://dx.doi.org/10.1530/JME-11-0123] [PMID: 22301947]

[354] Lee JH, Yoo JY, You YA, et al. Proteomic analysis of fetal programming-related obesity markers. Proteomics 2015; 15(15): 2669-77.
[http://dx.doi.org/10.1002/pmic.201400359] [PMID: 25886259]

[355] Manousopoulou A, Woo J, Woelk CH, et al. Are you also what your mother eats? Distinct proteomic portrait as a result of maternal high-fat diet in the cerebral cortex of the adult mouse. Int J Obes 2015; 39(8): 1325-8.
[http://dx.doi.org/10.1038/ijo.2015.35] [PMID: 25797609]

[356] You YA, Lee JH, Kwon EJ, et al. Proteomic analysis of one-carbon metabolism-related marker in liver of rat offspring. Mol Cell Proteomics 2015; 14(11): 2901-9.
[http://dx.doi.org/10.1074/mcp.M114.046888] [PMID: 26342040]

[357] Galata Z, Moschonis G, Makridakis M, *et al.* Plasma proteomic analysis in obese and overweight prepubertal children. Eur J Clin Invest 2011; 41(12): 1275-83.
[http://dx.doi.org/10.1111/j.1365-2362.2011.02536.x] [PMID: 21569026]

[358] Juonala M, Viikari JS, Kähönen M, *et al.* Childhood levels of serum apolipoproteins B and A-I predict carotid intima-media thickness and brachial endothelial function in adulthood: the cardiovascular risk in young Finns study. J Am Coll Cardiol 2008; 52(4): 293-9.
[http://dx.doi.org/10.1016/j.jacc.2008.03.054] [PMID: 18634985]

[359] Ernst E, Resch KL. Fibrinogen as a cardiovascular risk factor: a meta-analysis and review of the literature. Ann Intern Med 1993; 118(12): 956-63.
[http://dx.doi.org/10.7326/0003-4819-118-12-199306150-00008] [PMID: 8489110]

[360] Martini LA, Wood RJ. Vitamin D status and the metabolic syndrome. Nutr Rev 2006; 64(11): 479-86.
[http://dx.doi.org/10.1111/j.1753-4887.2006.tb00180.x] [PMID: 17131943]

[361] Martos-Moreno GÁ, Sackmann-Sala L, Barrios V, *et al.* Proteomic analysis allows for early detection of potential markers of metabolic impairment in very young obese children. Int J Pediatr Endocrinol 2014; 2014(1): 9.
[http://dx.doi.org/10.1186/1687-9856-2014-9] [PMID: 24949022]

[362] Jones SE, Jomary C. Clusterin. Int J Biochem Cell Biol 2002; 34(5): 427-31.
[http://dx.doi.org/10.1016/S1357-2725(01)00155-8] [PMID: 11906815]

[363] Won JC, Park CY, Oh SW, Lee ES, Youn BS, Kim MS. Plasma clusterin (ApoJ) levels are associated with adiposity and systemic inflammation. PLoS One 2014; 9(7): e103351.
[http://dx.doi.org/10.1371/journal.pone.0103351] [PMID: 25076422]

[364] Wassell J. Haptoglobin: function and polymorphism. Clin Lab 2000; 46(11-12): 547-52.
[PMID: 11109501]

[365] Reinehr T, Lass N, Toschke C, Rothermel J, Lanzinger S, Holl RW. Which Amount of BMI-SDS Reduction Is Necessary to Improve Cardiovascular Risk Factors in Overweight Children? J Clin Endocrinol Metab 2016; 101(8): 3171-9.
[http://dx.doi.org/10.1210/jc.2016-1885] [PMID: 27285295]

[366] Knop C, Singer V, Uysal Y, Schaefer A, Wolters B, Reinehr T. Extremely obese children respond better than extremely obese adolescents to lifestyle interventions. Pediatr Obes 2015; 10(1): 7-14.
[http://dx.doi.org/10.1111/j.2047-6310.2013.00212.x] [PMID: 24347523]

[367] Whitaker RC, Wright JA, Pepe MS, Seidel KD, Dietz WH. Predicting obesity in young adulthood from childhood and parental obesity. N Engl J Med 1997; 337(13): 869-73.
[http://dx.doi.org/10.1056/NEJM199709253371301] [PMID: 9302300]

[368] Reinehr T. Lifestyle intervention in childhood obesity: changes and challenges. Nat Rev Endocrinol 2013; 9(10): 607-14.
[http://dx.doi.org/10.1038/nrendo.2013.149] [PMID: 23897171]

[369] Bouwman FG, Claessens M, van Baak MA, *et al.* The physiologic effects of caloric restriction are reflected in the in vivo adipocyte-enriched proteome of overweight/obese subjects. J Proteome Res 2009; 8(12): 5532-40.
[http://dx.doi.org/10.1021/pr900606m] [PMID: 19827857]

[370] Bouwman FG, Wang P, van Baak M, Saris WH, Mariman EC. Obesity (Silver Spring). Increased β-oxidation with improved glucose uptake capacity in adipose tissue from obese after weight loss and maintenance. 2014; 22(3): pp. 819-27.

[371] Leggate M, Carter WG, Evans MJ, Vennard RA, Sribala-Sundaram S, Nimmo MA. Determination of inflammatory and prominent proteomic changes in plasma and adipose tissue after high-intensity intermittent training in overweight and obese males. J Appl Physiol (1985) 2012; 112(8): 1353-60.
[http://dx.doi.org/10.1152/japplphysiol.01080.2011] [PMID: 22267387]

[372] Renes J, Rosenow A, Roumans N, Noben JP, Mariman EC. Calorie restriction-induced changes in the secretome of human adipocytes, comparison with resveratrol-induced secretome effects. Biochim Biophys Acta 2014; 1844(9): 1511-22.
[http://dx.doi.org/10.1016/j.bbapap.2014.04.023] [PMID: 24802182]

[373] Sleddering MA, Markvoort AJ, Dharuri HK, *et al.* Proteomic analysis in type 2 diabetes patients before and after a very low calorie diet reveals potential disease state and intervention specific biomarkers. PLoS One 2014; 9(11): e112835.
[http://dx.doi.org/10.1371/journal.pone.0112835] [PMID: 25415563]

[374] Culnan DM, Cooney RN, Stanley B, Lynch CJ. Apolipoprotein A-IV, a putative satiety/antiatherogenic factor, rises after gastric bypass. Obesity (Silver Spring) 2009; 17(1): 46-52.
[http://dx.doi.org/10.1038/oby.2008.428] [PMID: 18948973]

[375] Dalmas E, Rouault C, Abdennour M, Rovere C, Rizkalla S, Bar-Hen A, *et al.* Variations in circulating inflammatory factors are related to changes in calorie and carbohydrate intakes early in the course of surgery-induced weight reduction
[http://dx.doi.org/10.3945/ajcn.111.013771]

[376] Gunta SS, Mak RH. Is obesity a risk factor for chronic kidney disease in children? Pediatr Nephrol 2013; 28(10): 1949-56.
[http://dx.doi.org/10.1007/s00467-012-2353-z] [PMID: 23150030]

[377] Suresh CP, Saha A, Kaur M, Kumar R, Dubey NK, Basak T, *et al.* Differentially expressed urinary biomarkers in children with idiopathic nephrotic syndrome. Clin Exp Nephrol 2015; 1-11.
[PMID: 26351173]

[378] Meier M, Kaiser T, Herrmann A, *et al.* Identification of urinary protein pattern in type 1 diabetic adolescents with early diabetic nephropathy by a novel combined proteome analysis. J Diabetes Complications 2005; 19(4): 223-32.
[http://dx.doi.org/10.1016/j.jdiacomp.2004.10.002] [PMID: 15993357]

[379] Klein J, Lacroix C, Caubet C, *et al.* Fetal urinary peptides to predict postnatal outcome of renal disease in fetuses with posterior urethral valves (PUV). Sci Transl Med 2013; 5(198): 198ra106.
[http://dx.doi.org/10.1126/scitranslmed.3005807] [PMID: 23946195]

[380] Boland CL, Harris JB, Harris KB. Pharmacological management of obesity in pediatric patients. Ann Pharmacother 2015; 49(2): 220-32.
[http://dx.doi.org/10.1177/1060028014557859] [PMID: 25366340]

[381] Rosenbaum M, Knight R, Leibel RL. The gut microbiota in human energy homeostasis and obesity. Trends Endocrinol Metab 2015; 26(9): 493-501.
[http://dx.doi.org/10.1016/j.tem.2015.07.002] [PMID: 26257300]

[382] Goulet O. Potential role of the intestinal microbiota in programming health and disease. Nutr Rev 2015; 73 (Suppl. 1): 32-40.
[http://dx.doi.org/10.1093/nutrit/nuv039] [PMID: 26175488]

[383] Lu CY, Ni YH. Gut microbiota and the development of pediatric diseases. J Gastroenterol 2015; 50(7): 720-6.
[http://dx.doi.org/10.1007/s00535-015-1082-z] [PMID: 25917564]

CHAPTER 4

Relationship Between Hormonal Milieu and Oxidative Stress in Childhood Obesity: A Physiopathological Basis for Antioxidant Treatment and Prevention of Cardiovascular Risk

Antonio Mancini[*]**, Francesco Leo, Chantal Di Segni, Sebastiano Raimondo** and **Aurora Natalia Rossodivita**

Departments of Medical Sciences and Pediatrics, Catholic University of the Sacred Heart, Rome, Italy

Abstract: The thrifty genotype, exposed to modern and industrialized societies, characterized by food availability and reduced physical activity, recently culminated in an epidemic obesity of giant proportions. Even more alarming than the figures regarding adult obesity is the increasing rate of obese children that has augmented almost 3-fold within the last 3 decades.

Obesity is associated with significant adverse effects on health, including metabolic, endocrine, cardiovascular, gastrointestinal, respiratory, neurologic, psychiatric, hematologic, and skeletal complications, and development of some types of malignancies. Studies strongly suggest that vascular, histopathological and metabolic changes begin in childhood. The development of metabolic problems associated with obesity during childhood track into adulthood increases the risk for type 2 diabetes, dyslipidemia and early cardiovascular disease.

In this paper, firstly we examine the numerous links between neuroendocrine peptides and cytokines, which contribute to inflammation and oxidative stress (OS) in obesity. A number of cytokine, mediators of inflammation, are produced by adipose tissue. In obese patients, increase in IL-6, C reactive protein (CRP), TNF-alpha and decrease in adiponectin and IL-10, induce pro-inflammatory stage, resulting in insulin resistance and endothelial dysfunction. Decreasing the levels of chronic inflammation and OS in childhood may prevent subsequent metabolic derangement along with increased cardiovascular morbidity and mortality in adulthood. OS has been proposed to be a potential mechanism linking obesity and endothelial dysfunction. In fact, oxidative reactions are critical in all the events which lead to atherogenesis. OS plays an important role in the pathogenesis of vascular alterations by either triggering exacerbating the biochemical processes accompanying endothelial dysfunction.

---

[*] **Corresponding author Antonio Mancini:** Department of Medical Sciences, Catholic University of the Sacred Heart, Rome, Italy; Tel: +39-06-30154440; Fax: +39-06-30157232; E-mail: mancini.giac@mclink.it

The production of Radical Oxygen species (ROS) and Radical Nitrogen Species (RNS) can occur at the cellular level in response to metabolic overload caused by an overabundance of macronutrients. Excessive generation of ROS in adipose tissue occurs by several interrelated pathophysiologic mechanisms, including nutrient metabolic overload, mitochondrial dysfunction, and endothelial reticulum stress. ROS generation is maintained by an inflammatory response, sustaining a vicious cycle. Puberty alters some of the inflammatory markers associated with endothelial dysfunction (adipocytokine levels, OS and insulin sensitivity) in obese children.

However, other than to inflammation, OS can be related to hormonal derangement in a reciprocal way. Some hormones influence antioxidant levels, but OS also can modify synthesis, activity and metabolism of hormones. Therefore, in the second section we examine some hormonal patterns which are influenced by obesity and their role in the regulation of antioxidant systems. In conclusion it seems that oxidative stress is certainly related to systemic inflammation but also to hormonal derangement.

Aside from the excess energy intake, nutrients have a specific role in the development of inflammation via the regulation of adipokine gene expression and secretion. In this way, it is possible to choose "non-inflammatory" or "anti-inflammatory" foods to minimize postprandial OS and inflammation. Therefore, lifestyle modifications, consisting in a reduction of caloric intake, a diet focused on particular macronutrient or micronutrient intake, and the encouragement of a regular exercise program with a personalized format, type and duration may reduce the consequences of childhood obesity. In particular we review the role of natural antioxidant in diet, as well as the administration of pharmacological antioxidants. Whether this approach is effective in improving vascular function in the short-term, but also in adult life remains to be established.

Keywords: Antioxidants, Childhood, Metabolic syndrome, Obesity, Oxidative stress.

INTRODUCTION

Obesity is a disease of body composition determined by a relative or absolute excess of body fat [1], which usually leads to an increase in body weight. The definition of overweight and obesity in childhood is still under debate. To date the definition of overweight and obesity in children is not based on the absolute value of body mass index (BMI), since it changes according to age, sex, height and weight of the child. Therefore to have an objective parameter, which is independent of age, the conditions of overweight and obesity in children are defined on the basis of the standard deviation of BMI.

The largest epidemiological transition of the 20th century concerned the shift of mortality and morbidity from infectious diseases to chronic diseases, particularly cardiovascular disease. This transition was primarily attributed to changes in social, economic and public health that occurred in the US during the first half of the century. The abundance of food brought not only better nutrition and improved health, but also an excess of positive energy balance, associated to a parallel increase of sedentary lifestyles in the population.

At the beginning of the millennium an augmented prevalence of obesity was thus generated with a consequential increase in related chronic disease [2]. Many studies in adults have shown the relationship between obesity and serious complications causing an increased risk of premature death in chronic diseases, such as diabetes mellitus type 2 (DM2), cholelithiasis, dyslipidemia, insulin resistance (IR), sleep apnea, coronary artery disease, hypertension and so on.

This phenomenon, spreading like wildfire across the planet, began to affect people more and more young, until obesity-related diseases appeared even in childhood.

Obesity is constantly increasing; in United States it progressed from 15% of overweight children in 1970 to nearly 30% in 2014. In Europe the percentage of overweight and obese children is slightly lower than in US. The difference can be seen especially in the age between 10 and 17, while 20% of overweight children in Europe are well below the 29% of American children. This does not reduce, however, the seriousness of a widespread problem, which is continuously increasing also in Europe: in particular the countries with higher prevalence of obese children are Greece (44% of obese males and 37% females), Italy (37% of obese males and 34% of females) and Spain (32% and 29%).

In Italy there are important differences between the North and the South of the country, in particular there is an higher prevalence in the South and in the islands, and also between different regions [3].

"Tracking" phenomenon is well known in pediatrics. It indicates any alteration occurred in childhood which is inclined to be present in adulthood. Therefore, when tracking occurs, like in obesity, it is useful to start a therapy to limit its future consequences as early as possible.

There are, in fact, clear epidemiological evidences of the risk of persistence of obesity of childhood onset into adulthood, with the worsening circumstance of a real storm of anticipation throughout the plethora of cardiovascular and metabolic complications (hyperlipidemia, DM 2, gallstones, liver disease) that characterize the status of adult obesity. It is not rare to find, in severely obese children, IR was very similar to that of an adult that anticipate, in effect, a state of full-blown diabetes.

The phenomenon of tracking appears to be related to several factors. First, the age in which obesity develops [4]. In fact, approximately 82% of males and 62% of females are inclined to maintain the state of overweight, if it is established before 10 years of age; on the contrary obese females have a greater probability to maintain the condition than males (78% *vs* 25%), if obesity appears, or becomes more severe, in the period of pubertal development. Adolescence is therefore a particularly critical period in which girls tend to become obese, because of increased body fat, keeping in time overweight, unlike the guys who tend to loose fat more easily due to enhanced muscle mass typical of this age.

Another factor in the maintenance of obesity in adulthood is the severity of obesity itself [5]. Among average children suffering from obesity in the first year of primary school (mean age 5.6 years), 47% will keep obesity at the fourteenth year. Among those with severe obesity (BMI to 99th percentile) in the first year of primary school, more than 70% remain obese at fourteen [6].

The persistence of adolescent obesity in adulthood appears to be also related to the presence of an obese parent. Among obese children at age 6, with an obese parent, 50% remain obese in adulthood, while among those aged 10-14 years with a relative obese, as 80% will remain obese as an adult [7].

Finally, knowing that only 1% of severely obese children spontaneously return to a normal BMI for adults, we can say that being overweight tends to keep from pediatric to adult and this association increases with age [8].

Obesity is a condition linked to metabolic syndrome (MetS), the clustering of abdominal obesity, dyslipidemia, hyperglycemia and hypertension, well studied in adults, but still discussed in children. After the publication of the first article on MetS in adolescents [9] a great debate has developed on its definition [10].

It is well known that obesity is associated to oxidative stress [11, 12], but despite a large number of studies for therapeutic strategies in adults, observations in children are still inconclusive, due to the difficulty to treat young patients especially in early infancy.

Due to the importance of this topic, but the lack of a clear physiopathological picture, we present a review on oxidative stress in childhood obesity (compared with adult obesity), focusing, on one side, on systemic inflammation and its vascular consequences and, on the other side, on the role of hormones in regulating antioxidant systems.

OBESITY AND OXIDATIVE STRESS

Oxidative Stress (OS) is defined as an unbalance between the production of radicals and antioxidant defenses. Recent papers suggest that mitochondrial reactive species work as signalling molecules for the production of pro-inflammatory cytokines, connecting, in this way, OS and inflammation. Different signals produced by the adipose tissue cause an increase of Radical Oxygen Species (ROS) and Radical Nitrogen Species (RNS). The dysregulation of such pathway could be a crucial characteristic of the obese people, who would perpetuate inflammation and OS in this way. Recent studies upgrade, both in children and adults, the adipose tissue as an endocrine organ producing different proteins (adipokines) with wide biologic activities. After the maturation from pre-adipocytes, the adipocytes gain, for instance, functions similar to the macrophages, including the ability to reply to the products of the bacterial wall, activation of cytokine cascade and their secretion [13]. Moreover, during weight gain or loss, the cellular composition of adipose tissue dynamically changes, both in size of each adipocyte and in the types of cell represented, like vascular cells and cells from immune system. These last ones, and especially the macrophages, dramatically increasing, play an important role in the pathogenesis of insulin resistance associated to obesity, through the production of Monocyte Chemoattractant Protein-1 (MCP-1) and the modulation of the spreading and the growth of the adipose tissue itself [14]. In the adipose tissue a bidirectional interaction between adipocyte and macrophages seems to be active. The enormous adipocyte number of the obese patient is able, through the release of free fatty acids, to stimulate Tumor Necrosis Factor (TNF) production in macrophages and, through the MCP-1 production, to cause their mobilization and chemotaxis, being responsible for the beginning of an inflammatory reaction, made stronger by a temporary presence of neutrophils and lymphocytes T. The same macrophages, finally, through the ROS production, seem to stimulate expression and release of MCP-1 within the adipocyte. In this way a vicious circle could be established and would promote a chronic inflammatory status with a gradually increasing intensity, typical of obesity and its complications. Finally, the macrophages regulate the remodelling of the adipose tissue during a chronic positive energetic balance. Depending on the activation of the macrophagic subtype M1 or M2, different cellular pathways will be activated, regulating the proliferation, the growth, and the survival of the adipocytes; therefore they will be responsible for the appearance of hypertrophic or hyperplastic obesity.

After a chronic positive energetic unbalance, in case of prevalence the M1 pro-inflammatory macrophagic subtype, the reduced survival and proliferation of the preadipocytes will cause an inadequate reserve; therefore the energetic backlog, through an excessive hypertrophy, will produce a dysfunctional adipose tissue, which will perpetuate an inflammatory condition and, in the long term, insulin resistance.

Conversely, if the M2 macrophagic subtype is prevalent, functional pool of preadipocytes will be favoured. These will differentiate into new adipocytes, contributing to the formation of an adequate hyperplastic adipose tissue with the maintenance of a normal cell function and insulin sensitivity [15].

Hormones and Inflammatory Molecules Produced by or Related to Adipose Tissue

Obesity is associated, therefore, to an increase in the secretion of pro-inflammatory cytokines (Leptin, TNF-α, IL-6, resistin) and to a decrease in the release of adipokines that downregulate inflammation (adiponectin, IL-10). Recent studies [16] show that not only the amount but also the kind of adipose tissue, as well as the kinds of fats in the diet, influence in different ways this chronic inflammatory state.

Among the inflammatory molecules produced by adipose tissue or indirectly connected to it, some play a key role in regulating appetite, the development of adipose tissue and the perpetuation of the vicious circle that, in the long term, determine the complications associated with obesity.

They are:

- **GHRELIN** It is a peptide of 28 aminoacids, mainly synthesized in the gastric fundus, but also in other organs such as the hypothalamus, the hippocampus, the cerebral cortex, the pituitary gland, the small intestine, the adrenal gland and the pancreas. Its receptor (GHS-R1a) is mainly expressed in the hypothalamus and it is a member of the family of receptors for Growth Hormone (GH). It can reach the hypothalamus from the bloodstream or through the vagus nerve and the nucleus of the solitary tract. The Ghrelin plays a role in regulating the short and long-term energy balance, appetite and weight gain. It increases gastric motility and gastric and pancreatic secretions, regulates lipid and glucose metabolism by stimulating cellular differentiation in adipose tissue and lipogenesis, while inhibiting apoptosis and adipocyte lipolysis. As orexigen hormone, it encourages a sense of hunger, so its endogenous levels increase immediately before a meal and are reduced in the following hours. Therefore in the long-term energy balance, it determines increased energy intake and reduced use of fat as fuel energy by promoting the deposition [17]. Several factors affect its blood concentration. Fasting and a restrictive diet are those that principally stimulate the secretion. Its serum level is inversely related to BMI. Ghrelin is used as a marker of IR in children. Its levels are related to insulin levels and to HOMA index regardless of BMI in obese adolescents with IR. In another study [18] about overweight and obese children a significant correlation between insulin sensitivity and decreased concentration of postprandial Ghrelin was demonstrated. The levels of Ghrelin vary also depending on the stage of puberty and may have a role in the regulation of reproductive physiology [19]. It decreases with the progress of the pubertal stage in children with IR.

- **OBESTATIN** It is a peptide derived from a post-translational processing of the precursor of Ghrelin. Also mainly produced in the stomach, acts as anorexigen hormone suppressing food intake, inhibiting the motility of the gastro-intestinal tract and reducing the body weight. Its action is expressed predominantly in a long-term regulation of body weight. Granata *et al*. [20] studied the functions of obestatin in mouse models and in humans, demonstrating its action on glucose and lipid metabolism through inhibition of lipolysis and increased glucose uptake. It stimulates the secretion of adiponectin and inhibits that of Leptin, thereby contributing to the reduction of insulin resistance and the related tissue inflammation.
- **LEPTIN** Leptin (LEP) is a protein of 167 aminoacids, weight of 16 Kd, produced mainly in white adipose tissue and secreted from the single adipocyte according to intracellular levels of triglycerides and their metabolites. It acts on receptors (LEPR) located on specific neuronal populations in the brain, located in the hypothalamus, the midbrain and brain stem and its main function is to oppose obesity [21]. Further studies have demonstrated the presence of LEPR in mice also in the placenta during gestation, suggesting a role as growth factor and modulator of development during the fetal growth. The same fetus, on the other hand, seems to produce leptin in cardiac, bone and cartilaginous structures, hematopoietic matrix and other Tissues too tissues, with interruption in adult life, as proof of the complex, and yet little known, functions that it could play [8]. The purely metabolic functions of this protein are expressed in the context of a network of signals involved in determining the energy balance of the individual. It acts as a long term regulator of the level of the body mass, especially of the fat mass, thus representing a true indicator of the energy status of the individual, with the delicate task of leading it towards structures and metabolic behaviours that intend to change the genetically and centrally-determined set-point. A recent study in overweight children and adolescents showed significantly higher values of Leptin in children with high BMI [22]. Reflecting the body fat reserves, Leptin plays a crucial role in the regulation of numerous neuroendocrine functions, from energetic homeostasis to a variety of processes related to reproduction [23, 24], bone function [25], cardiovascular system regulation [26] and immune function [27]. It is impossible, in fact, to dissociate the actions of Leptin from those of other substances such as insulin, glucocorticoids, catecholamines, even thyroid hormones, especially considering that mutual influences have been shown. There are various factors that influence the secretion of Leptin. The most important are the amount of subcutaneous fat and the state of energy reserves, being the Leptin gene mainly expressed in

adipose tissue. Its expression is also stimulated by the secretion of insulin, while the role of glucocorticoids is still under investigation, although some studies demonstrate their action in inducing hyperleptinemia, especially in situations of chronic hypercortisolism [28]. There is, in fact, a reciprocal stimulation of Leptin and cortisol, as demonstrated by the fact that Leptin increases blood levels of cortisol in humans [29]. Glucose and its metabolites have a permissive role in the Leptin secretion and expression, while the free fatty acids act as suppressors. There are also interactions between Leptin, sex hormones and growth hormone probably involved in the growth retardation of obese adolescents. Finally, infection, endotoxins and cytokines stimulate the synthesis of Leptin. Once entered into circulation, it binds to the transport protein Ob-Re (splice variant receptor Ob-R or LEPR); Leptin reaches its site of action. The main one has been found in the hypothalamic ventromedial (HVM) and lateral (HL) nucleus, where the highest concentration of Leptin receptors was found on peptidergic neurons, that would be, then, the central mediators of signal from peripheral nervous system, according to a feedback whose ramifications are still under investigation. Another subtype of Leptin transporter ensures the crossing of the blood-brain barrier, in order to create a precise balance between blood concentrations of the hormone and the cerebro-spinal fluid (CSF) levels, which are between 2 and 5% of serum values [8]. Once arriving in the central nervous system (CNS), the hormone acts depressing the activity of neurons using as a neurotransmitter neuropeptide Y (NPY), which are recognized as the "neurons of the hunger". In contrast, it stimulates nerve cells that synthesize peptides such as proopiomelanocortin (POMC) and the derived melanocortin, with the α-melanocyte-stimulating hormone (α-MSH) and cocaine-and-amphetamie-regulated-transcript (CART), associated with the functions of the "neurons of the satiety". Noteworthy is the correlation between Leptin and Ghrelin. The two hormones are secreted independently of one another, but they act on the same target in the hypothalamus in an antagonistic way. Recent evidences show that one of the major risk factors for the development of obesity is the inability of Leptin to perform its metabolic functions of appetite suppression and promotion of energy expenditure. Both in man and obese animal, however, higher blood levels of Leptin have been found, suggesting a mechanism of reduced sensibility, known as "Leptin Resistance". Then different pathophysiological mechanisms that would explain this phenomenon were studied. Among them, we recall the reduced transport of Leptin across the blood-brain barrier, the intracellular signal attenuation, mutations of the genes for Leptin or its receptor, intracellular OS and inflammation.

- ***ADIPONECTIN*** It is a protein highly expressed in adipose tissue; its levels decrease in obese patients, particularly in those with abdominal obesity, while they seem to increase during weight loss. Its clinical importance is due to its insulin-sensitizing activity and its anti-inflammatory and anti-atherogenic role; high blood levels are inversely related to obesity, IR, risk of type 2 diabetes mellitus, dyslipidemia, and cardiovascular disease. Recently the link between low levels of adiponectin and MetS has also been shown in obese children and adolescents [30]. It reduces the hepatic triglyceride content and the levels of free fatty acids into the bloodstream by increasing hepatic insulin sensitivity. Influencing the expression of key enzymes of gluconeogenesis, it regulates hepatic glucose production, and through the activation of intracellular kinases, it stimulates glucose uptake in adipocytes and muscles. Finally, through the inhibition of TNF-α secretion, it protects from atherosclerosis by modulating the proliferation of vascular smooth muscle cells [31]. Adiponectin has a special relationship with inflammatory cytokines produced within the adipose tissue and its expression and secretion is inhibited by TNF-α, IL-6 and dexamethasone.

- **KISSPEPTIN** Kisspeptin (Kp) is a component of a family of peptides derived from a precursor polypeptide of 145 amino acid product of transcription of the gene KISS1. It is released from anteroventral paraventricular hypothalamic and arcuate nuclei [32]. Its production is influenced by endogenous environmental and hormonal factors (sex steroids, Leptin) [33 - 36]. Kisspeptin receptor GPR54 acts, mainly, on hypothalamic GnRH-secreting neurons, so its primary function remains the stimulation of pubertal development [37]. Recently also other functions have been demonstrated such as the sexual differentiation of the brain during the fetal period and the regulation of the menstrual cycle in adult women. Finally, as recently proposed, an involvement in the regulation of antioxidant systems [38], through direct and indirect mechanisms, and metabolism [39], seems likely due to demonstrated direct production by adipose tissue [40, 41].
- **TNF-α** It is a pro-inflammatory cytokine, the main mediator of the acute inflammatory response, responsible of systemic complications that may occur during an inflammatory process. Mostly produced by macrophages and lymphocytes, it is also secreted by adipose tissue. Its production is not related to the amount of adipose tissue, but it is strictly dependent on the systemic effect of Leptin and other adipokines. One of its main clinical effects, in obese children, is in fact the induction of IR, being able to attenuate the signalling pathways associated with the insulin receptor, by directly acting on its tyrosine kinase activity. Another of the molecular mechanisms proposed to explain the role in the pathogenesis of IR is the stimulation of adipocyte lipolysis, causing the increase in the levels of fatty acids in the bloodstream. Through the activation of the transcription of nuclear factor kappa-light-chain-enhancer of activated B cells (NF-kB), together with IL-6, it determines a series of modifications on vascular tissue responsible of a chronic inflammatory state which, as known, leads to hypertension and atherosclerosis. Finally, as previously mentioned,

TNF-α inhibits, with autocrine or paracrine mechanisms, the expression of adiponectin, reducing, thus, the insulin sensitivity in different tissues.

- *IL-6* Interleukin 6 is a multifunctional cytokine with various roles in inflammation, defense against external agents and tissue damage. It is produced by many cell types and tissues, including cells of the immune system, fibroblasts, endothelial cells, skeletal muscle and adipose tissue. In particular, the portion produced by adipose tissue is significantly increased in obese subjects [42]. Like for TNF-α, IL-6 is responsible for the induction of IR and its complications too. The association between high levels of IL-6 and insulin has been demonstrated both in adults and children, so its blood levels can be considered important predictors of the onset of DM 2 and myocardial infarction.

- *IL-10* Activated macrophages and lymphocytes secrete this cytokine. Low capacity of production of IL-10 has been shown, however, in obesity, MetS and DM 2. It antagonizes the effects of TNF-α and IL-6, resulting in insulin sensitization and adversing chronic inflammation associated with obesity and endothelial damage. Low levels of IL-10 are in fact considered risk factors for atherosclerosis, acute coronary ischemia and insulin resistance.

- *RESISTIN* It is a peptide, also known as ADSF (adipose tissue-specific secretory factor) and FIZZ3 (found in inflammatory zone 3), expressed and secreted both by the adipocyte and the macrophage. Preliminary studies have suggested that Resistin has a significant effect on insulin action, connecting potentially obesity to IR. The ablation of the gene of Resistin in mice decreases the concentration of fasting glucose, through the reduction of gluconeogenesis, whereas administration of Resistin in the same mice increases hepatic glucose production. Therefore, a chronic "hyperresistinemia" compromises the insulin signalling pathway in all three target tissue: muscle, liver and adipose tissue. Resistin reduces sensitivity to insulin and may contribute, therefore, to the onset of IR and diabetes. Furthermore, recent investigations have shown that the protein is not produced by the adipocyte itself, but by other cells of the adipose tissue, which may be identified with the macrophages [43]. In humans, in particular, it seems that macrophages and blood monocytes are the main source of Resistin, compared to adipocytes.

- *VISFATIN* It is a hormone derived from fat cells, particularly in the visceral fat, whose blood concentration increases with the progression of obesity. However, it is not specifically expressed in adipose tissue. Its serum concentration is positively correlated to the blood triglycerides levels and down-regulated by hyper-nutrition. Antidiabetic properties were supposed. Such as insulin, Visfatin stimulates the uptake of glucose and suppresses the release of glucose by hepatocytes. It also induces the phosphorylation of transduction signal proteins that operate downstream the insulin receptor. Finally it has been shown that Visfatin binds to its specific receptor of insulin, without competing with it, suggesting that the two proteins may however have two different binding sites on the same receptor [44].

- **APELIN** It is a new peptide identified as the endogenous ligand of the orphan G-protein-coupled-receptor. It is expressed in a variety of tissues including the stomach, brain, heart, skeletal muscle and white adipose tissue. Its expression in adipose tissue is markedly influenced by nutritional status, since it is greatly reduced by fasting. Finally there is a strong relationship between Apelin and insulin, which has a positive effect on the direct adipocyte production of the peptide [45].
- **RETINOL-BINDING PROTEIN 4 (RBP4)** RBP4 is recently emerging as a new adipocytokine, connecting the adipocyte glucose uptake with systemic insulin sensitivity [46]. It modulates glucose homeostasis influencing the expression of the transporter GLUT4 in adipose tissue. Blood levels in obese children are considered not only as index of obesity and IR, but also of inflammation, being correlated with numerous factors associated with it.

A summary of these observations is reported in Table **1**.

Table 1. Main characteristics of hormones and inflammatory molecules produced by OS related to adipose tissue.

	MOLECULES	SITE OF PRODUCTION	ACTIONS
Proteins and hormones	GHRELIN	Gastric fundus, hypothalamus, hippocampus, cerebral cortex, gut, pancreas, adrenal gland.	Short- and long-term setting of energy balance, appetite and weight gain. It increases gastric motility and gastric- pancreatic secretions. It modulates lipidic and glucidic metabolism. It encourages a sense of hunger. Marker of insulin resistance in children.
	OBESTATIN	Mainly by the stomach.	Anorexigenic hormone: it suppresses food intake by inhibiting gastrointestinal motility and reducing body weight. Long- term weight regulator.
	ADIPONECTIN	Adipose Tissue.	It modulates certain metabolic processes, including the regulation of glucose and fatty acid catabolism. Insulin sensitizer. Anti-inflammatory properties

(Table 1) contd.....

MOLECULES		SITE OF PRODUCTION	ACTIONS
Proteins and hormones	**RETINOL-BINDING PROTEIN 4** (RBP4)	Liver, adipose tissue.	Directly correlates with systemic insulin sensitivity. It modulates glucose homeostasis. Its blood levels, in obese children, are indexes of insulin resistance and inflammation.
	LEPTIN (LEP)	White Adipose Tissue (Very sensitive to intracellular levels of triglycerides and their metabolites). Its secretion depends on the reserves of subcutaneous fat and the state of energy reserves.	It contrasts obesity. Long-term regulator of body mass, (mainly the fat one). Indicator of energy state. Regulates several neuroendocrine function: energy homeostasis, bone function, cardiovascular regulation and immune function.
	RESISTIN (ADSF)	Adipocytes and macrophages.	It reduces insulin sensitivity and may contributes to insulin resistance and diabetes.
	VISFATIN	Adipocytes (in particular by visceral fat). It increases with the development of obesity.	Anti-diabetes properties. It stimulates glucose uptake and it suppresses release by hepatocytes. It induces signal proteins' phosphorylation that work downstream of insulin receptor.
	APELIN	Stomach, brain, heart, skeletal muscle and white adipose tissue.	Modulates nutritional status.
Inflammatory molecules and cytokines	**TNF-α**	Mainly activated macrophages.	Main mediator of the inflammatory response. In obese children it induces insulin resistance.
	IL-6 (*Interleukin 6*)	Immune system, endothelial cells, skeletal muscle and adipose tissue.	It induces insulin resistance and increases complications associated with cardiovascular risk.
	IL-10(*Interleukin 10*)	Macrophages and activated lymphocytes.	It increases insulin sensitivity and reduces obesity, chronic inflammation and endothelial damage.

Oxidative Stress in Childhood Obesity

Only recently the aspect of OS was deepened even in childhood obesity. As well as in adults, higher levels of OS were encountered in obese children, compared to lean subjects, as demonstrated by the finding of much higher levels of peroxide radical [47]. In addition, the finding of tiger levels of malondialdehyde (MDA) in obese males than females [48] suggests a possible difference in exposure to sex dependent OS. The increase in oxidative parameters is also much more marked in children with actual metabolic complications. The accumulation of reactive species, in the child as well as in the adult, stimulates the production and the activation of antioxidant species, the levels of which will become therefore reduced. Molnar *et al* [49] reported levels of antioxidants and α-tocopherol significantly reduced in obese children with MetS.

Coenzyme Q_{10} (CoQ_{10}), the only liposoluble antioxidant synthetized in living organisms, is involved in energy metabolism due to the presence in mitochondrial respiratory chain. It has been studied in obese population and was found to be increased, both in adults and children [50, 51]. CoQ_{10} was markedly reduced by the biliopancreatic diversion [52]. Its importance is the strict relation with thyroid hormones (see below).

The importance of the amount of adipose tissue in the genesis of OS and alterations related to it have been demonstrated by Kelly *et al*. [53], who reported no improvement in the profile of adipokines or in markers of inflammation or OS after 8 weeks of exercise in the absence of weight loss. This indicates that the number of adipocytes and/or their activity are the primary factors in the production of free radicals and inflammatory cytokines [54].

The association between obesity, inflammation and adipokines in children has been described in depth, while there are few data that correlate OS to inflammation and endothelial damage. The levels of proinflammatory adipokines, Leptin, are strongly correlated with blood levels of MDA in prepubertal children, which also show an increase of homocysteine [55]. Studies in prepubertal children have also demonstrated the direct correlation between obesity, referred to as BMI, OS markers (8-isoprostane) and inflammatory markers (leukocyte count and IL-6) [56]. It was recently emphasized the distribution of adipose tissue and in particular a greater correlation between abdominal obesity and OS markers was proven.

OS, finally, has been proposed as a mechanism of connection between obesity and endothelial dysfunction since oxidative reactions are crucial in the series of events that lead to atherogenesis. Since the same pathogenic processes present in adult can be discovered in obese children, but with precocious exposition, the result is a sharp advance in the clinical manifestation of all the complications associated with obesity, including diabetes and MS [57, 58].

HORMONAL REGULATION OF ANTIOXIDANT SYSTEMS AND THEIR DERANGEMENT IN CHILDHOOD OBESITY

This section of the chapter is addressed to review hormone environment influence on antioxidant balance, with special focus on those who are involved in energy balance and OS modulation, also including recent data on hormones produced by adipose tissue. Since this aspect is relatively new there are no sufficient data in obesity. Most models are in *in vitro* or in experimental animals, therefore the topic of obesity is at moment speculative and requires further attention.

Then we summarize the main hormonal alterations observed in childhood obesity. Some of them seem to be adaptive to altered energy balance, but can be involved in pathological processes that, through a vicious circle, can contribute to worsen obesity itself.

Growth Hormone (GH)

GH and OS GH modulates functions and life cycle of defense cell systems. In human polymorphonuclear neutrophils (PMNs), cultured *in vitro*, GH pretreatment down-regulates Fas expression and inhibits apoptosis. However, it up-regulates reactive oxygen intermediate (ROI) production, stimulated by phorbol myristate acetate system [59]. This potentially harmful aspect is counterbalanced by enhanced life span, therefore the authors concluded that GH may improve host defense. ROI production is also increased in cultured monocytes; no effect was reported on apoptosis in monocytes or lymphocytes.

As concerns pathological model, the neutrophil O_2^- generating capacity was measured in a group of GHD adults and was found to be lower than controls; it was augmented by GH treatment [60].

In experimental rat models some data are proposed. Wistar rats were tested after caloric restriction during a 6 week period, resulting in decreased ROS generation and oxidative DNA damage in heart mitochondria; this was reverted by insulin treatment and by GH/insulin administration [61]. This datum could be particularly important in models of obesity. In fact, we remark that GH is decreased in obesity and therefore a putative hypothalamic protective role could be reduced. However, in the liver, GH and insulin decreased mitochondrial ROS generation, while increased oxidative damage to mitochondrial DNA. GH and insulin decreased three different markers of oxidative liver protein modifications, but increased lipoxidation-dependent markers, probably for the increase of phospholipid unsaturation. Therefore, GH seems to exert both prooxidant and protective effects, depending on parameters and tissue considered.

Ames dwarf mice (df/df), which are deficient in GH, PRL and TSH, live significantly longer, where transgenic mice with GH overexpression show premature ageing and reduced life-span. The evaluation of antioxidant systems [62] showed lower liver levels of glutathione and ascorbate in dwarf animals; by contrast, catalase activity in dwarf liver and kidney was higher than in the other groups, suggesting that GHD mice may contrast OS more efficiently than normal or GH-overexpressing mice.

This hypothesis was not in agreement with the study of Hauck *et al.* [63] in long-living GH receptor/binding protein gene knockout (GHR-KO) mouse. The authors discovered lower Superoxide Dismutase (SOD) and higher Glutathione Peroxidase (GPx) in kidney; Lipoperoxide (LP) was higher only in female mice. In the liver, female GHR-KO mice had lower GPx, while male GHR-KO mice had lower Catalase (CAT) and higher LP. GHR-KO males were also more susceptible to paraquat toxicity. Even if the authors concluded that the longevity in this experimental model was not due to an improved free-radical scavenging, at least in liver and kidney, their experiments showed an important sex-related modulation of these systems and a differential response of various tissues.

In the above cited study by Smith [60], adult GHD was associated by reduced lipid peroxidation, measured both as evaluation of lipid hydroperoxides in plasma – measured with ferrous oxidation with xylenol orange assay – and as susceptibility of LDL to peroxidation, by the copper-catalyzed lag phase. These data were coupled with a higher LDL and triglyceride and lower HDL cholesterol concentrations; the reduced lipid peroxidation and impaired polymorphonucleate 0_2^- generation were reversible with a 3-months recombinant GH treatment.

Mechanisms of OS have been studied, as human models, both in prepubertal and adult GH deficiency (GHD).

Prepubertal GHD showed significantly decreased lag phase and vitamin E, with a correlation between these parameters and IGF-1 or IGFBP-3; on the contrary MDA was significantly increased and inversely correlated with IGF-1/IGFBP-3 [64]. The study was repeated after 1 year of rGH therapy, which induced an increase in lag phase and a decrease in MDA, which reached normal levels.

When studying adult GHD, Scacchi *et al* found higher peroxide levels and lower lag phase, measured by a fluorescence kinetic method; no correlation was discovered, at baseline, with IGF-1 levels [65]. The patients were retested after a 4 months rGH treatment; peroxide levels decreased and Lag-time increased, reaching values of controls; a correlation with IGF-1 – direct in the case of Lag-time and indirect in the case of lipoperoxides – was restored. Therefore, the short-term GH administration ameliorated oxidative patterns, at a dose which increased, but not fully normalized, IGF-1 levels.

GH in Children Obesity Both in adults and children nutritional status affects GH levels [66], in particular high levels are associated with low trunk fat in undernourished girls [67] and on the contrary overweight adolescents may have low GH levels, which may be related to higher trunk fat and lipid levels.

It has been formulated the hypothesis that overweight adolescents would have lower GH and higher cortisol levels than normal-weight adolescents and that these hormonal alterations in overweight adolescents would be related to visceral adipose tissue (VAT) and intramyocellular lipid (IMCL) accumulation, higher lipid levels, and greater severity of IR.

In their study, Misra *et al* demonstrated a lower GH peak at GHRH-Arginine stimulation test in overweight adolescents (independently associated with higher regional fat mass) than in normal weight girls, consistent with reported inverse associations of GH with body weight [67]. However, overnight integrated GH secretion was the same in both groups, possibly as a consequence of differences in the object of different test: the dynamic test assesses maximal secretory capacity of GH to stimuli and it is used to diagnose GH deficiency, night time GH sampling reflects GH secretion, but it cannot be used for diagnostic purpose. Furthermore in overweight girls group, an inverse associations between GH concentrations and measures of body fat has been reported, consistent with similar findings in obese adults [68, 69] and with the greater truncal adiposity reported in GH-deficient children [70] and adults [71]. It remains unclear whether lower GH concentrations in overweight conditions lead to increased trunk fat accumulation or whether greater truncal adiposity leads to decreased GH secretion.

The same authors found an inverse association of GH and IGF-1 with Leptin in overweight girls, even if it is not clear if high Leptin levels cause a decrease in peak GH secretion or whether lower GH concentrations are associated with increased fat mass and, therefore, higher Leptin levels.

On the contrary mean IGF-1 levels were no different between obese and normal weight girls consistent with another study in overweight adolescents [72].

As night time GH sampling measures physiological GH secretion, it is possible that maximal secretory capacity of GH is decreased in overweight girls before physiological secretory capacity is affected. In fact, subjects in this study were certainly not as heavy as those in some other studies showing decreased overnight GH secretion [72, 73]. In addition, night time GH secretion is always higher than daytime GH secretion, thus influencing assessment of GH secretion over 24 h, and inducing a difference between the groups, with lower GH levels in overweight girls.

Within overweight girls, strong positive associations of IGF-1 with log peak GH on the GHRH-arginine test and log mean GH from frequent sampling overnight has been in summary described It is therefore possible that greater severity of overweight may be associated with lower IGF-1 levels in adolescents in association with lower GH levels. In addition, IGF-1 secretion is driven not only by GH status, but also by nutritional status, and differences attributable to low GH secretory capacity in overweight girls may not be manifest because of fulsome nutritional status. Over nutrition should be associated with higher IGF-1 levels, which may, by negative feedback, cause a decrease in GH secretion, which in turn may lower IGF-1 levels.

In conclusion, the decrease of GH amount could negatively influence antioxidant systems, even if this hypothesis is at this moment speculative.

Thyroid

Thyroid and OS: Review of thyroid role in regulation of antioxidant systems has been already reported [74]. Previous studies have shown that both hyperthyroidism and hypothyroidism are associated with enhanced OS involving enzymatic and non-enzymatic antioxidants [75]. Besides, some complications of hyperthyroidism are due just to the OS in target tissues [76]. Thyroid hormones *per se* can act as oxidants and produce DNA-damage (contrasted by catalase), probably through the phenolic group, similar to that of steroidal estrogens [77]. Many other mechanisms, reviewed by Venditti & Di Meo (2006), can be involved: enhanced Nitric Oxide Synthase (NOS) gene expression with NO overproduction; activation of hepatic nuclear factor-kB and following increase of cytokines stimulating ROS generation; uncoupling mechanisms involving Uncoupling Protein (UCP)-2 and UCP-3, regulated by thyroid hormones; increased turnover of mitochondrial proteins; mitoptosis, regulated by peroxisome proliferator-activated receptor gamma coactivator-1, which is upregulated by T3 administration. Thyroid hormones influence lipid composition of rat tissues and therefore the susceptibility to oxidative stress. However, there is specificity in tissue response, and discrepant effects of T3 and T4 are possible. In rat liver, T3-induced hyperthyroidism was found to be associated with altered lipid-peroxidation indices, including elevated levels of thiobarbituric reactive substances (TBARS) and hydroperoxides [78 - 81]. On the contrary, no change in TBARS was found in homogenized livers from rats made hyperthyroid by administration of T4 over a 4-week period [82]. As regards testis, no significant change (TBARS or hydroperoxides) was observed in lipid peroxidation of hyperthyroid adult rats, but hyperthyroidism promoted protein oxidation rate as indicated by an enhanced content of protein-bound carbonyls [83]. In conclusion, we should emphasize the fact of a tissue-linked variability in the effects of hyperthyroidism on the activity of antioxidant enzymes (Mn-SOD or Cu, Zn-SOD, catalase, glutathione-peroxidase) with differential effects of the two thyroid hormones [84].

At a systemic level, also in humans, hyperthyroidism has been associated with reduced circulating levels of alpha-tocopherol [85, 86] and CoQ_{10} [87]. CoQ_{10} showed a trend to increase in hypothyroidism [87]; it appeared to be a sensitive index of tissue effect of thyroid hormones, in situations in which drug interference, such as amiodarone [88], or systemic illness inducing a low-T3 conditions [89] complicate the interpretation of thyroid hormone levels.

However, data on hypothyroidism in humans are conflicting. Baskol *et al* showed in a group of 33 patients with primary hypothyroidism elevated MDA and NO levels and low paraoxonase (PON)-1 activity, while superoxide dismutase (SOD) was not different from controls. Interestingly, thyroid treatment decreased MDA and increased PON1, without reaching levels observed in controls [90]. They concluded that a prooxidant environment in hypothyroidism could play a role in the pathogenesis of atherosclerosis in such patients. Elevated MDA levels were also shown in subclinical hypothyroidism [91]; the increased in OS was attributed to lack of antioxidants but also to altered lipid metabolism, since MDA showed a correlation with LDL-cholesterol, total cholesterol and triglycerides. Total antioxidant status (TAS) was similar in overt hypothyroidism, subclinical hypothyroidism and controls.

Different studies confirmed the NO elevation [92, 93]. Data on other parameters are more conflicting. As PON-1 is concerned, a decreased activity was observed both in hypo- and hyperthyroidism [94], while not significant differences with controls were shown in other studies [92].

Another study [95] showed increased levels of TBARS, but also of antioxidants, such as SOD, CAT and Vitamin E. All these parameters correlated with T3; moreover the correlation between T3 and CAT remained significant also when corrected with total cholesterol. While TBARS elevation was shown also in some studies [93, 96], other studies did not confirm the datum in overt hypothyroidism [92] and in subclinical hypothyroidism [97].

We showed low Total Antioxidant Capacity (TAC) levels in hypothyroid patients [98] and increased CoQ_{10} levels also in secondary hypothyroidism (mainly due to its metabolic role in mitochondrial respiratory chain and therefore underutilized in hypothyroid tissue). In the last case, hypothyroidism has a predominant effect on other conditions influencing CoQ_{10} in opposite direction, such as acromegaly and hypoadrenalism [98, 99].

Finally, new perspectives concern DUOX (Dual OXidase) genes expression, which is crucial for H_2O_2 generation essential for thyroid peroxidase (TPO)-catalyzed thyroid hormone synthesis [100]. Two oxidases of such family are present in thyroid (DUOX1 and DUOX2) and work together maturation factors (DUOXA1 and DUOXA2), which allow DUOX proteins to translocate to the follicular cell membrane and exert their enzymatic activity (OHYE). Cases of hypothyroidism due to mutation of DUOX or DUOXA genes have been presented in literature [100, 101]. While defects of this system interfere with thyroid hormone synthesis, another new intracellular ROS generating system has been demonstrated in the human thyroid gland: NADPH oxidase 4 (NOX4) [102]; defects in such a system could be associated with thyroid cancer (via activation by H-Ras oncogene) and Hashimoto's thyroiditis (in such a situation increased extracellular production cause an increased Intercellular Adhesion Molecule 1 (ICAM-1) expression and cytokine release) [103].

Thyroid in Children Obesity: Different studies, as reviewed by Reinehr [104] and Pacifico [105] show a slightly increased TSH level both in adult and childhood obesity. TSH is significantly correlated with BMI as demonstrated by cross-sectional and longitudinal studies as reviewed by Pacifico [105]. In our experience a group of 27 children showed a mean ± ES TSH level of 2,86 ± 0,52mcU/ml significantly greater than normal weight controls (2 ± 0,87) [106]. A positive correlation between weight gain during five years and progressive TSH increase has been observed [107] suggesting that small differences in thyroid function can influence BMI due to the effect of thyroid hormones on energy balance. However other studies suggest that obesity *per se* can induce an alteration of pituitary-thyroid axis [108]. Different studies have explored the TSH modifications after weight loss, obtained by diet or different bariatric surgery techniques (bilio-pancreatic diversion, Roux-en-Y gastric by-pass, vertical gastroplasty). Studies in obese children are less numerous, but seem to confirm that normalization of thyroid hormones follows weight loss [109 - 112]. It is important to underline that, despite changes in TSH do not always correlate with weight loss or modification of body composition [113, 114], decrease in TSH, predict an improvement of insulin resistance [114].

TSH alterations are coupled with normal T4 levels and T3 levels slightly elevated or in the upper normal range. Among the causes of TSH increase, subclinical hypothyroidism seems to be infrequent. It could be related to autoimmunity or iodine deficiency which exhibits low prevalence [115]. Similarly higher prevalence of TSH elevation in absence of Thyroid auto-antibodies has been reported [116, 117]. The TSH response to TRH has been found low [118], normal or exaggerated [115, 119]. Pretreatment with pyridostigmine, an inhibitor of acetylcholinesterase, is able to increase the TSH response to TRH in adults but not in children, suggesting a differential modulation of somatostatinergic tone in different ages [118]. Other possible explanations for TSH levels in obesity include:

- Reduced TSH bio-activity;
- Alterations in TSH R-gene;
- Thyroid hormone resistance;
- Alterations of central control of TSH;

The last one could be explained by different mechanisms: a special role could be exerted by Leptin. Many data support this hypothesis:

- Direct correlation between TSH and Leptin;
- Presence of Leptin receptors in arterial pituitary gland;
- Similar circadian rhythms;
- Altered pattern of TSH secretion in Leptin deficient adults.

However this relationship seems to be reciprocal, since TSH induces differentiations and proliferation of adipocytes and stimulates Leptin secretion by adipose tissue.

Whatever the mechanisms involved the modifications of pituitary thyroid axis could express a compensatory phenomenon. The increase in T3 can lead to increased energy expenditure, as expected due to the role of thyroid hormones in basal metabolic rate. However an unfavorable consequence could be an increase of radical production due to overstimulation of mitochondrial respiratory chain and therefore increase in OS.

Adrenal Glands

Adrenals and OS Redox balance is strictly related to adrenal gland physiology. The physiological formation of free radicals during steroidogenesis is under investigation, concerning glucocorticoids, androgens and estrogens. An unpaired electron is localized at position 20 in glucocorticoids, whereas it is at position 3 in the other steroid hormones [120]. The pathway of biosynthesis involves a sequence of transformations catalyzed by cytochrome P450 enzymes. It has been hypothesized that interaction of P450 enzymes with certain steroids acting as pseudosubstrates may cause a damage appearing as a steroidogenic enzyme deficiency. The high content of ascorbate may serve to protect P450 enzymes from the damaging effects of ROS formed as results of P450/pseudosubstrate interactions [121].

Ascorbic acid (Asc) is a cofactor required both in catecholamine synthesis and adrenal steroidogenesis: an overview of *in vitro* and *in vivo* studies on the role of vitamin C in adrenal cortex was published [122]. The authors also studied a model of mutant mice lacking the plasma membrane transporter SVCT2, which, for the severity of decrease in tissue levels of Asc, die soon after birth, with evidence of depletion of catecholamines storage vesicles and decreased plasma levels of corticosterone.

Asc probably participates also in steroidogenic monoxygenase system in the adrenal cortex with the aid of regenerating system including outer mitochondrial membrane cytochrome b. In mutants rats unable to synthesize Asc, increase in aldosterone concentration after Na-deficiency was selectively suppressed. Other data suggest that enhanced aldosterone formation (catalized by P450-aldo) may be supported by Asc with its regenerating system [123]. Tissue Asc level is affected during the estrous phase and by contraceptive steroid therapy, ovariectomy [124]. These data could potentially have a relation with dietary antioxidants.

Hyperaldosteronism, on the other hand, plays a permissive role in leading to altered redox state. Among the involved mechanisms, a PTH mediated intracellular Ca^{++} overloading leads to OS, which can be prevented with anti-aldosteronic drugs, Ca-channel blockers or antioxidants [125].

Aldosterone concentrations are inappropriately high in many patients with hypertension. Besides causing sodium retention and increasing blood pressure, mineralocorticoid receptor (MR) activation induces OS, endothelial dysfunction, inflammation and subsequently fibrosis. MR may be activated by aldosterone and cortisol or via transactivation by AT1 receptor through a mechanism involving Epidermal Growth Factor Receptor (EGFR) and Mitogen-activated protein kinase (MAPK). These mechanisms, together with rapid non-genomic effects of aldosterone on heart and vascular system [126], contribute to the increased cardiovascular risk in these patients. Moreover, aldosterone-induced OS plays a role in impairing insulin signaling [127]. In the cardiometabolic syndrome, the activation of renin-angiotensin-aldosterone system contributes to the alteration of insulin/IGF-1 signaling pathways and to ROS formation inducing endothelial dysfunction and cardiovascular disease [128]. In turn ROS, also induced by adipokines such as TNF-α, non-esterified fatty acids, angiotensinogen, *etc.*, can activate MR receptors, in an aldosterone-independent way, as demonstrated in rats [129]. Finally, OS is implicated in the physiopathology of cardiac dysfunction leading to heart failure. In this case an addictive effect of several components of neuro-hormonal activation (catecholamines, angiotensin, aldosterone, TNF-α, endothelin, cytokines) to enhance OS has been hypothesized, since it can cause cardiomyocyte apoptosis, ventricular remodeling, mechano-electric uncoupling and endothelial dysfunction [130].

All the reported data can assume relevance considering the interrelationships between obesity and hypertension, even in young people.

As regards DHEAS, some data are available on exogenous DHEA, that can exert a dual effect (antioxidant or prooxidant) depending on the dose and tissue specificity [131, 132]. It prevents oxidative injury in obstructive jaundice in rats. When administered to male Wistar rats it produces significant differences in some parameters of OS in rats hearts, suggesting a prooxidant answer in this model [133].

The main knowledge about cortisol and OS comes from the animal model of adrenalectomized (Adx) rat. Removal of both adrenal glands significantly reduced the content of MDA in gastric tissue and erythrocytes in comparison with sham-operated rats, suggesting a factor in the adrenal gland that may predispose to MDA production. However data in literature on lipid peroxidation associated with adrenalectomy in different rat tissues are controversial [134]. Toleikis found that *in vitro* lipid peroxidation decreased in liver, lung and kidney homogenates of Wistar rats after adrenalectomy [135]. On the contrary, an *in vivo* study by Hidalgo showed that TBARS in liver tissue were higher in Adx group than in sham-operated one [136]. In the same study, liver TBARs levels were lower in corticosterone-administered Adx group. In a study by Yildirim gastric tissue MDA levels in Adx rats treated with prednisolone were higher than in Adx-alone rats. In contrast, in Adx rats treated with epinephrine, erythrocyte MDA concentration was higher than in Adx rats, suggesting an organ-specific effect of adrenal hormones on lipid peroxidation may be present. Toleikis also showed a significant increase in erythrocyte GSH levels in Adx rats [134].

An increase in lipid peroxidation and a decrease in blood plasma tocopherol was described in patients with chronic adrenocortical failure, suggesting the inclusion of antioxidants in the therapeutic approach to these patients [137].

A link was found between exercise-induced cortisol increase, muscle enzyme levels and antioxidant systems [138]. Moreover, OS is increased in genetic syndromes with hypoadrenalism, such as X-linked adrenoleukodystrophy [139]. Therefore, it can be hypothesized some metabolic alterations in adrenal failure (surprisingly similar to those observed in the chronic fatigue syndrome) can be related to CoQ_{10} deficiency [140].

Indexes of oxidative stress (MDA and levels of SOD) were present in patients with Cushing's syndrome (CS), joint to markers of endothelial dysfunction (ICAM-1). However increased ICAM-1 concentrations persisted after operation and the most pronounced impairment of microvascular activity was present in patients with hypertension and diabetes mellitus [141].

Relative incompetence of blood α-tocopherol (with absence of increasing age-related levels as in normal subjects) accompanied by its decreased levels in the red blood cells was described [142].

Finally, a significant lowering in plasma thiol levels (even when corrected for albumin), consistent with OS, were shown in animal models (equine Cushing's disease) [143].

Since cardiovascular disease is the major cause of morbidity and mortality in CS, mechanisms underlying this phenomenon are under investigation [144], together with changes induced by short-term cortisol administration in normotensive healthy men. Among the candidate mechanisms, by which cortisol could contribute to elevate blood pressure, are the inhibition of the vasodilator NO system and an increase in vasoconstrictor erythropoietin concentration [145].

Glucocorticoid excess triggers overproduction of ROS, which contribute to disrupt NO availability in endothelium, leading to vascular complications and also acting to modify kidney structure and function [146].

Physical and psychological stressors, which activate hypothalamic-hypophyseal-adrenal (HHA) axis, also cause oxidative damage. What is the role of adrenal hormones? A study was performed in restrain stress in rats, evaluating the effect of low, intermediate and high doses of corticosterone on antioxidant defenses. A coordinate decreases of activities in the brain, liver and heart of free-radical scavenging enzymes SOD, CAT, glutathione S-transferase (GST) and glutathione-reductase (GR), as well as the non-enzymatic antioxidants GSH and serum urate. Lipid peroxidation and protein carbonyl contents significantly increased in brain, liver, heart. This study is very important since suggests that stress hormones have a causal role in impacting oxidative processes induced during the adaptive response.

On the other hand, adaptation to stress induces a panel of stress-response proteins at cellular level. For example, thioredoxin (TRX) is significantly induced under oxidative conditions [147]. Either antisense TRX expression or cellular treatment with H_2O_2 negatively modulates glucocorticoid receptor (GR) function and decreases glucocorticoid-inducible gene expression. Impaired cellular response to glucocorticoids is rescued by overexpression of TRX: not only the ligand binding domain but also the DNA binding domain of the GR is a target of TRX. Therefore cellular glucocorticoid responsiveness is coordinately modulated by the redox state and TRX level, suggesting the importance of the cross-talk between neuroendocrine control of stress response and cellular antioxidant systems [148].

Common pathophysiological pathways in stress related diseases were described, involving stress hormones (cortisol, NE) on one hand and NO activity on the other hand [149]. Similarly OS and inflammation are traditionally associated with fatigue and impaired recovery from exercise, and antioxidant supplementation has a positive effect on alteration in markers of inflammation (cytokines, C Reactive Protein or CRP) joint to cortisol response [150]. However, supplementation of Vitamin E to improve performance and minimizing exercise-induced muscle damage is debated because of unclear evidences, at least in humans [151].

Due to the importance of oxidative stress in physiopathology of adrenal gland, we performed studies evaluating both TAC and CoQ_{10}. A further rationale for studying CoQ_{10} in pituitary-adrenal disease was the common biosynthetic pathway of cholesterol and ubiquinone.

We have therefore assayed plasma CoQ_{10} levels in different conditions with increased or defective activity of pituitary-adrenal axis (3 subjects with ACTH-dependent adrenal hyperplasia, 2 cases of Cushing's disease and 1 case of 17---hydroxylase deficiency; 10 subjects with secondary hypoadrenalism, including three subjects with also secondary hypothyroidism) [152]. CoQ_{10} levels were significantly lower in isolated hypoadrenalism than in patients with adrenal hyperplasia and multiple pituitary deficiencies (mean ± SEM: 0.57±0.04 vs 1.08±0.08 and 1.10±0.11 µg/ml, respectively). When corrected for cholesterol levels, the same trend was observed, but not reaching the statistical significance. These data indicate that secretion of adrenal hormones is in some way related to CoQ_{10} levels, both in augmented and reduced conditions. However in secondary hypoadrenalism, some other pituitary dependent axes can be affected. Therefore we compared patients with post-surgical isolated hypoadrenalism with those who presented also hypothyroidism. Since thyroid hormones have an important role in modulating CoQ_{10} levels and metabolism, when coexistent, thyroid deficiency seems to play a prevalent role instead of adrenal deficiency.

Studies performed in adrenal disease should be particularly important to understand physiopathology in childhood obesity. Despite CS is relatively uncommon, the modifications of pituitary-adrenal axis related to dietary habits or stress could be relevant, in such critical period, for the dysregulation in adult age.

Adrenals in Childhood Obesity Obesity symptoms and signs could be often confused with CS and, *de facto*, obese children are relatively hypercortisolemic [153, 154] (pseudo-CS) [155].

Obese non-Cushingoid children show normal basal plasma, salivary and urinary free cortisol concentrations (UFC), normal basal ACTH concentrations and diurnal variation and the response to dexamethasone is maintained. In other reports UFC (a measure of cortisol excess) was higher in overweight than in normal-weight girls. Mean serum cortisol concentrations (an integrated measure of cortisol secretion overnight) were also higher but did not reach significant differences. Within overweight girls, log mean cortisol concentrations were inversely and independently associated with subcutaneous adipose tissue. Finally, there are evidences that body fat mass correlates with total excretion of glucocorticoid metabolites and consequently increased cortisol secretion and turnover.

The biochemical effects of steroid explain phenotypic characteristics: high cortisol levels have antilipolytic effects [156] and are associated with increased trunk fat [157, 158]. Higher cortisol levels in overweight adolescents may also contribute to increased trunk fat and higher lipid levels [153]. Moreover they can predict the degree of insulin resistance and lipid elevations [153].

CS is a rare entity, especially in children [159], but the presentation is characterized by weight gain associated to growth failure. Therefore the differential diagnosis with simple obesity is mandatory. Most common causes in children include exogenous glucocorticoid administration or ACTH production by pituitary gland [160]. Some features are different from the adult disease: the prevalence in males, the predominance of mixed androgen and cortisol secreting adrenocortical tumors, the association with genetic disorders such as McCune-Albright Syndrome [161].

However, recently new relationships between cortisol and adipose tissue have been discovered: the alteration of enzymes which metabolize cortisone to cortisol (hydroxy-steroid-dehydrogenase Type 1) [162] are responsible for increased cortisol production at adipose tissue, so justifying the term "CS of the omentum" [163]. Another new field, to be explored in childhood obesity, is the activation of mineralocorticoid receptor, with effects on differentiation of preadipocytes, induction of cytokines, down regulation of uncoupling protein 1 [162, 164].

No associations of cortisol with Adiponectin, which was associated inversely only with measures of body fat, was found. Although similar associations have been reported in prepubertal children [165], there are no previous reports of associations of cortisol with insulin resistance and lipids in pubertal children, showing a modulation related to dietary habits and age maturation, which requires further investigation.

In summary, the increased activation of pituitary-adrenal axis could be a factor inducing OS in obese children.

Gonads

Gonads and OS Sex differences in antioxidant modulation can be related to genetic background or to the milieu of circulating hormones, especially after puberty, which, as it has been reported above, can be anticipated in obese children. Despite the focus of the review concerns childhood obesity and therefore the role of steroids should be irrelevant, we report data on both male and female sex hormones, due to the relevance for cardiovascular risk.

Male Sex Hormones Different models seem to suggest a prooxidant effect of testosterone. It activates lipid peroxidation (LPO), counterbalanced by estrogen, in the aorta of rats both *in vitro* and *in vivo*, irrespective of dose and duration of treatment [166]. In male spontaneous hypertensive rats (SHR), that exhibit a blunted pressure-natriuresis relationship, enhanced oxidative stress was observed, compared with female SHR. In fact, male SHR had enhanced urinary excretion of H_2O_2 which decreased after gonadectomy. In inner kidney medullary, male SHR had a testosterone-dependent increase in SOD activity. Both intact and gonadectomized males had high levels of catalase activity, which are interpreted as compensatory to the increase in whole body ROS production [167].

On the other hand, protective effects of androgens on OS were investigated in other models, such as neuronal cells [168, 169].

More important are the studies investigating gonadal steroids, OS and cardiovascular risk. In an animal model, castration increased aortic atheroma formation and testosterone replacement reduced this effect [170]. In addition, testosterone has direct vasoactive properties, which are a direct effect on the vascular smooth muscle, not mediated by the nuclear androgen receptor, because the effect is too rapid and is not reduced by flutamide, a nuclear androgen receptor blocker [171 - 173]. Many other studies, with comparative effects of androgens and estrogens are reported below, in the section of female sex hormones.

Recent studies have shown men with coronary artery disease (CAD) have significantly lower concentrations of bioavailable testosterone than men with normal angiograms [174], and prevalence of hypogonadism in a group of men with CAD is about twice than observed in general population [175]. Hypotestosteronemia is associated with an atherogenic lipid profile (elevated low density lipoproteins and triglycerides, decreased high density lipoprotein), high fibrinogen with a hypercoagulable state, an increase in insulin resistance and hyperinsulinaemia, and higher systolic and diastolic blood pressure [176]. When testosterone is instilled into the left coronary artery, vasodilatation ensues and coronary flow increases [177]. More importantly, acute administration of intravenous testosterone improves exercise tolerance and reduces angina threshold in men with CAD [178, 179]. Non-genomic effects of testosterone on vascular smooth muscle cells were more extensively studied [180, 181].

OS can underlie the above mentioned clinical conditions. Low testosterone and androgen deficiency were demonstrated by statistical meta-analysis to be associated with increased risk for developing the metabolic syndrome over time [182], even if pathophysiological details of these changes in atherosclerosis [183] and implications in testosterone replacement therapy [184] are still under investigation.

In a recent work, Total Antioxidant Capacity (TAC) was determined during cardiovascular bypass surgery in patients with CAD: TAC decreased during surgery, but no further decrease in TAC was observed during reperfusion, indicating that it is a relatively stable index of the antioxidant barrier of the body [185]. Finally, a relationship between sex hormones and plasmatic TAC was observed, using a novel automatized measurement method [186]. TAC, expressed as millimole Trolox equivalent/L significantly correlated with total testosterone in male subjects and also with estradiol in a group of pre- and post-menopausal women [187].

To investigate the role of gonadal steroids in systemic antioxidant regulation, we determined plasma CoQ_{10} and Total Antioxidant Capacity (TAC) in post-surgical hypopituitaric patients. Twenty-six patients, aged 28-55 yrs, were studied 6 to 12 months after operation. Sixteen patients presented low testosterone values and were also studied after treatment with testosterone enantate. CoQ_{10} levels were significantly lower in isolated hypogonadism than in normogonadism. Testosterone treatment induced a significant change both in CoQ_{10} level and TAC. CoQ_{10} and TAC values significantly correlated, suggesting an inter-relationship between different antioxidants [188]. Our data suggest that hypogonadism could represent a condition of OS, in turn related with augmented cardiovascular risk. Further studies are needed to clarify if precocious onset of OS can anticipate or worsen this phenomenon.

Female Sex Hormones Also in case of estrogens, literature is enormous and not fully unequivocal. Both pro-oxidant and anti-oxidant effects are reported depending on the kind of estrogen and different models studied.

There is evidence that 17-β-Estradiol (E2) induces ROS production in mitochondria as signal-transducing messengers. In this way it activates the binding of three oxidant-sensitive transcription factors: Activator Protein 1 (AP-

1), cAMP-response-element Binding Protein (CREB) and Nuclear Respiratory Factor 1 [189]. However, the production of ROS seems to exert negative effect and explain a sex-related differential longevity [190]. It was shown mitochondria from female rats generate half the amount of hydrogen peroxide than those from males and have higher levels of mitochondrial reduced glutathione. Estrogens bind to E-receptors and, via activation of MAP kinase and NfKb pathways, resulting in an up-regulation of antioxidant enzymes. Moreover, the 16S rRNA expression, which decreases significantly with aging, is 4 times higher in mitochondria from females than age-matched males. On the contrary, the oxidative damage of mitochondrial DNA is fourfold higher in males than females. Finally, ovariectomy abolishes these sex differences and estrogen replacement rescues the effect of ovariectomy. ROS produced during moderate exercise, as during training, up-regulate the expression of antioxidants in muscle stress. Findings in transgenic animal overexpressing Mn-SOD or catalase strongly support this view [191]. Also sex differences in severity of inflammatory diseases (atherosclerosis, neurological disorders, rheumatoid arthritis, periodontitis, *etc.*) can be attributed to female sex hormones [192].

Estrogens and anti-estrogens, like tamoxifene and toremifene, have shown to have strong membrane antioxidant properties *in vitro*, not due to scavenging of free radicals, also confirmed in living organisms [193]. 17-β-E2, like some other antioxidants, activate membrane-bound guanylate cyclase, in PC12 cells, as model of developing neurons [194].

In other models (rat liver microsomes, with lipid peroxidation determined by measuring TBARS after exposure to various prooxidants) catecholestrogens appeared to be the most strong antioxidants, even if estrogens and catecholestrogens interact with the peroxidative process at different levels [138]. In microsomes from rat liver estradiol and 2-hydroxyestradiol were able to inhibit the initial stage of microsomal LP [195]. The same study showed LP of erythrocyte membranes exhibited different patterns of biochemical interactions promoted by these two estrogens.

Protective effects of estrogens on ter-butylhydroperoxide-induced hepatocyte damage were studied *in vitro*, suggesting that this protection may be related not only to their antioxidant activity against free radicals, but also to the maintenance of the normal redox status of cells, which partially restores intracellular GSH levels [196]. Even if these models could appear very specific it must be kept in mind the precocious onset of non-alcoholic fatty liver disease in childhood. Another model of hepatotoxicity is the effect of ferrylmyoglobin, with early lipid peroxidation and further decrease in GSH and ATP.

Neutrophil granulocytes play an important role in atherogenesis also through their free radical generation. Despite the conflicting results in literature [197 - 200], a suppressive effect on superoxide anion production of human neutrophil granulocytes by 17-β-E2, progesterone and testosterone was demonstrated [201]. This *in vitro* investigation also showed an effect of weak estrogens, like estrone and estriol, on superoxide anion production in human neutrophil granulocytes similar to that of estradiol.

In ovariectomized Wistar rats, administration of estradiol reduced MDA, together with a slight decline in catalase and SOD, with no modification of Vitamins A and E. The addition of medroxyprogesterone did not further modify these results [202]. In rat uterus of the same animal model, a linear correlation between estradiol and LPO was found. This phenomenon was in part modulated by the inverse correlation between uterine catalase and uterine MDA [203].

As far as vascular system is concerned, estrogen depletion after ovariectomy in rats induced, via OS, the activation of heme-oxygenase 1 (HO-1), an inducible stress protein. NO/iNOS system contributes to the induction of HO-1, which may subsequently suppress iNOS activity. Estradiol replacement reversed these effects [204].

A dual modulation of permeability in endothelial cells, by eNOS- and iNOS-related mechanisms, is exerted by estrogens, as shown in cultures of human umbilical vein endothelial cells [205].

In an experiment with three cellular cultures (bovine aortic endothelial cells, placental trophoblasts and macrophages), opposite effects of estrogens and progestins were found on the protection from LDL oxidation [206]. Progestins promoted LDL oxidation and conjointly endothelial cells cytotoxicity, while estrogens had antioxidant and cytoprotective effects. Moreover, progestins (especially medroxyprogesterone acetate and levonorgestrel) opposed the effects of estrogens when given in combination [207].

An interesting review on the cellular and molecular mechanisms underlying vasculoprotective action of estrogens [208] explains how E2 can act through a non-genomic stimulation of membrane/intracellular mediators and/or the classical genomic pathway. In this way E2 improves vasomotion modulating vasoconstrictor and vasodilator systems, affects remodeling of the vascular wall and modulates vascular inflammatory response.

Estradiol is so effective as α-tocopherol in terms of defense against fatty acid peroxidation, but far more effective against cholesterol peroxidation [209]. However, oxidability of lipoproteins *in vitro* and inhibition of this phenomenon by antioxidants *in vivo* is still under investigation [210].

As human studies are concerned, erythrocyte GPx is influenced during the menstrual cycle: higher GPx activity was found from the later follicular to early luteal phase. A significant correlation was observed between E2 and GSH-Px cycle-related changes, while no significant cycle phase-dependent variation was found in pyruvate kinase activity [211].

The above reported experimental data support the controversies on estrogen replacement therapy and cardioprotection [212]. Initially attributed to LDL lowering and HDL increasing, this protective effect is centered on decreased LDL oxidation. A direct effect on arterial tissue and a modulation of vascular reactivity through NO and prostaglandin synthesis, based on both receptoral and immediate non-genomic mechanisms, are also involved. Recently another mechanism was hypothesized implicating the esterification of estrogens in HDL and the transfer to LDL. Despite these mechanisms, recent placebo-controlled studies in women with CHD failed to show beneficial effects of hormone replacement therapy on coronary events, even if mutations in thrombogenic genes may represent an important confounding factor [212, 213].

Postmenopausal women develop visceral obesity and insulin resistance and show an increase risk for type 2 diabetes [213]. This matter can also be inserted in the general field of the interaction between exercise and diet to modulate endogenous antioxidant defense [214] and, once again, the role of childhood onset of OS and its prevention remains to be established.

Gonads in Children Obesity According to Lee *et al.*, in children between 36 and 54 months and overweight between 3 and 9 years of age, overweight increases the risks of precocious thelarche and may reduce the age of menarche [215]. The mechanism underlying this observation could be related with Leptin, which in normal weight children rises transiently before the onset of puberty, thus promoting gonadotropin secretion. In obesity as above described plasma Leptin levels are high and this fact can produce early sex maturation, especially in girls. Often both obese boys and girls show premature adrenarche rather than a true puberty and teenage obese girls develop more often than normal weight girls ovarian hyperandrogenism with mild hirsutism, acne, anovulation and menstrual irregularity.

In these girls there is an excess of IGF-1 which acts in synergy with adrenocorticotropic hormone (ACTH), which stimulates the adrenocortical cells, and with luteinizing hormone (LH), which stimulates ovarian theca cells with a following higher androgen secretion. These effects are mediated through induction of P450c 17α-hydroxylase activity. The bioavailability of androgens is increased due to the suppression of hepatic expression of sex hormone binding globulin (SHBG) and its reduced plasma concentration operated by high level of insulin. Low levels of SHBG in turn increase free androgens and consequently frequency of gonadotropin-releasing hormone (GnRH) pulses and the ratio of LH to follicle-stimulating hormone (FSH), thereby exacerbating thecal androgen production. The increase in free androgens may also induce precocious adrenarche in prepubertal girls and boys and may cause anovulation and hirsutism in adolescent girls and young women [216, 217].

For what concern obese boys, total and free testosterone is generally normal but may decline with weight gain (in association with a fall in gonadotropin concentrations) and reverse with weight loss. Furthermore aromatization of androstenedione in adipose tissue increases plasma estrone concentrations, causing gynecomastia in adolescent boys.

As above stated, hypotestosteronemia could be included among the constellation of MetS. Due to protective effect of testosterone via antioxidants, this could be another factor inducing OS in obese children.

Adipose tissue (Leptin and Kisspeptin)

Since these peptides have been extensively described before, we only remark some their possible correlation with OS. Different Leptin actions are well known, including regulation of appetite, energy homeostasis, neuroendocrine influences, and regulation of hypothalamic-pituitary-gonadal axis. More recently, the role of Leptin in cardiovascular system has been investigated: Leptin has been shown to exert a vasodilator effect via endothelial-cell (EC)-dependent and independent mechanisms [218]. For instance, Leptin (at concentrations observed in obesity) is capable of expanding rat and dog coronary arterioles [219]. Such an effect is prevented by EC denudation and NO synthase inhibition. Other evidences of effect on NO release from EC and the underlying biochemical mechanisms have been reported [220]. Evidence in humans are less strong [218], however taken together these studies underlie a possible role of hyperleptinemia in redox balance of endothelial cells.

Another new field concerns a possible role of Kisspeptin. A very recent study explored the model of mice KO for the gene of Kisspeptin Receptor (Kiss1rKO). In comparison with wild type animals adult females Kiss1rKO showed a marked increase in body weight and in Leptin concentrations and compromising of glucose tolerance. On the contrary males Kiss1rKO had normal body weight and glucose metabolism, suggesting a sex related differential modulation of metabolic Kisspeptin actions. Surprisingly females Kiss1rKO also showed decreased full food intake, but also motor activity and energetic expenditure. The bases for these findings are related to the capacity of Kisspeptin to modulate the sense of satiety and to the connections between Kisspeptin neurons and neurons secreting Pro-opio-melanocortin (POMC) and NPY [221].

In our context it seems particularly relevant to underline that metabolic Kisspeptin actions can in turn be joined to a modulatory role on oxidative stress at cellular levels, especially in liver [38]. The administration of Kisspeptin-10 can increase activity of antioxidant enzymes, such as SOD and Catalase with concomitant reduction of MDA, total antioxidant capacity and aspartic-amino transferase suggesting a protective antioxidant role at least in hepatic tissue.

ANTIOXIDANT-ENRICHED DIET AS A TREATMENT FOR OBESITY

As regards the topic of a possible role of antioxidant in the diet and treatment of obesity, a great number of studies is reported in literature concerning these two points: 1) dietary habits and cardiovascular risk; 2) effects of antioxidant supplementation on plasmatic parameters and on clinical course of MS and its complications.

As far as the first point is concerned, different epidemiological studies in non-diabetic people showed an inverse correlation between the degree of IR and circulating levels of several carotenoids [222, 223], which appeared further reduced in glucose intolerance and DM2 [224]. A decreased dietary intake of antioxidants has been shown in IR individuals in some studies [225] but not in others [226]. Some recent meta-analyses reached contrasting results: an inverse correlation between intake of salad/vegetables (but not fruit) was observed with the risk of diabetes [225]; however in other study the total antioxidant intake (rather than simply fruit and vegetables) was related to a protective effect from DM2 [226].

A diet rich in fruit and vegetables has been shown to protect from DM2 and Cardiovascular Disease (CVD), as demonstrated in prospective cohort studies [227, 228]. A reduced risk for DM2 has been also related to the intake of green leafy or dark yellow vegetables and coffee [229, 230].

Finally, as second aspect, a lot of studies investigated the effects of antioxidant enriched diet. Some data concern animal studies: in chronic renal failure rats, the administration of vitamin E, C and cathechin increased antioxidant activity and reduction of OS markers, also decreasing HOMA index [231]. Linoleic acid supplementations to Zucker obese rats improved the insulin sensitivity in several studies [232], probably acting as Peroxisome Proliferator-activated Receptor (PPAR) gamma agonist, and taurine showed a significant insulin-sensitizing effect both in acute [233] and chronic [234] conditions in animals and humans

[235]. In a rat model of diet-induced obesity and hypercholesterolemia, augmented carotenoid intake induces a significant decrease in oxidative stress markers and increase in SOD, catalase and GPX [236]. As human studies is concerned, dietary antioxidants decrease LDL oxidation in hyperlipemic patients [237, 238]. A cross-sectional study in 486 healthy women showed an inverse correlation between fruit and vegetables intake and plasma CRP levels; the prevalence of MetS was lower in high consumers of such kinds of diet [239].

Antioxidant enriched diet seems to be beneficial in independent way in respect to body weight reduction, as documented by the reduction in MDA after an 8-week moderately hypocaloric diet (based on specific seafood rich in omega3 fatty acids and taurine) [240] and some clinical trials [52, 241], even if not all studies confirm the results [242 - 244]. Moreover, is no clear association between antioxidant intake and modification of OS parameters and/or antioxidant system [245, 246]. In fact, after biliopancreatic diversion, the amelioration of IR is not accompanied by an augmented TAC in plasma [247]. In addition, the difficulty in measuring ROS, different methods of TAC determination, the still unknown relationship between plasma and intracellular redox status really complicate the interpretation of results of this study. However, in our opinion, the main reason is that antioxidants work as a strictly related network, and different pattern can be observed in different antioxidants, considered as a single parameter.

A recent paper of our group demonstrated that a natural antioxidant enriched diet is capable of reducing hyperinsulinemia in MetS and to enhance metformin effect in such patients [248]. Metformin affects gluconeogenesis, but it is also capable of augmenting insulin sensitivity through Insulin-related Substrate (IRS) mechanism [249]. An especially important role could be attributed to flavonoid, which was markedly increased in enriched diet, according to recent literature data [250 - 252].

Literature about antioxidant status and obesity in childhood is less extensive. Previous studies showed decreased levels of vitamins in plasma of obese children [50, 51, 253]. An important study showed in a group of 18 obese with mean age of 9.18 is a significant decrease of Vitamin E and lag phase (index of susceptibility of LDL to *in vitro* oxidation) (cancellato *and*) a significant increase in MDA when compared with healthy controls [12]. All altered indexes of oxidant status ameliorated with a 6 months period of dietary restriction, but returned to baseline after another 6-months period of free diet. These data indicate the reversibility of the status, correlated with hypocaloric diet. In our preliminary unpublished study total antioxidant capacity in children is significantly correlated with percent of fat mass (p=0,035) but mean levels are lower than those reached in adult age, suggesting that the maturation of antioxidants could not be complete and therefore children are especially exposed to OS.

It has been shown that OS is strictly linked to birth weight [254 - 256]. Park demonstrated a negative correlation between birth weight, IR, Ghrelin and CoQ_{10} level; a positive correlation was instead found between BMI and Leptin and finally a negative correlation between BMI and α-tocopherol and lycopene [257]. Interestingly classifying children by tertiles of birth weight, the higher tertile group showed an increased OS (decreased CoQ_{10} and catalase activity). The literature on CoQ_{10} is not unequivocal: in fact in obese patients with metabolic syndrome increased plasma total CoQ_{10} and ubiquinol concentrations were described [258] and CoQ_{10} was increased also in childhood obesity [259]. We described a lowering of CoQ_{10} after weight loss induced by bilio-pancreatic diversion [247]. However the interpretation of plasmatic levels of CoQ_{10} is complex due to different roles of this parameter involved in oxidant status but also in energy metabolism and strictly related to thyroid hormones as above discussed.

When considering the composition of the diet, it has been shown that children with chronic constipation, with low intake of dietary fibers, were twice as likely to be obese [260]. In a crossover study with obese children, 15 g/day of dietary fiber plus an hypocaloric diet resulted in a greater mean weight loss [261]. A review of nutraceutical in early infancy is reported by Pignatelli [262].

Many interventional studies are focused on metabolic consequences of obesity, in particular Non Alcoholic Fatty Liver Disease (NAFLD) and again were not fully in agreement. Moreover the period of observation is short ranging from 1 to 24 months. They mainly concern the administration of Vitamin E, alone or combined with Vitamin C and lifestyle intervention [263 - 268]. Vitamin E has been shown to lower aminotransferase levels in a pilot study in obese children with NAFLD [269], while another of these studies [268] showed greater efficacy of lifestyle in comparison with Vitamin E. A decrease in OS markers and an increase in antioxidants has been observed in hypercholesterolemic non obese children who consumed mandarin juice [270]. Based on these experiences same authors explored the effects of a supplemented hypocaloric diet with mandarin juice which is rich in Vitamin C, flavonoids and carotenoids in comparison with simple hypocaloric diet [271]. The supplemented group showed a decrease in products of OS, such as MDA and Carbonil groups and an increase in both α-tocopherol and in intracellular glutathione. However due to the short period of observation (four weeks) these data need a further confirmation.

Another trial was performed with a combination of Vitamin E and C with selenium for a period of 4 months, in a programme of lifestyle intervention, again in obese children and adolescents. Interestingly, this treatment induced significant changes in OS parameters (increase in α-tocopherol, ascorbic acid and selenium, with decrease of 8-iso-prostaglandin $F_{2\alpha}$), but a partial response in liver enzymes and no variation in parameters of systemic inflammation [272]. The discrepancy of effects *in vivo* and *in vitro* could be explained by the complex interrelationships between different status of single antioxidants, other hormone adaptive responses, the duration of treatment and the difficulty to evaluate the real compliance to diet intervention, physical exercises and other factors influencing energetic balance, especially in the population of prepubertal patients.

In summary, the composition of the diet and the enrichment with natural antioxidants seem to be particularly important, also considering that some studies claimed an increase in markers of OS and major compromising of endothelial function after different diets used in treating obesity [273].

CONCLUSION

All the reported studies underline the risk connected to childhood obesity. In addition to excess energy intake, nutrients have a specific role in the development of inflammation via the regulation of adipokine gene expression and secretion. In this way, it is possible to choose non-inflammatory or anti-inflammatory foods to minimize postprandial oxidative stress and inflammation. Therefore, lifestyle modifications, consisting of a reduction in caloric intake, a diet focused on particular macronutrient or micronutrient intake, and the encouragement of a regular exercise program with a personalized format, type and duration may reduce the consequences of childhood obesity. Hormonal pattern modified by the condition of obesity should be remarked in these inter relationships. Some hormonal changes appeared as a consequence of augmented body weight/fat mass, expressing in most cases compensatory mechanisms. However hormone themselves influence the oxidative status of the body especially thyroid hormones, other pituitary dependent axis and, as more recently evidenced, also adipocytokines, with a vicious circle (Fig. **1**).

Insufficient data are reported on antioxidant modulation by endocrine system in childhood. Most papers concern *in vitro* studies or, in case of studies in humans, models referring to cardiovascular disease and endocrine disorders in adult people. Studies in ageing are abundant especially in relation to degenerative disorders or cancer. However, from the analysis of such literature, as reported in the present chapter, it appears that oxidative stress in childhood obesity is the consequence of both phenomena: systemic inflammation and hormonal pattern changes. However the strategies of intervention can be directed on the two extreme of these self-reinforcing chains: lifestyle and antioxidant diet.

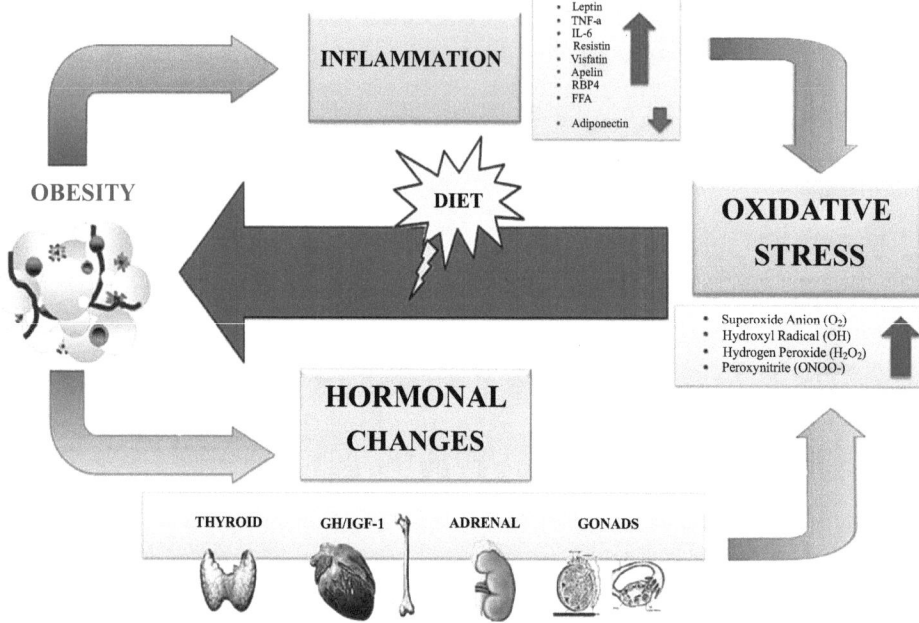

Fig. (1). Hypothetical model of interrelationship between dietary, inflammatory and hormonal consequences and OS.

Therefore we have reviewed the role of natural antioxidants in diet, as well as the administration of pharmacological antioxidants as a possible tool to reverse this pathological circle. Whether this approach is successful in improving vascular function not only in the short-term, but also in adult life remains to be established.

CONFLICT OF INTEREST

The authors confirm that they have no conflict of interest to declare for this publication.

ACKNOWLEDGEMENTS

Declared none.

REFERENCES

[1] Hellerstein MK, Parks EJ. Obesity and Overweight. In: McGraw-Hill, Ed. Greenspan's basic & clinical endocrinology. New York 2007; pp. 796-816.

[2] Kimm SY, Obarzanek E. Childhood Obesity: A New Pandemic of the New Millennium. Pediatrics 2002; 110(5): 1003-10007.
[http://dx.doi.org/10.1542/peds.110.5.1003]

[3]   Vieno A, Santinello M, Martini MC. Epidemiology of overweight and obesity among Italian early adolescents: relation with physical activity and sedentary behaviour. Epidemiol Psichiatr Soc 2005; 14: 100-7.
[http://dx.doi.org/10.1017/S1121189X00006308]

[4]   Parsons TJ, Power C, Logan S, Summerbell CD. Childhood predictors of adult obesity: a systematic review. Int J Obes Relat Metab Disord 1999; 23 (Suppl. 8): S1-S107.
[PMID: 10641588]

[5]   Power C, Lake JK, Cole TJ. Measurement and long-term health risks of child and adolescent fatness. Int J Obes Relat Metab Disord 1997; 21(7): 507-26.
[http://dx.doi.org/10.1038/sj.ijo.0800454] [PMID: 9226480]

[6]   Cunningham SA, Kramer MR, Narayan KM. Incidence of childhood obesity in the United States. N Engl J Med 2014; 370(5): 403-11.
[http://dx.doi.org/10.1056/NEJMoa1309753] [PMID: 24476431]

[7]   Whitaker RC, Wright JA, Pepe MS, Seidel KD, Dietz WH. Predicting obesity in young adulthood from childhood and parental obesity. N Engl J Med 1997; 337(13): 869-73.
[http://dx.doi.org/10.1056/NEJM199709253371301] [PMID: 9302300]

[8]   Bernasconi S, Iughetti L. L'obesità in età evolutiva. Milano 2005.

[9]   Cook S, Weitzman M, Auinger P, Nguyen M, Dietz WH. Prevalence of a metabolic syndrome phenotype in adolescents: findings from the third National Health and Nutrition Examination Survey, 19881994. Arch Pediatr Adolesc Med 2003; 157(8): 821-7.
[http://dx.doi.org/10.1001/archpedi.157.8.821] [PMID: 12912790]

[10] Pacifico L, Anania C, Martino F, Poggiogalle E, Chiarelli F, Arca M, *et al.* Management of metabolic syndrome in children and adolescents Nutr Metab Cardiovasc Dis Elsevier Ltd; 2011 Jun 2011; 21(6): 455-66.
[http://dx.doi.org/10.1016/j.numecd.2011.01.011] [PMID: 21565479]

[11] Codoñer-Franch P, Boix-García L, Simó-Jordá R, Del Castillo-Villaescusa C, Maset-Maldonado J, Valls-Bellés V. Is obesity associated with oxidative stress in children? Int J Pediatr Obes 2010; 5(1): 56-63.
[http://dx.doi.org/10.3109/17477160903055945] [PMID: 19565402]

[12] Mohn A, Catino M, Capanna R, Giannini C, Marcovecchio M, Chiarelli F. Increased oxidative stress in prepubertal severely obese children: effect of a dietary restriction-weight loss program. J Clin Endocrinol Metab 2005; 90(5): 2653-8.
[http://dx.doi.org/10.1210/jc.2004-2178] [PMID: 15705920]

[13] Gregor MF, Hotamisligil GS. Adipocyte stress: the endoplasmic reticulum and metabolic disease. J Lipid Res 2009; 48: 1905-14.

[14] Weisberg SP, McCann D, Desai M, Rosenbaum M, Leibel RL, Ferrante AW Jr. Obesity is associated with macrophage accumulation in adipose tissue. J Clin Invest 2003; 112(12): 1796-808.
[http://dx.doi.org/10.1172/JCI200319246] [PMID: 14679176]

[15] Sorisky A, Molgat AS, Gagnon A. Macrophage-induced adipose tissue dysfunction and the preadipocyte: should I stay (and differentiate) or should I go? Adv Nutr 2013; 4(1): 67-75.
[http://dx.doi.org/10.3945/an.112.003020] [PMID: 23319125]

[16] Iyer A, Fairlie DP, Prins JB, Hammock BD, Brown L. Inflammatory lipid mediators in adipocyte function and obesity. Nat Rev Endocrinol 2010; 6(2): 71-82.
[http://dx.doi.org/10.1038/nrendo.2009.264] [PMID: 20098448]

[17] Cummings DE, Purnell JQ, Frayo RS, Schmidova K, Wisse BE, Weigle DS. A preprandial rise in plasma ghrelin levels suggests a role in meal initiation in humans. Diabetes 2001; 50(8): 1714-9.
[http://dx.doi.org/10.2337/diabetes.50.8.1714] [PMID: 11473029]

[18] Galli-Tsinopoulou A, Stylianou C, Farmakiotis D, Rousso I, Karamouzis M, Nousia-Arvanitakis S. Ghrelin serum levels during oral glucose tolerance test in prepubertal obese children with insulin resistance. J Pediatr Endocrinol Metab 2007; 20(10): 1085-92.
[http://dx.doi.org/10.1515/JPEM.2007.20.10.1085] [PMID: 18051927]

[19] Wang XM, Jiang YJ, Liang L, Du LZ. Changes of ghrelin following oral glucose tolerance test in obese children with insulin resistance. World J Gastroenterol 2008; 14(12): 1919-24.
[http://dx.doi.org/10.3748/wjg.14.1919] [PMID: 18350633]

[20] Granata R, Gallo D, Luque RM, Baragli A, Scarlatti F, Grande C, et al. Obestatin regulates adipocyte function and protects against diet-induced insulin resistance and inflammation. Faseb J 2012; 26(8): 3393-411.
[http://dx.doi.org/10.1096/fj.11-201343] [PMID: 22601779]

[21] Pan H, Guo J, Su Z. Physiology & Behavior Advances in understanding the interrelations between Leptin resistance and obesity. Physiol Behav Elsevier Inc; 2014 2014; 130: 157-69.

[22] Antunes H, Santos C, Carvalho S. Serum leptin levels in overweight children and adolescents. Br J Nutr 2009; 101(8): 1262-6.
[http://dx.doi.org/10.1017/S0007114508055682] [PMID: 18755049]

[23] Donato J Jr, Cravo RM, Frazão R, Elias CF. Hypothalamic sites of leptin action linking metabolism and reproduction. Neuroendocrinology 2011; 93(1): 9-18.
[http://dx.doi.org/10.1159/000322472] [PMID: 21099209]

[24] Bjørbaek C. Central leptin receptor action and resistance in obesity. J Investig Med 2009; 57(7): 789-94.
[http://dx.doi.org/10.2310/JIM.0b013e3181bb0d49] [PMID: 20029269]

[25] Wong IP, Nguyen AD, Khor EC, et al. Neuropeptide Y is a critical modulator of leptins regulation of cortical bone. J Bone Miner Res 2013; 28(4): 886-98.
[http://dx.doi.org/10.1002/jbmr.1786] [PMID: 23044938]

[26] Patel SB, Reams GP, Spear RM, Freeman RH, Villarreal D. Leptin: linking obesity, the metabolic syndrome, and cardiovascular disease. Curr Hypertens Rep 2008; 10(2): 131-7.
[http://dx.doi.org/10.1007/s11906-008-0025-y] [PMID: 18474180]

[27] Wauman J, Tavernier J. Leptin receptor signaling: pathways to Leptin resistance. Front Biosci (Landmark Ed) 2011; 16: 2771-93.
[PMID: 21622208] [http://dx.doi.org/10.2741/3885]

[28] Liu Y, Zhang X, Shi D, Cheng Z, Meng H. Association between plasma Leptin level and periodontal parameters in patients with aggressive periodontitis. Zhonghua Kou Qiang Yi Xue Za Zhi 2013; 48: 3-6.
[PMID: 23534512]

[29] Barkan D, Jia H, Dantes A, Vardimon L, Amsterdam A, Rubinstein M. Leptin modulates the glucocorticoid-induced ovarian steroidogenesis. Endocrinology 1999; 140(4): 1731-8.
[PMID: 10098510]

[30] Jeffery AN, Murphy MJ, Metcalf BS, et al. Adiponectin in childhood. Int J Pediatr Obes 2008; 3(3): 130-40.
[http://dx.doi.org/10.1080/17477160801954538] [PMID: 19086185]

[31] Arslan N, Erdur B, Aydin A. Hormones and cytokines in childhood obesity. Indian Pediatr 2010; 47(10): 829-39.
[http://dx.doi.org/10.1007/s13312-010-0142-y] [PMID: 21048235]

[32] Oakley AE, Clifton DK, Steiner RA. Kisspeptin signaling in the brain. Endocr Rev 2009; 30(6): 713-43.
[http://dx.doi.org/10.1210/er.2009-0005] [PMID: 19770291]

[33]   Welt CK, Chan JL, Bullen J, et al. Recombinant human leptin in women with hypothalamic amenorrhea. N Engl J Med 2004; 351(10): 987-97.
[http://dx.doi.org/10.1056/NEJMoa040388] [PMID: 15342807]

[34]   Fernández-Fernández R, Navarro VM, Barreiro ML, et al. Effects of chronic hyperghrelinemia on puberty onset and pregnancy outcome in the rat. Endocrinology 2005; 146(7): 3018-25.
[http://dx.doi.org/10.1210/en.2004-1622] [PMID: 15790726]

[35]   Luque RM, Kineman RD, Tena-Sempere M. Regulation of hypothalamic expression of KiSS-1 and GPR54 genes by metabolic factors: analyses using mouse models and a cell line. Endocrinology 2007; 148(10): 4601-11.
[http://dx.doi.org/10.1210/en.2007-0500] [PMID: 17595226]

[36]   Hiney JK, Srivastava VK, Pine MD, Les Dees W. Insulin-like growth factor-I activates KiSS-1 gene expression in the brain of the prepubertal female rat. Endocrinology 2009; 150(1): 376-84.
[http://dx.doi.org/10.1210/en.2008-0954] [PMID: 18703622]

[37]   Navarro VM, Tena-Sempere M. Kisspeptins and the neuroendocrine control of reproduction. Front Biosci (Schol Ed) 2011; 3: 267-75.
[http://dx.doi.org/10.2741/s150] [PMID: 21196375]

[38]   Aydin M, Oktar S, Yonden Z, Ozturk OH, Yilmaz B. Direct and indirect effects of kisspeptin on liver oxidant and antioxidant systems in young male rats. Cell Biochem Funct 2010; 28(4): 293-9.
[http://dx.doi.org/10.1002/cbf.1656] [PMID: 20517893]

[39]   Tolson KP, Garcia C, Yen S, et al. Impaired kisspeptin signaling decreases metabolism and promotes glucose intolerance and obesity. J Clin Invest 2014; 124(7): 3075-9.
[http://dx.doi.org/10.1172/JCI71075] [PMID: 24937427]

[40]   Cockwell H, Wilkinson DA, Bouzayen R, Imran SA, Brown R, Wilkinson M. KISS1 expression in human female adipose tissue. Arch Gynecol Obstet 2013; 287(1): 143-7.
[http://dx.doi.org/10.1007/s00404-012-2514-0] [PMID: 22899305]

[41]   Brown RE, Imran SA, Ur E, Wilkinson M. KiSS-1 mRNA in adipose tissue is regulated by sex hormones and food intake. Mol Cell Endocrinol 2008; 281(1-2): 64-72.
[http://dx.doi.org/10.1016/j.mce.2007.10.011] [PMID: 18069123]

[42]   Fried SK, Bunkin DA, Greenberg AS. Omental and subcutaneous adipose tissues of obese subjects release interleukin-6: depot difference and regulation by glucocorticoid. J Clin Endocrinol Metab 1998; 83(3): 847-50.
[PMID: 9506738]

[43]   Zou C, Shao J. Role of adipocytokines in obesity-associated insulin resistance. J Nutr Biochem 2008; 19(5): 277-86.
[PMID: 18054218]

[44]   Fukuhara A, Matsuda M, Nishizawa M, et al. Visfatin: a protein secreted by visceral fat that mimics the effects of insulin. Science 2005; 307(5708): 426-30.
[http://dx.doi.org/10.1126/science.1097243] [PMID: 15604363]

[45]   Boucher J, Masri B, Daviaud D, et al. Apelin, a newly identified adipokine up-regulated by insulin and obesity. Endocrinology 2005; 146(4): 1764-71.
[http://dx.doi.org/10.1210/en.2004-1427] [PMID: 15677759]

[46]   Yang Q, Graham TE, Mody N, et al. Serum retinol binding protein 4 contributes to insulin resistance in obesity and type 2 diabetes. Nature 2005; 436(7049): 356-62.
[http://dx.doi.org/10.1038/nature03711] [PMID: 16034410]

[47]   Atabek ME, Vatansev H, Erkul I. Oxidative stress in childhood obesity. J Pediatr Endocrinol Metab 2004; 17(8): 1063-8.
[http://dx.doi.org/10.1515/JPEM.2004.17.8.1063] [PMID: 15379416]

[48] Lima SC, Arrais RF, Almeida MG, Souza ZM, Pedrosa LF. [Plasma lipid profile and lipid peroxidation in overweight or obese children and adolescents]. J Pediatr (Rio J) 2004; 80(1): 23-8.
[http://dx.doi.org/10.2223/JPED.1129] [PMID: 14978545]

[49] Molnár D, Decsi T, Koletzko B. Reduced antioxidant status in obese children with multimetabolic syndrome. Int J Obes Relat Metab Disord 2004; 28(10): 1197-202.
[http://dx.doi.org/10.1038/sj.ijo.0802719] [PMID: 15314634]

[50] Decsi T, Molnár D, Koletzko B. Reduced plasma concentrations of alpha-tocopherol and beta-carotene in obese boys. J Pediatr 1997; 130(4): 653-5.
[http://dx.doi.org/10.1016/S0022-3476(97)70253-1] [PMID: 9108867]

[51] Kuno T, Hozumi M, Morinobu T, Murata T, Mingci Z, Tamai H. Antioxidant vitamin levels in plasma and low density lipoprotein of obese girls. Free Radic Res 1998; 28(1): 81-6.
[http://dx.doi.org/10.3109/10715769809097878] [PMID: 9554835]

[52] Singh U, Devaraj S, Jialal I. Vitamin E, oxidative stress, and inflammation. Annu Rev Nutr 2005; 25: 151-74.
[http://dx.doi.org/10.1146/annurev.nutr.24.012003.132446] [PMID: 16011463]

[53] Kelly AS, Steinberger J, Olson TP, Dengel DR. In the absence of weight loss, exercise training does not improve adipokines or oxidative stress in overweight children. Metabolism 2007; 56(7): 1005-9.
[http://dx.doi.org/10.1016/j.metabol.2007.03.009] [PMID: 17570265]

[54] Codoñer-Franch P, Valls-Bellés V, Arilla-Codoñer A, Alonso-Iglesias E. Oxidant mechanisms in childhood obesity: the link between inflammation and oxidative stress. Transl Res 2011; 158(6): 369-84.
[http://dx.doi.org/10.1016/j.trsl.2011.08.004] [PMID: 22061044]

[55] Ustundag B, Gungor S, Aygün AD, Turgut M, Yilmaz E. Oxidative status and serum leptin levels in obese prepubertal children. Cell Biochem Funct 2007; 25(5): 479-83.
[http://dx.doi.org/10.1002/cbf.1334] [PMID: 16874844]

[56] Oliver SR, Rosa JS, Milne GL, *et al.* Increased oxidative stress and altered substrate metabolism in obese children. Int J Pediatr Obes 2010; 5(5): 436-44.
[http://dx.doi.org/10.3109/17477160903545163] [PMID: 20233149]

[57] Skilton MR, Celermajer DS. Endothelial dysfunction and arterial abnormalities in childhood obesity. Int J Obes (Lond) 2006; 30(7): 1041-9.
[http://dx.doi.org/10.1038/sj.ijo.0803397] [PMID: 16801941]

[58] Matsuda M, Shimomura I. Increased oxidative stress in obesity: Implications for metabolic syndrome, diabetes, hypertension, dyslipidemia, atherosclerosis, and cancer. Obes Res Clin Pract Asia Oceania Assoc for the Study of Obesity 2013; 7(5): e330-41.

[59] Matsuda T, Saito H, Inoue T, Fukatsu K, Han I, Furukawa S, *et al.* Growth hormone inhibits apoptosis and up-regulates reactive oxygen intermediates production by human polymorphonuclear neutrophils. JPEN J Parenter Enter Nutr 1998; 22: 368-74.
[http://dx.doi.org/10.1177/0148607198022006368] [PMID: 9829610]

[60] Smith JC, Lang D, McEneny J, *et al.* Effects of GH on lipid peroxidation and neutrophil superoxide anion-generating capacity in hypopituitary adults with GH deficiency. Clin Endocrinol (Oxf) 2002; 56(4): 449-55.
[http://dx.doi.org/10.1046/j.1365-2265.2002.01493.x] [PMID: 11966737]

[61] Sanz A, Gredilla R, Pamplona R, *et al.* Effect of insulin and growth hormone on rat heart and liver oxidative stress in control and caloric restricted animals. Biogerontology 2005; 6(1): 15-26.
[http://dx.doi.org/10.1007/s10522-004-7380-0] [PMID: 15834660]

[62] Brown-Borg HM, Bode AM, Bartke A. Antioxidative mechanisms and plasma growth hormone levels: potential relationship in the aging process. Endocrine 1999; 11(1): 41-8.
[http://dx.doi.org/10.1385/ENDO:11:1:41] [PMID: 10668640]

[63] Hauck SJ, Aaron JM, Wright C, Kopchick JJ, Bartke A. Antioxidant enzymes, free-radical damage, and response to paraquat in liver and kidney of long-living growth hormone receptor/binding protein gene-disrupted mice. Horm Metab Res 2002; 34(9): 481-6.
[http://dx.doi.org/10.1055/s-2002-34787] [PMID: 12384824]

[64] Mohn A, Marzio D, Giannini C, Capanna R, Marcovecchio M, Chiarelli F. Alterations in the oxidant-antioxidant status in prepubertal children with growth hormone deficiency: effect of growth hormone replacement therapy. Clin Endocrinol (Oxf) 2005; 63(5): 537-42.
[http://dx.doi.org/10.1111/j.1365-2265.2005.02378.x] [PMID: 16268806]

[65] Scacchi M, Valassi E, Pincelli AI, *et al.* Increased lipid peroxidation in adult GH-deficient patients: effects of short-term GH administration. J Endocrinol Invest 2006; 29(10): 899-904.
[http://dx.doi.org/10.1007/BF03349194] [PMID: 17185899]

[66] Misra M, Miller KK, Bjornson J, *et al.* Alterations in growth hormone secretory dynamics in adolescent girls with anorexia nervosa and effects on bone metabolism. J Clin Endocrinol Metab 2003; 88(12): 5615-23.
[http://dx.doi.org/10.1210/jc.2003-030532] [PMID: 14671143]

[67] Misra M, Miller KK, Almazan C, Worley M, Herzog DB, Klibanski A. Hormonal determinants of regional body composition in adolescent girls with anorexia nervosa and controls. J Clin Endocrinol Metab 2005; 90(5): 2580-7.
[http://dx.doi.org/10.1210/jc.2004-2041] [PMID: 15713709]

[68] Kim KR, Nam SY, Song YD, Lim SK, Lee HC, Huh KB. Low-dose growth hormone treatment with diet restriction accelerates body fat loss, exerts anabolic effect and improves growth hormone secretory dysfunction in obese adults. Horm Res 1999; 51(2): 78-84.
[PMID: 10352397]

[69] Pijl H, Langendonk JG, Burggraaf J, *et al.* Altered neuroregulation of GH secretion in viscerally obese premenopausal women. J Clin Endocrinol Metab 2001; 86(11): 5509-15.
[http://dx.doi.org/10.1210/jcem.86.11.8061] [PMID: 11701729]

[70] Roemmich JN, Huerta MG, Sundaresan SM, Rogol AD. Alterations in body composition and fat distribution in growth hormone-deficient prepubertal children during growth hormone therapy. Metabolism 2001; 50(5): 537-47.
[http://dx.doi.org/10.1053/meta.2001.22510] [PMID: 11319714]

[71] Burger AG, Monson JP, Colao AM, Klibanski A. Cardiovascular risk in patients with growth hormone deficiency: effects of growth hormone substitution. Endocr Pract 2006; 12(6): 682-9.
[http://dx.doi.org/10.4158/EP.12.6.682] [PMID: 17229667]

[72] Ballerini MG, Ropelato MG, Doméné HM, Pennisi P, Heinrich JJ, Jasper HG. Differential impact of simple childhood obesity on the components of the growth hormone-insulin-like growth factor (IGF)-IGF binding proteins axis. J Pediatr Endocrinol Metab 2004; 17(5): 749-57.
[http://dx.doi.org/10.1515/JPEM.2004.17.5.749] [PMID: 15237710]

[73] Heptulla R, Smitten A, Teague B, Tamborlane WV, Ma YZ, Caprio S. Temporal patterns of circulating leptin levels in lean and obese adolescents: relationships to insulin, growth hormone, and free fatty acids rhythmicity. J Clin Endocrinol Metab 2001; 86(1): 90-6.
[PMID: 11231983]

[74] Mancini A, Giacchi E, Raimondo S, Di Segni C, Silvestrini A, Meucci E. Hypothyroidism, Oxidative Stress and Reproduction. Hypothyroidism - Influences and Treatments, InTech Open Access 2012; 117-34.

[75] Resch U, Helsel G, Tatzber F, Sinzinger H. Antioxidant status in thyroid dysfunction. Clin Chem Lab Med 2002; 40(11): 1132-4.
[http://dx.doi.org/10.1515/cclm.2002.198] [PMID: 12521231]

[76] Asayama K, Kato K. Oxidative muscular injury and its relevance to hyperthyroidism. Free Radic Biol Med 1990; 8(3): 293-303.
[http://dx.doi.org/10.1016/0891-5849(90)90077-V] [PMID: 2187767]

[77] Dobrzyńska MM, Baumgartner A, Anderson D. Antioxidants modulate thyroid hormone- and noradrenaline-induced DNA damage in human sperm. Mutagenesis 2004; 19(4): 325-30.
[http://dx.doi.org/10.1093/mutage/geh037] [PMID: 15215333]

[78] Venditti P, Balestrieri M, Di Meo S, De Leo T. Effect of thyroid state on lipid peroxidation, antioxidant defences, and susceptibility to oxidative stress in rat tissues. J Endocrinol 1997; 155(1): 151-7.
[http://dx.doi.org/10.1677/joe.0.1550151] [PMID: 9390017]

[79] Fernández V, Barrientos X, Kipreos K, Valenzuela A, Videla LA. Superoxide radical generation, NADPH oxidase activity, and cytochrome P-450 content of rat liver microsomal fractions in an experimental hyperthyroid state: relation to lipid peroxidation. Endocrinology 1985; 117(2): 496-501.
[http://dx.doi.org/10.1210/endo-117-2-496] [PMID: 2990853]

[80] Venditti P, Daniele MC, Masullo P, Di Meo S. Antioxidant-sensitive triiodothyronine effects on characteristics of rat liver mitochondrial population. Cell Physiol Biochem 1999; 9(1): 38-52.
[http://dx.doi.org/10.1159/000016301] [PMID: 10352343]

[81] Huh K, Kwon TH, Kim JS, Park JM. Role of the hepatic xanthine oxidase in thyroid dysfunction: effect of thyroid hormones in oxidative stress in rat liver. Arch Pharm Res 1998; 21(3): 236-40.
[http://dx.doi.org/10.1007/BF02975281] [PMID: 9875437]

[82] Asayama K, Dobashi K, Hayashibe H, Megata Y, Kato K. Lipid peroxidation and free radical scavengers in thyroid dysfunction in the rat: a possible mechanism of injury to heart and skeletal muscle in hyperthyroidism. Endocrinology 1987; 121(6): 2112-8.
[http://dx.doi.org/10.1210/endo-121-6-2112] [PMID: 2824181]

[83] Choudhury S, Chainy GB, Mishro MM. Experimentally induced hypo- and hyper-thyroidism influence on the antioxidant defence system in adult rat testis. Andrologia 2003; 35(3): 131-40.
[http://dx.doi.org/10.1046/j.1439-0272.2003.00548.x] [PMID: 12780529]

[84] Venditti P, Di Meo S. Thyroid hormone-induced oxidative stress. Cell Mol Life Sci 2006; 63(4): 414-34.
[http://dx.doi.org/10.1007/s00018-005-5457-9] [PMID: 16389448]

[85] Ademoğlu E, Gökkuşu C, Yarman S, Azizlerli H. The effect of methimazole on the oxidant and antioxidant system in patients with hyperthyroidism. Pharmacol Res 1998; 38(2): 93-6.
[http://dx.doi.org/10.1006/phrs.1998.0336] [PMID: 9721594]

[86] Bianchi G, Solaroli E, Zaccheroni V, Grossi G, Bargossi AM, Melchionda N, et al. Oxidative stress and anti-oxidant metabolites in patients with hyperthyroidism: effect of treatment. Hormone and metabolic research = Hormon- und Stoffwechselforschung = Hormones et metabolisme 1999.
[http://dx.doi.org/10.1055/s-2007-978808]

[87] Mancini A, De Marinis L, Calabrò F, Fiumara C, Goglia A, Littarru GP. Physiopathological relevance of coenzyme Q10 in thyroid disorders: CoQ10 concentrations in normal and diseased human thyroid tissue. Biomedical and Clinical Aspects of Coenzyme Q. Amsterdam: Elsevier 1991; pp. 441-8.

[88] Mancini A, De Marinis L, Calabrò F, et al. Evaluation of metabolic status in amiodarone-induced thyroid disorders: plasma coenzyme Q10 determination. J Endocrinol Invest 1989; 12(8): 511-6.
[http://dx.doi.org/10.1007/BF03350748] [PMID: 2592737]

[89] Mancini A, Corbo GM, Gaballo A, et al. Relationships between plasma CoQ10 levels and thyroid hormones in chronic obstructive pulmonary disease. Biofactors 2005; 25(1-4): 201-4.
[http://dx.doi.org/10.1002/biof.5520250124] [PMID: 16873947]

[90] Baskol G, Atmaca H, Tanriverdi F, Baskol M, Kocer D, Bayram F. Oxidative stress and enzymatic antioxidant status in patients with hypothyroidism before and after treatment. Exp Clin Endocrinol

Diabetes 2007; 115(8): 522-6.
[http://dx.doi.org/10.1055/s-2007-981457] [PMID: 17853336]

[91] Torun AN, Kulaksizoglu S, Kulaksizoglu M, Pamuk BO, Isbilen E, Tutuncu NB. Serum total antioxidant status and lipid peroxidation marker malondialdehyde levels in overt and subclinical hypothyroidism. Clin Endocrinol (Oxf) 2009; 70(3): 469-74.
[http://dx.doi.org/10.1111/j.1365-2265.2008.03348.x] [PMID: 18727709]

[92] Coria MJ, Pastrán AI, Gimenez MS. Serum oxidative stress parameters of women with hypothyroidism. Acta Biomed 2009; 80(2): 135-9.
[PMID: 19848051]

[93] Erdamar H, Demirci H, Yaman H, et al. The effect of hypothyroidism, hyperthyroidism, and their treatment on parameters of oxidative stress and antioxidant status. Clin Chem Lab Med 2008; 46(7): 1004-10.
[http://dx.doi.org/10.1515/CCLM.2008.183] [PMID: 18605962]

[94] Azizi F, Raiszadeh F, Solati M, Etemadi A, Rahmani M, Arabi M. Serum paraoxonase 1 activity is decreased in thyroid dysfunction. J Endocrinol Invest 2003; 26(8): 703-9.
[http://dx.doi.org/10.1007/BF03347350] [PMID: 14669822]

[95] Santi A, Duarte MM, Moresco RN, et al. Association between thyroid hormones, lipids and oxidative stress biomarkers in overt hypothyroidism. Clin Chem Lab Med 2010; 48(11): 1635-9.
[http://dx.doi.org/10.1515/CCLM.2010.309] [PMID: 20704527]

[96] Nanda N, Bobby Z, Hamide A, Koner BC, Sridhar MG. Association between oxidative stress and coronary lipid risk factors in hypothyroid women is independent of body mass index. Metabolism 2007; 56(10): 1350-5.
[http://dx.doi.org/10.1016/j.metabol.2007.05.015] [PMID: 17884444]

[97] Kebapcilar L, Akinci B, Bayraktar F, et al. Plasma thiobarbituric acid-reactive substance levels in subclinical hypothyroidism. Med Princ Pract 2007; 16(6): 432-6.
[http://dx.doi.org/10.1159/000107747] [PMID: 17917442]

[98] Mancini A, Festa R, Di Donna V, et al. Hormones and antioxidant systems: role of pituitary and pituitary-dependent axes. J Endocrinol Invest 2010; 33(6): 422-33.
[http://dx.doi.org/10.1007/BF03346615] [PMID: 20631494]

[99] Mancini A, Leone E, Silvestrini A, et al. Evaluation of antioxidant systems in pituitary-adrenal axis diseases. Pituitary 2010; 13(2): 138-45.
[http://dx.doi.org/10.1007/s11102-009-0213-z] [PMID: 20012698]

[100] Ohye H, Sugawara M. Dual oxidase, hydrogen peroxide and thyroid diseases. Exp Biol Med (Maywood) 2010; 235(4): 424-33.
[http://dx.doi.org/10.1258/ebm.2009.009241] [PMID: 20407074]

[101] Varela V, Rivolta CM, Esperante SA, Gruñeiro-Papendieck L, Chiesa A, Targovnik HM. Three mutations (p.Q36H, p.G418fsX482, and g.IVS192A>C) in the dual oxidase 2 gene responsible for congenital goiter and iodide organification defect. Clin Chem 2006; 52(2): 182-91.
[http://dx.doi.org/10.1373/clinchem.2005.058321] [PMID: 16322276]

[102] Weyemi U, Caillou B, Talbot M, et al. Intracellular expression of reactive oxygen species-generating NADPH oxidase NOX4 in normal and cancer thyroid tissues. Endocr Relat Cancer 2010; 17(1): 27-37.
[http://dx.doi.org/10.1677/ERC-09-0175] [PMID: 19779036]

[103] Sharma R, Traore K, Trush MA, Rose NR, Burek CL. Intracellular adhesion molecule-1 up-regulation on thyrocytes by iodine of non-obese diabetic.H2[h4] mice is reactive oxygen species-dependent. Clin Exp Immunol 2008; 152(1): 13-20.
[http://dx.doi.org/10.1111/j.1365-2249.2008.03590.x] [PMID: 18241232]

[104] Reinehr T. Obesity and thyroid function. Mol Cell Endocrinol 2010; 316(2): 165-71.
[http://dx.doi.org/10.1016/j.mce.2009.06.005] [PMID: 19540303]

[105] Pacifico L, Anania C, Ferraro F, Andreoli GM, Chiesa C. Thyroid function in childhood obesity and metabolic comorbidity. Clin Chim Acta 2012; 413(3-4): 396-405.
[http://dx.doi.org/10.1016/j.cca.2011.11.013] [PMID: 22130312]

[106] Leo F, Rossodivita AN, Di Segni C, *et al.* Frailty of Obese Children: Evaluation of Plasma Antioxidant Capacity in Pediatric Obesity. Exp Clin Endocrinol Diabetes 2016; 124(8): 481-6.
[http://dx.doi.org/10.1055/s-0042-105280] [PMID: 27169687]

[107] Knudsen N, Laurberg P, Rasmussen LB, *et al.* Small differences in thyroid function may be important for body mass index and the occurrence of obesity in the population. J Clin Endocrinol Metab 2005; 90(7): 4019-24.
[http://dx.doi.org/10.1210/jc.2004-2225] [PMID: 15870128]

[108] Rotondi M, Magri F, Chiovato L. Thyroid and obesity: not a one-way interaction. J Clin Endocrinol Metab 2011; 96(2): 344-6.
[http://dx.doi.org/10.1210/jc.2010-2515] [PMID: 21296993]

[109] Reinehr T, de Sousa G, Andler W. Hyperthyrotropinemia in obese children is reversible after weight loss and is not related to lipids. J Clin Endocrinol Metab 2006; 91(8): 3088-91.
[http://dx.doi.org/10.1210/jc.2006-0095] [PMID: 16684827]

[110] Reinehr T, Isa A, de Sousa G, Dieffenbach R, Andler W. Thyroid hormones and their relation to weight status. Horm Res 2008; 70(1): 51-7.
[http://dx.doi.org/10.1159/000129678] [PMID: 18493150]

[111] Grandone A, Santoro N, Coppola F, Calabrò P, Perrone L, Del Giudice EM. Thyroid function derangement and childhood obesity: an Italian experience. BMC Endocr Disord 2010; 10: 8.
[http://dx.doi.org/10.1186/1472-6823-10-8] [PMID: 20441588]

[112] Marras V, Casini MR, Pilia S, *et al.* Thyroid function in obese children and adolescents. Horm Res Paediatr 2010; 73(3): 193-7.
[http://dx.doi.org/10.1159/000284361] [PMID: 20197672]

[113] Reinehr T, Andler W. Thyroid hormones before and after weight loss in obesity. Arch Dis Child 2002; 87(4): 320-3.
[http://dx.doi.org/10.1136/adc.87.4.320] [PMID: 12244007]

[114] Aeberli I, Jung A, Murer SB, *et al.* During rapid weight loss in obese children, reductions in TSH predict improvements in insulin sensitivity independent of changes in body weight or fat. J Clin Endocrinol Metab 2010; 95(12): 5412-8.
[http://dx.doi.org/10.1210/jc.2010-1169] [PMID: 20843953]

[115] Stichel H, lAllemand D, Grüters A. Thyroid function and obesity in children and adolescents. Horm Res 2000; 54(1): 14-9.
[http://dx.doi.org/10.1159/000063431] [PMID: 11182630]

[116] Bhowmick SK, Dasari G, Levens KL, Rettig KR. The prevalence of elevated serum thyroid-stimulating hormone in childhood/adolescent obesity and of autoimmune thyroid diseases in a subgroup. J Natl Med Assoc 2007; 99(7): 773-6.
[PMID: 17668643]

[117] Dekelbab BH, Abou Ouf HA, Jain I. Prevalence of elevated thyroid-stimulating hormone levels in obese children and adolescents. Endocr Pract 2010; 16(2): 187-90.
[http://dx.doi.org/10.4158/EP09176.OR] [PMID: 19833586]

[118] Mancini A, Fiumara C, Conte G, *et al.* Pyridostigmine effects on TSH response to TRH in adult and children obese subjects. Horm Metab Res 1993; 25(6): 309-11.
[http://dx.doi.org/10.1055/s-2007-1002106] [PMID: 8344646]

[119] Donders SH, Pieters GF, Heevel JG, Ross HA, Smals AG, Kloppenborg PW. Disparity of thyrotropin (TSH) and prolactin responses to TSH-releasing hormone in obesity. J Clin Endocrinol Metab 1985; 61(1): 56-9.

[http://dx.doi.org/10.1210/jcem-61-1-56] [PMID: 3923032]

[120] Kodama M, Inoue F, Saito H, Oda T, Sato Y. Formation of free radicals from steroid hormones: possible significance in environmental carcinogenesis. Anticancer Res 1997; 17(1A): 439-44.
[PMID: 9066691]

[121] Hornsby PJ. Cytochrome P-450/pseudosubstrate interactions and the role of antioxidants in the adrenal cortex. Endocr Res 1986; 12(4): 469-94.
[http://dx.doi.org/10.3109/07435808609035451] [PMID: 3549274]

[122] Patak P, Willenberg HS, Bornstein SR. Vitamin C is an important cofactor for both adrenal cortex and adrenal medulla. Endocr Res 2004; 30(4): 871-5.
[http://dx.doi.org/10.1081/ERC-200044126] [PMID: 15666839]

[123] Mitani F, Ogishima T, Mukai K, Suematsu M. Ascorbate stimulates monooxygenase-dependent steroidogenesis in adrenal zona glomerulosa. Biochem Biophys Res Commun 2005; 338(1): 483-90.
[http://dx.doi.org/10.1016/j.bbrc.2005.08.156] [PMID: 16168385]

[124] Das PC, Das KP, Bagchi K, Dey CD. Evaluation of tissue ascorbic acid status in different hormonal states of female rat. Life Sci 1993; 52(18): 1493-8.
[http://dx.doi.org/10.1016/0024-3205(93)90111-F] [PMID: 8483380]

[125] Sun Y, Ahokas RA, Bhattacharya SK, Gerling IC, Carbone LD, Weber KT. Oxidative stress in aldosteronism. Cardiovasc Res 2006; 71(2): 300-9.
[http://dx.doi.org/10.1016/j.cardiores.2006.03.007] [PMID: 16631148]

[126] Marney AM, Brown NJ. Aldosterone and end-organ damage. Clin Sci 2007; 113(6): 267-78.
[http://dx.doi.org/10.1042/CS20070123] [PMID: 17683282]

[127] Lastra-Gonzalez G, Manrique-Acevedo C, Sowers JR. The role of aldosterone in cardiovascular disease in people with diabetes and hypertension: an update. Curr Diab Rep 2008; 8(3): 203-7.
[http://dx.doi.org/10.1007/s11892-008-0035-9] [PMID: 18625117]

[128] Cooper SA, Whaley-Connell A, Habibi J, Wei Y, Lastra G, Manrique C, et al. Renin-angiotensi--aldosterone system and oxidative stress in cardiovascular insulin resistance. Am J Physiol Hear Circ Physiol 2007; 293: H2009-23.
[http://dx.doi.org/10.1152/ajpheart.00522.2007] [PMID: 17586614]

[129] Fujita T. Aldosterone in salt-sensitive hypertension and metabolic syndrome. J Mol Med 2008; 86(6): 729-34.
[http://dx.doi.org/10.1007/s00109-008-0343-1] [PMID: 18437332]

[130] Korantzopoulos P, Galaris D, Papaioannides D, Siogas K. The possible role of oxidative stress in heart failure and the potential of antioxidant intervention. Med Sci Monit 2003; 9(6): RA120-5.
[PMID: 12824962]

[131] Celebi F, Yilmaz I, Aksoy H, Gümüş M, Taysi S, Oren D. Dehydroepiandrosterone prevents oxidative injury in obstructive jaundice in rats. J Int Med Res 2004; 32(4): 400-5.
[http://dx.doi.org/10.1177/147323000403200408] [PMID: 15303771]

[132] Kim SK, Novak RF. The role of intracellular signaling in insulin-mediated regulation of drug metabolizing enzyme gene and protein expression. Pharmacol Ther 2007; 113(1): 88-120.
[http://dx.doi.org/10.1016/j.pharmthera.2006.07.004] [PMID: 17097148]

[133] Jacob MH, Janner D da R, Belló-Klein A, Llesuy SF, Ribeiro MF. Dehydroepiandrosterone modulates antioxidant enzymes and Akt signaling in healthy Wistar rat hearts. J Steroid Biochem Mol Biol 2008; 112(1-3): 138-44.
[http://dx.doi.org/10.1016/j.jsbmb.2008.09.008] [PMID: 18848627]

[134] Yildirim A, Sahin YN, Suleyman H, Yilmaz A, Yildirim S. The role of prednisolone and epinephrine on gastric tissue and erythrocyte antioxidant status in adrenalectomized rats. J Physiol Pharmacol 2007; 58(1): 105-16.
[PMID: 17440230]

[135] Toleikis PM, Godin DV. Alteration of antioxidant status following sympathectomy: differential effects of modified plasma levels of adrenaline and noradrenaline. Mol Cell Biochem 1995; 152(1): 39-49.
[PMID: 8609910]

[136] Hidalgo J, Gasull T, Garcia A, Blanquez A, Armario A. Role of glucocorticoids and catecholamines on hepatic thiobarbituric acid reactants in basal and stress conditions in the rat. Horm Metab Res 1991; 23(3): 104-9.
[http://dx.doi.org/10.1055/s-2007-1003626] [PMID: 1650747]

[137] Zelinskiĭ BA, Vlasenko MV. [Lipid peroxidation in patients with chronic adrenal cortex failure]. Probl Endokrinol (Mosk) 1990; 36(1): 37-40.
[PMID: 2330359]

[138] Vargas CR, Wajner M, Sirtori LR, Goulart L, Chiochetta M, Coelho D, *et al*. Evidence that oxidative stress is increased in patients with X-linked adrenoleukodystrophy. Biochim Biophys Acta - Mol Basis Dis 2004; 1688: 26-32.

[139] Di Biase A, Salvati S, Varí R, *et al*. Susceptibility to oxidation of plasma low-density lipoprotein in X-linked adrenoleukodystrophy: effects of simvastatin treatment. Mol Genet Metab 2000; 71(4): 651-5.
[http://dx.doi.org/10.1006/mgme.2000.3100] [PMID: 11136559]

[140] Baschetti R. Chronic fatigue syndrome: an endocrine disease off limits for endocrinologists? Eur J Clin Invest 2003; 33(12): 1029-31.
[http://dx.doi.org/10.1111/j.1365-2362.2003.01272.x] [PMID: 14636284]

[141] Prázný M, Jezková J, Horová E, *et al*. Impaired microvascular reactivity and endothelial function in patients with Cushings syndrome: influence of arterial hypertension. Physiol Res 2008; 57(1): 13-22.
[PMID: 17223725]

[142] Tishenina R. Alpha-tocopherol concentration of the blood plasma and erythrocytes in patients with symptomatic obesity due to hypothalamo-hypophyseal-adrenal disease. Probl Endokrinol (Mosk) 1986.

[143] Keen JA, McLaren M, Chandler KJ, McGorum BC. Biochemical indices of vascular function, glucose metabolism and oxidative stress in horses with equine Cushings disease. Equine Vet J 2004; 36(3): 226-9.
[http://dx.doi.org/10.2746/0425164044877215] [PMID: 15147129]

[144] Whitworth JA, Williamson PM, Mangos G, Kelly JJ. Cardiovascular consequences of cortisol excess. Vasc Health Risk Manag 2005; 1(4): 291-9.
[http://dx.doi.org/10.2147/vhrm.2005.1.4.291] [PMID: 17315601]

[145] Whitworth JA, Mangos GJ, Kelly JJ. Cushing, cortisol, and cardiovascular disease. Hypertension 2000; 36(5): 912-6.
[http://dx.doi.org/10.1161/01.HYP.36.5.912] [PMID: 11082166]

[146] Benghuzzi H, Tucci M, Hughes J, Lyon R, Adams S. Glomerular response to adrenocortical hormone alone or in combination with selenomethionine. Biomed Sci Instrum 2005; 41: 74-9.
[PMID: 15850085]

[147] Tanaka H, Makino Y, Okamoto K. Thioredoxin in the endocrine response to stress. Vitam Horm 1999; 57: 153-75.
[http://dx.doi.org/10.1016/S0083-6729(08)60643-3] [PMID: 10232049]

[148] Makino Y, Okamoto K, Yoshikawa N, *et al*. Thioredoxin: a redox-regulating cellular cofactor for glucocorticoid hormone action. Cross talk between endocrine control of stress response and cellular antioxidant defense system. J Clin Invest 1996; 98(11): 2469-77.
[http://dx.doi.org/10.1172/JCI119065] [PMID: 8958209]

[149] Esch T, Stefano GB, Fricchione GL, Benson H. Stress-related diseases a potential role for nitric oxide. Med Sci Monit 2002; 8(6): RA103-18.
[PMID: 12070451]

[150] Peake JM, Suzuki K, Coombes JS. The influence of antioxidant supplementation on markers of inflammation and the relationship to oxidative stress after exercise. J Nutr Biochem 2007; 18(6): 357-71.
[http://dx.doi.org/10.1016/j.jnutbio.2006.10.005] [PMID: 17156994]

[151] Tiidus PM, Houston ME. Vitamin E status and response to exercise training. Sports Med 1995; 20(1): 12-23.
[http://dx.doi.org/10.2165/00007256-199520010-00002] [PMID: 7481276]

[152] Mancini A, Bianchi A, Fusco A, et al. Coenzyme Q10 evaluation in pituitary-adrenal axis disease: preliminary data. Biofactors 2005; 25(1-4): 197-9.
[http://dx.doi.org/10.1002/biof.5520250123] [PMID: 16873946]

[153] Misra M, Bredella MA, Tsai P, Mendes N, Miller KK, Klibanski A. Lower growth hormone and higher cortisol are associated with greater visceral adiposity, intramyocellular lipids, and insulin resistance in overweight girls. Am J Physiol Endocrinol Metab 2008; 295(2): E385-92.

[154] Weigensberg MJ, Toledo-Corral CM, Goran MI. Association between the metabolic syndrome and serum cortisol in overweight Latino youth. J Clin Endocrinol Metab 2008; 93(4): 1372-8.
[http://dx.doi.org/10.1210/jc.2007-2309] [PMID: 18252788]

[155] Mårin P, Kvist H, Lindstedt G, Sjöström L, Björntorp P. Low concentrations of insulin-like growth factor-I in abdominal obesity. Int J Obes Relat Metab Disord 1993; 17(2): 83-9.
[PMID: 8384169]

[156] Ottosson M, Lönnroth P, Björntorp P, Edén S. Effects of cortisol and growth hormone on lipolysis in human adipose tissue. J Clin Endocrinol Metab 2000; 85(2): 799-803.
[PMID: 10690893]

[157] Epel ES, McEwen B, Seeman T, et al. Stress and body shape: stress-induced cortisol secretion is consistently greater among women with central fat. Psychosom Med 2000; 62(5): 623-32.
[http://dx.doi.org/10.1097/00006842-200009000-00005] [PMID: 11020091]

[158] Garrapa GG, Pantanetti P, Arnaldi G, Mantero F, Faloia E. Body composition and metabolic features in women with adrenal incidentaloma or Cushings syndrome. J Clin Endocrinol Metab 2001; 86(11): 5301-6.
[PMID: 11701696]

[159] Magiakou MA, Mastorakos G, Oldfield EH, et al. Cushings syndrome in children and adolescents. Presentation, diagnosis, and therapy. N Engl J Med 1994; 331(10): 629-36.
[http://dx.doi.org/10.1056/NEJM199409083311002] [PMID: 8052272]

[160] Stratakis CA. Cushing syndrome in pediatrics. Endocrinol Metab Clin North Am 2012; 41(4): 793-803.
[http://dx.doi.org/10.1016/j.ecl.2012.08.002] [PMID: 23099271]

[161] Chan LF, Storr HL, Grossman AB, Savage MO. Pediatric Cushings syndrome: clinical features, diagnosis, and treatment. Arq Bras Endocrinol Metabol 2007; 51(8): 1261-71.
[http://dx.doi.org/10.1590/S0004-27302007000800012] [PMID: 18209864]

[162] Kargi AY, Iacobellis G. Adipose tissue and adrenal glands: novel pathophysiological mechanisms and clinical applications. Int J Endocrinol 2014; 614074.
[http://dx.doi.org/10.1155/2014/614074]

[163] Bujalska IJ, Kumar S, Stewart PM. Does central obesity reflect Cushings disease of the omentum? Lancet 1997; 349(9060): 1210-3.
[http://dx.doi.org/10.1016/S0140-6736(96)11222-8] [PMID: 9130942]

[164] Zennaro M-C, Caprio M, Fève B. Mineralocorticoid receptors in the metabolic syndrome. Trends Endocrinol Metab 2009; 20(9): 444-51.
[http://dx.doi.org/10.1016/j.tem.2009.05.006] [PMID: 19800255]

[165] Barat P, Gayard-Cros M, Andrew R, *et al.* Truncal distribution of fat mass, metabolic profile and hypothalamic-pituitary adrenal axis activity in prepubertal obese children. J Pediatr 2007; 150(5): 535-539, 539.e1.
[http://dx.doi.org/10.1016/j.jpeds.2007.01.029] [PMID: 17452232]

[166] Karachentsev AN, Melchenko IA. [Effect of sex hormones on lipid peroxidation in the rat aorta]. Eksp Klin Farmakol 1997; 60(6): 13-6.
[PMID: 9460589]

[167] Sullivan JC, Sasser JM, Pollock JS. Sexual dimorphism in oxidant status in spontaneously hypertensive rats. Am J Physiol Regul Integr Comp Physiol 2007; 292(2): R764-8.
[http://dx.doi.org/10.1152/ajpregu.00322.2006] [PMID: 16917021]

[168] Ahlbom E, Grandison L, Bonfoco E, Zhivotovsky B, Ceccatelli S. Androgen treatment of neonatal rats decreases susceptibility of cerebellar granule neurons to oxidative stress *in vitro* Eur J Neurosci 1999; 11(4): 1285-91.
[http://dx.doi.org/10.1046/j.1460-9568.1999.00529.x] [PMID: 10103123]

[169] Chisu V, Manca P, Lepore G, Gadau S, Zedda M, Farina V. Testosterone induces neuroprotection from oxidative stress. Effects on catalase activity and 3-nitro-L-tyrosine incorporation into alpha-tubulin in a mouse neuroblastoma cell line. Arch Ital Biol 2006; 144(2): 63-73.
[PMID: 16642786]

[170] Alexandersen P, Haarbo J, Byrjalsen I, Lawaetz H, Christiansen C. Natural androgens inhibit male atherosclerosis: a study in castrated, cholesterol-fed rabbits. Circ Res 1999; 84(7): 813-9.
[http://dx.doi.org/10.1161/01.RES.84.7.813] [PMID: 10205149]

[171] English KM, Jones RD, Jones TH, Morice AH, Channer KS. Gender differences in the vasomotor effects of different steroid hormones in rat pulmonary and coronary arteries. Horm Metab Res 2001; 33(11): 645-52.
[http://dx.doi.org/10.1055/s-2001-18689] [PMID: 11733866]

[172] English KM, Jones RD, Jones TH, Morice AH, Channer KS. Testosterone acts as a coronary vasodilator by a calcium antagonistic action. J Endocrinol Invest 2002; 25(5): 455-8.
[http://dx.doi.org/10.1007/BF03344037] [PMID: 12035943]

[173] Deenadayalu VP, White RE, Stallone JN, Gao X, Garcia AJ. Testosterone relaxes coronary arteries by opening the large-conductance, calcium-activated potassium channel. Am J Physiol Heart Circ Physiol 2001; 281(4): H1720-7.
[PMID: 11557563]

[174] English KM, Mandour O, Steeds RP, Diver MJ, Jones TH, Channer KS. Men with coronary artery disease have lower levels of androgens than men with normal coronary angiograms. Eur Heart J 2000; 21(11): 890-4.
[http://dx.doi.org/10.1053/euhj.1999.1873] [PMID: 10806012]

[175] Morris P, Pugh PJ, Hall J. The relationship between smoking, statin therapy and testosterone in men with coronary artery disease. Endocr Abstr 2002; p. 248.

[176] English KM, Steeds R, Jones TH, Channer KS. Testosterone and coronary heart disease: is there a link? QJM 1997; 90(12): 787-91.
[http://dx.doi.org/10.1093/qjmed/90.12.787] [PMID: 9536344]

[177] Webb CM, Adamson DL, de Zeigler D, Collins P. Effect of acute testosterone on myocardial ischemia in men with coronary artery disease. Am J Cardiol 1999; 83(3): 437-439, A9.
[http://dx.doi.org/10.1016/S0002-9149(98)00880-7] [PMID: 10072236]

[178] Rosano GM, Leonardo F, Pagnotta P, *et al.* Acute anti-ischemic effect of testosterone in men with coronary artery disease. Circulation 1999; 99(13): 1666-70.
[http://dx.doi.org/10.1161/01.CIR.99.13.1666] [PMID: 10190874]

[179] Webb CM, McNeill JG, Hayward CS, de Zeigler D, Collins P. Effects of testosterone on coronary vasomotor regulation in men with coronary heart disease. Circulation 1999; 100(16): 1690-6.
[http://dx.doi.org/10.1161/01.CIR.100.16.1690] [PMID: 10525487]

[180] Jones RD, Pugh PJ, Jones TH, Channer KS. The vasodilatory action of testosterone: a potassium-channel opening or a calcium antagonistic action? Br J Pharmacol 2003; 138(5): 733-44.
[http://dx.doi.org/10.1038/sj.bjp.0705141] [PMID: 12642373]

[181] Jones RD, Ruban LN, Morton IE, et al. Testosterone inhibits the prostaglandin F2alpha-mediated increase in intracellular calcium in A7r5 aortic smooth muscle cells: evidence of an antagonistic action upon store-operated calcium channels. J Endocrinol 2003; 178(3): 381-93.
[http://dx.doi.org/10.1677/joe.0.1780381] [PMID: 12967331]

[182] Kupelian V, Page ST, Araujo AB, Travison TG, Bremner WJ, McKinlay JB. Low sex hormone-binding globulin, total testosterone, and symptomatic androgen deficiency are associated with development of the metabolic syndrome in nonobese men. J Clin Endocrinol Metab 2006; 91(3): 843-50.
[http://dx.doi.org/10.1210/jc.2005-1326] [PMID: 16394089]

[183] Von Eckardstein A, Wu FC. Testosterone and atherosclerosis. Growth Horm IGF Res 2003; 13 (Suppl. A): S72-84.

[184] Nieschlag E, Behre HM, Bouchard P, et al. Testosterone replacement therapy: current trends and future directions. Hum Reprod Update 2004; 10(5): 409-19.
[http://dx.doi.org/10.1093/humupd/dmh035] [PMID: 15297434]

[185] Kedziora-Kornatowska K, Bartosz M, Mussur M, Zasłonka J, Kedziora J, Bartosz G. The total antioxidant capacity of blood plasma during cardiovascular bypass surgery in patients with coronary heart disease. Cell Mol Biol Lett 2003; 8(4): 973-7.
[PMID: 14668920]

[186] Erel O. A novel automated method to measure total antioxidant response against potent free radical reactions. Clin Biochem 2004; 37(2): 112-9.
[http://dx.doi.org/10.1016/j.clinbiochem.2003.10.014] [PMID: 14725941]

[187] Demirbag R, Yilmaz R, Erel O. The association of total antioxidant capacity with sex hormones. Scand Cardiovasc J 2005; 39(3): 172-6.
[http://dx.doi.org/10.1080/14017430510035862] [PMID: 16146980]

[188] Mancini A, Leone E, Festa R, et al. Effects of testosterone on antioxidant systems in male secondary hypogonadism. J Androl 2008; 29(6): 622-9.
[http://dx.doi.org/10.2164/jandrol.107.004838] [PMID: 18641414]

[189] Felty Q, Xiong WC, Sun D, et al. Estrogen-induced mitochondrial reactive oxygen species as signal-transducing messengers. Biochemistry 2005; 44(18): 6900-9.
[http://dx.doi.org/10.1021/bi047629p] [PMID: 15865435]

[190] Borras C, Gambini J, Vina J. Mitochondrial oxidant generation is involved in determining why females live longer than males. Front Biosci 2007; 12: 1008-13.
[http://dx.doi.org/10.2741/2120] [PMID: 17127355]

[191] Vina J, Borras C, Gomez-Cabrera M, Orr W. Part of the series: from dietary antioxidants to regulators in cellular signalling and gene expression. Role of reactive of reactive oxygen species and (phyto)oestrogens in the modulation of adaptive response to stress. Free Rad Res 2006; 40: 111-9.

[192] Nilsson BO. Modulation of the inflammatory response by estrogens with focus on the endothelium and its interactions with leukocytes. Inflamm Res 2007; 56(7): 269-73.
[http://dx.doi.org/10.1007/s00011-007-6198-z] [PMID: 17659431]

[193] Ahotupa M, Mäntylä E, Kangas L. Antioxidant properties of the triphenylethylene antiestrogen drug toremifene. Naunyn Schmiedebergs Arch Pharmacol 1997; 356(3): 297-302.
[http://dx.doi.org/10.1007/PL00005054] [PMID: 9303565]

[194] Chen ZJ, Che D, Chang CH. Antioxidants, vitamin C and dithiothreitol, activate membrane-bound guanylate cyclase in PC12 cells. J Pharm Pharmacol 2001; 53(2): 243-7.
[http://dx.doi.org/10.1211/0022357011775262] [PMID: 11273022]

[195] Miura T, Muraoka S, Ogiso T. Inhibition of lipid peroxidation by estradiol and 2-hydroxyestradiol. Steroids 1996; 61(6): 379-83.
[http://dx.doi.org/10.1016/0039-128X(96)00044-X] [PMID: 8776801]

[196] Leal AM, Begoña Ruiz-Larrea M, Martínez R, Lacort M. Cytoprotective actions of estrogens against tert-butyl hydroperoxide-induced toxicity in hepatocytes. Biochem Pharmacol 1998; 56(11): 1463-9.
[http://dx.doi.org/10.1016/S0006-2952(98)00248-2] [PMID: 9827578]

[197] Arnal JF, Douin-Echinard V, Brouchet L, et al. Understanding the oestrogen action in experimental and clinical atherosclerosis. Fundam Clin Pharmacol 2006; 20(6): 539-48.
[http://dx.doi.org/10.1111/j.1472-8206.2006.00445.x] [PMID: 17109647]

[198] Buyon JP, Korchak HM, Rutherford LE, Ganguly M, Weissmann G. Female hormones reduce neutrophil responsiveness in vitro Arthritis Rheum 1984; 27(6): 623-30.
[http://dx.doi.org/10.1002/art.1780270604] [PMID: 6329234]

[199] Laloraya M, Jain S, Thomas M, Kopergaonkar S, Pradeep Kumar G. Estrogen surge: a regulatory switch for superoxide radical generation at implantation. Biochem Mol Biol Int 1996; 39(5): 933-40.
[PMID: 8866010]

[200] Roy D, Liehr JG. Temporary decrease in renal quinone reductase activity induced by chronic administration of estradiol to male Syrian hamsters. Increased superoxide formation by redox cycling of estrogen. J Biol Chem 1988; 263(8): 3646-51.
[PMID: 2831197]

[201] Békési G, Kakucs R, Várbíró S, et al. In vitro effects of different steroid hormones on superoxide anion production of human neutrophil granulocytes. Steroids 2000; 65(12): 889-94.
[http://dx.doi.org/10.1016/S0039-128X(00)00183-5] [PMID: 11077087]

[202] Gomez-Zubeldia M, Hernandez R, Viguera J, Arbues J, Aparicio A, Millan J. Cytochrome P-450/pseudosubstrate interactions and the role of antioxidants in the adrenal cortex. Endocr Res 2000; (26): 97-107.
[PMID: 10711726]

[203] Gómez-Zubeldia MA, Hinchado G, Arbués JJ, Nogales AG, Millán JC. Influence of estradiol on oxidative stress in the castrated rat uterus. Gynecol Oncol 2001; 80(2): 227-32.
[http://dx.doi.org/10.1006/gyno.2000.6057] [PMID: 11161864]

[204] Lee YM, Cheng PY, Hong SF, et al. Oxidative stress induces vascular heme oxygenase-1 expression in ovariectomized rats. Free Radic Biol Med 2005; 39(1): 108-17.
[http://dx.doi.org/10.1016/j.freeradbiomed.2005.02.033] [PMID: 15925283]

[205] Cho MM, Ziats NP, Pal D, Utian WH, Gorodeski GI. Estrogen modulates paracellular permeability of human endothelial cells by eNOS- and iNOS-related mechanisms. Am J Physiol 1999; 276(2 Pt 1): C337-49.
[PMID: 9950761]

[206] Zhu X, Bonet B, Gillenwater H, Knopp RH. Opposing effects of estrogen and progestins on LDL oxidation and vascular wall cytotoxicity: implications for atherogenesis. Proc Soc Exp Biol Med 1999; 222(3): 214-21.
[http://dx.doi.org/10.1046/j.1525-1373.1999.d01-138.x] [PMID: 10601880]

[207] Zhu X, Bonet B, Knopp RH. Estradiol 17beta inhibition of LDL oxidation and endothelial cell cytotoxicity is opposed by progestins to different degrees. Atherosclerosis 2000; 148(1): 31-41.
[http://dx.doi.org/10.1016/S0021-9150(99)00219-1] [PMID: 10580168]

[208] Joswig M, Hach-Wunderle V, Ziegler R, Nawroth PP. Postmenopausal hormone replacement therapy and the vascular wall: mechanisms of 17 beta-estradiols effects on vascular biology. Exp Clin

Endocrinol Diabetes 1999; 107(8): 477-87.
[http://dx.doi.org/10.1055/s-0029-1232556] [PMID: 10612478]

[209] Ayres S, Tang M, Subbiah MT. Estradiol-17beta as an antioxidant: some distinct features when compared with common fat-soluble antioxidants. J Lab Clin Med 1996; 128(4): 367-75.
[http://dx.doi.org/10.1016/S0022-2143(96)80008-4] [PMID: 8833885]

[210] Cynshi O, Stocker R. Inhibition of lipoprotein lipid oxidation. Handbook Exp Pharmacol 2005; 170(170): 563-90.
[http://dx.doi.org/10.1007/3-540-27661-0_21] [PMID: 16596815]

[211] Massafra C, De Felice C, Gioia D, Buonocore G. Variations in erythrocyte antioxidant glutathione peroxidase activity during the menstrual cycle. Clin Endocrinol (Oxf) 1998; 49(1): 63-7.
[http://dx.doi.org/10.1046/j.1365-2265.1998.00441.x] [PMID: 9797848]

[212] Subbiah MT. Estrogen replacement therapy and cardioprotection: mechanisms and controversies. Braz J Med Biol Res 2002; 35(3): 271-6.
[http://dx.doi.org/10.1590/S0100-879X2002000300001] [PMID: 11887204]

[213] Parthasarathy S, Khan-Merchant N, Penumetcha M, Santanam N. Oxidative stress in cardiovascular disease. J Nucl Cardiol 2001; 8(3): 379-89.
[http://dx.doi.org/10.1067/mnc.2001.114150] [PMID: 11391309]

[214] Pansini F, Mollica G, Bergamini CM. Management of the menopausal disturbances and oxidative stress. Curr Pharm Des 2005; 11(16): 2063-73.
[http://dx.doi.org/10.2174/1381612054065819] [PMID: 15974959]

[215] Lee JM, Appugliese D, Kaciroti N, Corwyn RF, Bradley RH, Lumeng JC. Weight status in young girls and the onset of puberty. Pediatrics 2007; 119(3): e624-30.
[http://dx.doi.org/10.1542/peds.2006-2188] [PMID: 17332182]

[216] Sam S. Obesity and Polycystic Ovary Syndrome. Obes Manag 2007; 3(2): 69-74.
[http://dx.doi.org/10.1089/obe.2007.0019]

[217] Chang RJ. The reproductive phenotype in polycystic ovary syndrome. Nat Clin Pract Endocrinol Metab 2007; 3(10): 688-95.
[http://dx.doi.org/10.1038/ncpendmet0637] [PMID: 17893687]

[218] Leung YM, Kwan CY. Dual vascular effects of leptin via endothelium: hypothesis and perspective. Chin J Physiol 2008; 51(1): 1-6.
[PMID: 18551989]

[219] Knudson JD, Dincer UD, Zhang C, *et al.* Leptin receptors are expressed in coronary arteries, and hyperLeptinemia causes significant coronary endothelial dysfunction. Am J Physiol Hear Circ Physiol 2005; 289: H48-56.
[http://dx.doi.org/10.1152/ajpheart.01159.2004]

[220] Vecchione C, Maffei A, Colella S, *et al.* Leptin effect on endothelial nitric oxide is mediated through Akt-endothelial nitric oxide synthase phosphorylation pathway. Diabetes 2002; 51(1): 168-73.
[http://dx.doi.org/10.2337/diabetes.51.1.168] [PMID: 11756337]

[221] Stengel A, Wang L, Goebel-Stengel M, Taché Y. Centrally injected kisspeptin reduces food intake by increasing meal intervals in mice. Neuroreport 2011; 22(5): 253-7.
[http://dx.doi.org/10.1097/WNR.0b013e32834558df] [PMID: 21386700]

[222] Sugiura M, Nakamura M, Ikoma Y, *et al.* The homeostasis model assessment-insulin resistance index is inversely associated with serum carotenoids in non-diabetic subjects. J Epidemiol 2006; 16(2): 71-8.
[http://dx.doi.org/10.2188/jea.16.71] [PMID: 16537987]

[223] Ylönen K, Alfthan G, Groop L, Saloranta C, Aro A, Virtanen SM. Dietary intakes and plasma concentrations of carotenoids and tocopherols in relation to glucose metabolism in subjects at high risk of type 2 diabetes: the Botnia Dietary Study. Am J Clin Nutr 2003; 77(6): 1434-41.
[PMID: 12791620]

[224] Ford ES, Will JC, Bowman BA, Narayan KM. Diabetes mellitus and serum carotenoids: findings from the Third National Health and Nutrition Examination Survey. Am J Epidemiol 1999; 149(2): 168-76.
[http://dx.doi.org/10.1093/oxfordjournals.aje.a009783] [PMID: 9921962]

[225] Hodge AM, English DR, ODea K, Giles GG. Dietary patterns and diabetes incidence in the Melbourne Collaborative Cohort Study. Am J Epidemiol 2007; 165(6): 603-10.
[http://dx.doi.org/10.1093/aje/kwk061] [PMID: 17220476]

[226] Hamer M, Chida Y. Intake of fruit, vegetables, and antioxidants and risk of type 2 diabetes: systematic review and meta-analysis. J Hypertens 2007; 25(12): 2361-9.
[http://dx.doi.org/10.1097/HJH.0b013e3282efc214] [PMID: 17984654]

[227] Rimm EB, Ascherio A, Giovannucci E, Spiegelman D, Stampfer MJ, Willett WC. Vegetable, fruit, and cereal fiber intake and risk of coronary heart disease among men. JAMA 1996; 275(6): 447-51.
[http://dx.doi.org/10.1001/jama.1996.03530300031036] [PMID: 8627965]

[228] Liu S, Manson JE, Lee IM, *et al.* Fruit and vegetable intake and risk of cardiovascular disease: the Womens Health Study. Am J Clin Nutr 2000; 72(4): 922-8.
[PMID: 11010932]

[229] Dauchet L, Amouyel P, Hercberg S, Dallongeville J. Fruit and vegetable consumption and risk of coronary heart disease: a meta-analysis of cohort studies. J Nutr 2006; 136(10): 2588-93.
[PMID: 16988131]

[230] Kris-Etherton PM, Hecker KD, Bonanome A, *et al.* Bioactive compounds in foods: their role in the prevention of cardiovascular disease and cancer. Am J Med 2002; 113 (Suppl. 9B): 71S-88S.
[http://dx.doi.org/10.1016/S0002-9343(01)00995-0] [PMID: 12566142]

[231] Korish AA, Arafah MM. Catechin combined with vitamins C and E ameliorates insulin resistance (IR) and atherosclerotic changes in aged rats with chronic renal failure (CRF). Arch Gerontol Geriatr 2008; 46(1): 25-39.
[http://dx.doi.org/10.1016/j.archger.2007.02.006] [PMID: 17418908]

[232] Houseknecht KL, Vanden Heuvel JP, Moya-Camarena SY, *et al.* Dietary conjugated linoleic acid normalizes impaired glucose tolerance in the Zucker diabetic fatty fa/fa rat. Biochem Biophys Res Commun 1998; 244(3): 678-82.
[http://dx.doi.org/10.1006/bbrc.1998.8303] [PMID: 9535724]

[233] Haber CA, Lam TK, Yu Z, *et al.* N-acetylcysteine and taurine prevent hyperglycemia-induced insulin resistance *in vivo*: possible role of oxidative stress. Am J Physiol Endocrinol Metab 2003; 285(4): E744-53.
[http://dx.doi.org/10.1152/ajpendo.00355.2002] [PMID: 12799318]

[234] Nakaya Y, Minami A, Harada N, Sakamoto S, Niwa Y, Ohnaka M. Taurine improves insulin sensitivity in the Otsuka Long-Evans Tokushima Fatty rat, a model of spontaneous type 2 diabetes. Am J Clin Nutr 2000; 71(1): 54-8.
[PMID: 10617946]

[235] Xiao C, Giacca A, Lewis GF. Oral taurine but not N-acetylcysteine ameliorates NEFA-induced impairment in insulin sensitivity and beta cell function in obese and overweight, non-diabetic men. Diabetologia 2008; 51(1): 139-46.
[http://dx.doi.org/10.1007/s00125-007-0859-x] [PMID: 18026714]

[236] Shih CK, Chang JH, Yang SH, Chou TW, Cheng HH. beta-Carotene and canthaxanthin alter the pro-oxidation and antioxidation balance in rats fed a high-cholesterol and high-fat diet. Br J Nutr 2008; 99(1): 59-66.
[http://dx.doi.org/10.1017/S0007114507781497] [PMID: 17640418]

[237] Inami S, Takano M, Yamamoto M, *et al.* Tea catechin consumption reduces circulating oxidized low-density lipoprotein. Int Heart J 2007; 48(6): 725-32.
[http://dx.doi.org/10.1536/ihj.48.725] [PMID: 18160764]

[238] Bose KS, Agrawal BK. Effect of lycopene from cooked tomatoes on serum antioxidant enzymes, lipid peroxidation rate and lipid profile in coronary heart disease. Singapore Med J 2007; 48(5): 415-20.
[PMID: 17453080]

[239] Esmaillzadeh A, Kimiagar M, Mehrabi Y, Azadbakht L, Hu FB, Willett WC. Fruit and vegetable intakes, C-reactive protein, and the metabolic syndrome. Am J Clin Nutr 2006; 84(6): 1489-97.
[PMID: 17158434]

[240] Parra D, Bandarra NM, Kiely M, Thorsdottir I, Martínez JA. Impact of fish intake on oxidative stress when included into a moderate energy-restricted program to treat obesity. Eur J Nutr 2007; 46(8): 460-7.
[http://dx.doi.org/10.1007/s00394-007-0686-3] [PMID: 18026868]

[241] Azadbakht L, Kimiagar M, Mehrabi Y, Esmaillzadeh A, Hu FB, Willett WC. Soy consumption, markers of inflammation, and endothelial function: a cross-over study in postmenopausal women with the metabolic syndrome. Diabetes Care 2007; 30(4): 967-73.
[http://dx.doi.org/10.2337/dc06-2126] [PMID: 17392557]

[242] Czernichow S, Couthouis A, Bertrais S, *et al.* Antioxidant supplementation does not affect fasting plasma glucose in the Supplementation with Antioxidant Vitamins and Minerals (SU.VI.MAX) study in France: association with dietary intake and plasma concentrations. Am J Clin Nutr 2006; 84(2): 395-9.
[PMID: 16895889]

[243] Dietary supplementation with n-3 polyunsaturated fatty acids and vitamin E after myocardial infarction: results of the GISSI-Prevenzione trial. Gruppo Italiano per lo Studio della Sopravvivenza nellInfarto miocardico. Lancet 1999; 354(9177): 447-55.
[http://dx.doi.org/10.1016/S0140-6736(99)07072-5] [PMID: 10465168]

[244] Antoniades C, Tousoulis D, Tentolouris C, Toutouzas P, Stefanadis C. Oxidative stress, antioxidant vitamins, and atherosclerosis. From basic research to clinical practice. Herz 2003; 28(7): 628-38.
[http://dx.doi.org/10.1007/s00059-003-2417-8] [PMID: 14689123]

[245] Weinberg RB, VanderWerken BS, Anderson RA, Stegner JE, Thomas MJ. Pro-oxidant effect of vitamin E in cigarette smokers consuming a high polyunsaturated fat diet. Arterioscler Thromb Vasc Biol 2001; 21(6): 1029-33.
[http://dx.doi.org/10.1161/01.ATV.21.6.1029] [PMID: 11397715]

[246] Collins R, Armitage J, Parish S, Sleight P, Peto R. MRC/BHF Heart Protection Study of antioxidant vitamin supplementation in 20,536 high-risk individuals: a randomised placebo-controlled trial. Lancet 2002; 360(9326): 23-33.
[http://dx.doi.org/10.1016/S0140-6736(02)09328-5] [PMID: 12114037]

[247] Mancini A, Leone E, Festa R, Grande G, Di Donna V, De Marinis L, *et al.* Evaluation of antioxidant systems (coenzyme Q10 and total antioxidant capacity) in morbid obesity before and after biliopancreatic diversion. Metabolism 2008; 57: 1384-9.

[248] Mancini A. Oxidative stress and metabolic syndrome: effects of a natural antioxidants enriched diet on insulin resistance. Clin Nutrition ESPEN 10: e52-60.

[249] Yusuf S, Dagenais G, Pogue J, Bosch J, Sleight P. Vitamin E supplementation and cardiovascular events in high-risk patients. N Engl J Med 2000; 342(3): 154-60.
[http://dx.doi.org/10.1056/NEJM200001203420302] [PMID: 10639540]

[250] Shaw LM. The insulin receptor substrate (IRS) proteins: at the intersection of metabolism and cancer. Cell Cycle 2011; 10(11): 1750-6.
[http://dx.doi.org/10.4161/cc.10.11.15824] [PMID: 21597332]

[251] Shabrova EV, Tarnopolsky O, Singh AP, Plutzky J, Vorsa N, Quadro L. Insights into the molecular mechanisms of the anti-atherogenic actions of flavonoids in normal and obese mice. PLoS One 2011; 6(10): e24634.

[http://dx.doi.org/10.1371/journal.pone.0024634] [PMID: 22016761]

[252] Curtis PJ, Sampson M, Potter J, Dhatariya K, Kroon PA, Cassidy A. Chronic ingestion of flavan-3-ols and isoflavones improves insulin sensitivity and lipoprotein status and attenuates estimated 10-year CVD risk in medicated postmenopausal women with type 2 diabetes: a 1-year, double-blind, randomized, controlled trial. Diabetes Care 2012; 35(2): 226-32.
[http://dx.doi.org/10.2337/dc11-1443] [PMID: 22250063]

[253] Strauss RS. Comparison of serum concentrations of alpha-tocopherol and beta-carotene in a cross-sectional sample of obese and nonobese children (NHANES III). National Health and Nutrition Examination Survey. J Pediatr 1999; 134(2): 160-5.
[http://dx.doi.org/10.1016/S0022-3476(99)70409-9] [PMID: 9931523]

[254] Chiavaroli V, Giannini C, DAdamo E, de Giorgis T, Chiarelli F, Mohn A. Insulin resistance and oxidative stress in children born small and large for gestational age. Pediatrics 2009; 124(2): 695-702.
[http://dx.doi.org/10.1542/peds.2008-3056] [PMID: 19651586]

[255] Mohn A, Chiavaroli V, Cerruto M, *et al.* Increased oxidative stress in prepubertal children born small for gestational age. J Clin Endocrinol Metab 2007; 92(4): 1372-8.
[http://dx.doi.org/10.1210/jc.2006-1344] [PMID: 17264184]

[256] Hillestrøm PR, Weimann A, Jensen CB, Storgaard H, Vaag AA, Poulsen HE. Consequences of low birthweight on urinary excretion of DNA markers of oxidative stress in young men. Scand J Clin Lab Invest 2006; 66(5): 363-70.
[http://dx.doi.org/10.1080/00365510600696402] [PMID: 16901847]

[257] Park E. Birth weight was negatively correlated with plasma ghrelin, insulin resistance, and coenzyme Q10 levels in overweight children. Nutr Res Pract 2010; 4(4): 311-6.
[http://dx.doi.org/10.4162/nrp.2010.4.4.311] [PMID: 20827347]

[258] Miles MV, Morrison JA, Horn PS, Tang PH, Pesce AJ. Coenzyme Q10 changes are associated with metabolic syndrome. Clin Chim Acta 2004; 344(1-2): 173-9.
[http://dx.doi.org/10.1016/j.cccn.2004.02.016] [PMID: 15149886]

[259] Menke T, Niklowitz P, de Sousa G, Reinehr T, Andler W. Comparison of coenzyme Q10 plasma levels in obese and normal weight children. Clin Chim Acta 2004; 349(1-2): 121-7.
[http://dx.doi.org/10.1016/j.cccn.2004.06.015] [PMID: 15469864]

[260] Pashankar DS, Loening-Baucke V. Increased prevalence of obesity in children with functional constipation evaluated in an academic medical center. Pediatrics 2005; 116(3): e377-80.
[http://dx.doi.org/10.1542/peds.2005-0490] [PMID: 16140681]

[261] Gropper SS, Acosta PB. The therapeutic effect of fiber in treating obesity. J Am Coll Nutr 1987; 6(6): 533-5.
[http://dx.doi.org/10.1080/07315724.1987.10720213] [PMID: 2826563]

[262] Pignatelli P, Basili S. Nutraceuticals in the early infancy. Cardiovasc Ther 2010; 28(4): 236-45.
[http://dx.doi.org/10.1111/j.1755-5922.2010.00194.x] [PMID: 20553293]

[263] Lavine JE. Vitamin E treatment of nonalcoholic steatohepatitis in children: a pilot study. J Pediatr 2000; 136(6): 734-8.
[http://dx.doi.org/10.1016/S0022-3476(00)05040-X] [PMID: 10839868]

[264] Kugelmas M, Hill DB, Vivian B, Marsano L, McClain CJ. Cytokines and NASH: a pilot study of the effects of lifestyle modification and vitamin E. Hepatology 2003; 38(2): 413-9.
[http://dx.doi.org/10.1053/jhep.2003.50316] [PMID: 12883485]

[265] Vajro P, Mandato C, Franzese A, *et al.* Vitamin E treatment in pediatric obesity-related liver disease: a randomized study. J Pediatr Gastroenterol Nutr 2004; 38(1): 48-55.
[http://dx.doi.org/10.1097/00005176-200401000-00012] [PMID: 14676594]

[266] Nobili V, Marcellini M, Devito R, *et al.* NAFLD in children: a prospective clinical-pathological study and effect of lifestyle advice. Hepatology 2006; 44(2): 458-65.

[http://dx.doi.org/10.1002/hep.21262] [PMID: 16871574]

[267] Wang C-L, Liang L, Fu J-F, *et al.* Effect of lifestyle intervention on non-alcoholic fatty liver disease in Chinese obese children. World J Gastroenterol 2008; 14(10): 1598-602.
[http://dx.doi.org/10.3748/wjg.14.1598] [PMID: 18330955]

[268] Nobili V, Manco M, Devito R, *et al.* Lifestyle intervention and antioxidant therapy in children with nonalcoholic fatty liver disease: a randomized, controlled trial. Hepatology 2008; 48(1): 119-28.
[http://dx.doi.org/10.1002/hep.22336] [PMID: 18537181]

[269] Reinehr T, Andler W. Changes in the atherogenic risk factor profile according to degree of weight loss. Arch Dis Child 2004; 89(5): 419-22.
[http://dx.doi.org/10.1136/adc.2003.028803] [PMID: 15102630]

[270] Zimmet P, Alberti KG, Kaufman F, *et al.* The metabolic syndrome in children and adolescents - an IDF consensus report. Pediatr Diabetes 2007; 8(5): 299-306.
[http://dx.doi.org/10.1111/j.1399-5448.2007.00271.x] [PMID: 17850473]

[271] Codoñer-Franch P, López-Jaén AB, De La Mano-Hernández A, Sentandreu E, Simó-Jordá R, Valls-Bellés V. Effects of hypocaloric very-low- carbohydrate diet vs. Mediterranean diet on endothelial function in obese women. Eur J Clin Invest 2009 May; 39(5): 339-47.
[http://dx.doi.org/10.1111/j.1651-2227.2010.01903.x] [PMID: 19302563]

[272] Murer SB, Aeberli I, Braegger CP, *et al.* Antioxidant supplements reduced oxidative stress and stabilized liver function tests but did not reduce inflammation in a randomized controlled trial in obese children and adolescents. J Nutr 2014; 144(2): 193-201.
[http://dx.doi.org/10.3945/jn.113.185561] [PMID: 24353344]

[273] Buscemi S, Verga S, Tranchina MR, Cottone S, Cerasola G. Effects of hypocaloric very-low-carbohydrate diet vs. Mediterranean diet on endothelial function in obese women. Eur J Clin Invest 2009 May; 39(5): 339-47.
[PMID: 19302563]

CHAPTER 5

The Role of Gut Microflora in Obesity - Does the Data Provide an Option for Intervention?

Parth J. Parekh[1], Edward C. Oldfield, IV[2], Amrit Lamba[3] and David A. Johnson[4],*

[1] Department of Internal Medicine, Division of Gastroenterology and Hepatology, Tulane University, New Orleans, LA, USA

[2] Department of Internal Medicine, Eastern Virginia Medical School, Norfolk, VA, USA

[3] Department of Internal Medicine, Tulane University, New Orleans, LA, USA

[4] Department of Internal Medicine, Division of Gastroenterology and Hepatology, Eastern Virginia Medical School, Norfolk, VA, USA

Abstract: The obesity epidemic has proven to have a significant burden on the current of state of healthcare. At an individual level, obesity and its sequelae have numerous effects on the state of health and quality of life. On a global perspective, treatment of obesity and its sequelae come at a high cost. Obesity, in terms of intestinal dysbiosis, is a complicated disequilibrium that offers many unclear complications. Thus, restoration of the commensal microflora serves a potential therapeutic option in combatting the obesity epidemic be it *via* antibiotic therapy, probiotics, prebiotics, symbiotics (combination of prebiotic and probiotic therapy), or fecal microbiota transplant. This manuscript will review the role of intestinal dysbiosis in the pathogenesis of obesity and the potential role for microflora manipulation as therapy.

Keywords: Antibiotics, Butyrate, Dysbiosis, Fecal Microbiota Transplant, FFAR, Fiaf, Metabolic Endotoxemia, Microbiota, Obesity, Prebiotics, Probiotics, Proprionate, SCFAs, Symbiotics.

INTRODUCTION

The commensal microbiota is the largest immune system in the body, which is host to approximately 10^{14} microorganisms and comprised of greater than 1,000 distinct bacterial species [1]. The gut microbiota is also thought to play a pivotal role in metabolic programming, and thus recent research efforts have focused on the role of intestinal dysbiosis in the pathogenesis of obesity [1, 2].

---

* **Corresponding author David A. Johnson:** Division of Gastroenterology and Hepatology, Eastern Virginia Medical School, Norfolk, VA 23510, USA; Tel: (757)466-0615; Fax: (757) 466-9082; E-mail: dajevms@aol.com

Atta-ur-Rahman and M. Iqbal Choudhary (Eds.)
All rights reserved-© 2017 Bentham Science Publishers

Through recent advances in pyrosequencing technologies, researchers have gained further insight into the symbiotic relationship between the intestinal microbiota and the mammalian host, and how this dynamic interrelationship can have significant impact on regulating metabolic function. This then raises the question as to whether or not manipulating the commensal microbiota is potential for therapy in combating the obesity epidemic, which currently afflicts more than 1/3 of the adult population in the United States [1]. Here, we review the current literature relating to the gut microbiota, provide an overview on the role of intestinal dysbiosis on the pathogenesis of obesity, and discuss approaches to manipulate this symbiotic relationship as a potential for therapy.

OBESITY AND THE MICROFLORA: A BRIEF OVERVIEW

Initial studies in mice demonstrated that transfer of gut microflora from conventionally raised, genetically obese mice into germ-free mice resulted in phenotypically obese mice, suggesting obesity is a transmissible trait through the microbiota [3 - 6]. These studies led to further investigation into the underlying mechanisms at play. There are several ways by which the commensal microflora is thought modulate host energy metabolism, which ultimately contribute to the pathogenesis of obesity. These include bile acid metabolism, fermentation of dietary polysaccharides, and chronic inflammation (see Fig. **1**).

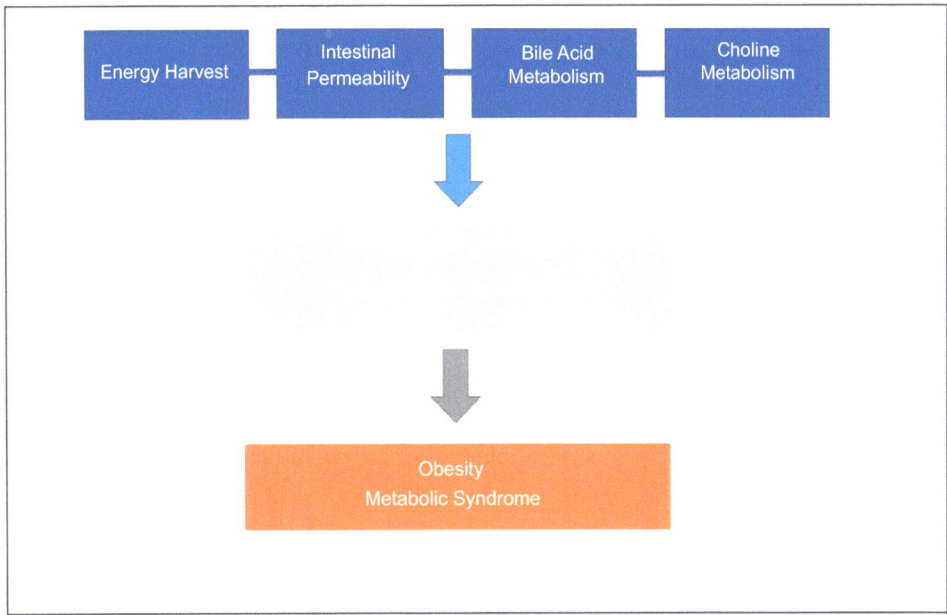

Fig. (1). Intestinal dysbiosis and the underlying mechanisms in the pathogenesis of obesity and the metabolic syndrome [1, 7 - 9].

Recent studies have demonstrated that microbiota-mediated changes in the bile acid metabolism contribute to the pathogenesis of obesity [7 - 9]. Bile acids are signaling molecules that act as a natural ligand for nuclear hormone receptors, namely farsenoid X receptor (FXR), which are expressed at high levels in the intestine [10]. Most recently, Parséus et al. investigated the role of the gut microflora in modulating obesity and associated phenotypes through FXR [11]. Germ-free mice, conventionally raised wild-type, and FXR -/- mice were fed a high-fat diet for 10 days, during which their weight gain, glucose metabolism, gut microflora composition, and bile acid composition were closely monitored. In addition, gut microflora was transferred from wild-type and FXR -/- mice to germ-free mice. After a 10-week high-fat diet, conventionally raised wild-type mice gained significantly more weight than germ-free mice, which occurred in association with increased fasting glucose and insulin levels in addition to impaired glucose and insulin tolerance. In the absence of intact FXR signaling, the gut microflora did not affect weight gain, however these mice did exhibit increased fasting glucose and insulin levels and impaired glucose and insulin tolerance similar to that seen in conventionally raised wild-type mice. Conversely in FXR -/- mice, the presence of the gut microflora did not affect fasting insulin or insulin tolerance. They also noted that the bile acid composition differed between FXR -/- and wild-type mice. Pyrosequencing demonstrated decreased levels of *Firmicutes* and increased levels of *Bacteroidetes* in FXR -/- mice compared to wild-type mice after being fed a high-fat diet for ten weeks. Lastly, the authors investigated the role of altered gut microbiota and its impact on metabolic differences between conventionally raised wild-type mice and FXR -/- mice. Microflora from FXR -/- mice fed a high-fat diet and conventionally raised wild-type mice were transferred into germ-free mice and after ten weeks on a high-fat diet, mice colonized with the microflora from FXR -/- gained less weight than mice that were colonized with microflora from conventionally raised wild-type mice. This led the authors to conclude that intestinal dysbiosis promotes diet-induced obesity through FXR and that FXR alters the microbial composition, which may contribute to increased adiposity.

Another way by which the gut microflora contributes to the pathogenesis of obesity is through its role in energy harvest, namely the fermentation of dietary polysaccharides [2, 6]. Through a complex process involving methanogens in the gut (primarily the distal small intestine), the commensal microflora ferments dietary polysaccharides to form its metabolites, namely monosaccharides and short chain fatty acids (SCFAs), which regulates energy homeostasis in the host [2]. The three main SCFAs produced are acetate, propionate, and butyrate, all of which have been shown to have protective effects against diet-induced obesity and insulin resistance; acetate and propionate are the main metabolites produced by *Bacteroidetes*, whereas butyrate is the main metabolite produced by *Firmicutes*

[1, 12, 13]. After being produced in the colon, the three SCFAs are absorbed through gut epithelial cells, but each has different roles in metabolic function. Acetate, which is readily absorbed, enters hepatic portal circulation and is subsequently distributed throughout the body as a substrate for cholesterol synthesis [14]. Similar to acetate, propionate also enters hepatic portal circulation, however it is primarily stored in the liver where its utilized in gluconeogenesis [14]. Butyrate is not as readily absorbed compared to acetate and propionate, and thus is primarily oxidized by colonocytes ultimately acting as an energy source [14, 15]. Studies have demonstrated there to be increased fermentation activity by the gut microflora and as a result a greater concentration of fecal SCFAs in obese cohorts compared to overweight and lean subjects [16, 17].

Free fatty acid receptors (FFAR) 2 and 3, which are G-protein coupled receptors, mediate the signaling cascades of acetate (which has an affinity for FFAR 2), propionate (which has an affinity for FFAR 3), and butyrate (which has an affinity for FFAR 3) [1, 2, 18]. FFAR 2 and FFAR 3 work in tandem to regulate satiety and intestinal motility [19]. Quantitative studies have demonstrated an increased expression of FFAR 2 and 3 in glucagon-like peptide-1 secreting cells, which modulate satiety *via* production of digestive enzymes [16, 20]. Additionally, mice models have shown that FFAR2 and FFAR3-deficient mice have increased energy expenditure, lean body mass, and significantly lower fat body mass when compared to wild-type mice [21, 22].

Fasting-induced adipocyte factor (Fiaf), also referred to as angiopoietin-like-4, is a protein that is predominately secreted by the liver that has been shown to suppress the production of adipocyte-LPL (lipoprotein lipase) [1, 2]. The primary function of LPL is to hydrolyze triglycerides into two free fatty acids and one monoacylglycerol molecule, which are then able to enter the adipocyte where they are then re-esterified into triglycerides and stored as fat [12, 23]. Hypothalamic expression of Fiaf is regulated *via* physiologic appetite regulators, which ultimately induce an anorexigenic effect through inhibition of AMP-activated protein kinase (AMPK) activity, suggesting a central regulatory role of Fiaf in energy homeostasis [1, 2, 15]. Bäckhead and colleagues were able to demonstrate an increase in LPL activity in adipose tissue with an accompanying decrease in Fiaf expression with a net result being phenotypically obese mice upon conventionalization of germ-free mice [3]. A subsequent study by Bäckhead *et al.* demonstrated that germ-free Fiaf-deficient mice were not resistant to high-fat western diet-induced obesity when compared to germ-free wild-type mice, which suggests that the gut microflora suppresses Fiaf expression as a regulatory mechanism, thereby increasing LPL activity and fat deposition in adipocytes [4]. In the same study, Bäckhead *et al.* also demonstrated that conventionalization of germ-free mice resulted in decreased expression of skeletal and hepatic levels of

AMPK [4]. In addition, there was increased fatty acid oxidation and elevated levels of AMP and NAD+ in skeletal muscle and liver, respectively, in the germ-free population when subjected to a high-fat western diet. This led authors to conclude that the microflora has a suppressive effect on fatty acid oxidation and AMPK, which predisposes the host to obesity [1, 2, 4].

The commensal microbiota also serves a critical role in the development of the innate immune system and host energy metabolism that starts even before birth and thus is dependent on maternal-fetal interactions. It has been well documented that the gut microbiota undergoes significant changes throughout the first several years of life, with constant variation in the predominate taxa ranging from *Escherichia, Clostridium, Bacteroides,* or *Bifidobacterium*; these changes in the gut microbiota likely reflect the changes needed for optimization of energy harvest and nutrient extraction from the changing composition of breast during this time [24 - 27]. Additionally, differences in the microbiota are impacted by the composition of breast milk and formula compositions, again suggesting a role of the gut microbiota in the regulation of metabolism [27, 28]. Furthermore, these microbial changes have been linked to the pathogenesis of pediatric obesity [28], however further investigation is necessary before any definitive conclusion can be drawn about the relationship between childhood obesity and the gut microbiota.

Lastly, intestinal dysbiosis resulting in obesity is associated with a low-grade inflammatory state that impacts energy homeostasis. This may be the result of several mechanisms working in concert. The first of which is the effect of metabolic endotoxemia on the pro-inflammatory cascade. Lipopolysaccharides (LPS), or bacterial endotoxins, trigger metabolic endotoxemia and ultimately drive the pro-inflammatory cascade [1, 2]. This is thought to occur as intestinal dysbiosis disrupts intestinal permeability and reduces the expression of genes coding for proteins of the tight junctions and ultimately triggering the pro-inflammatory cascade [29]. Vors *et al*. recently evaluated whether fat amounts can modulate postprandial dynamics and handling of LPS by varying postprandial lipidemia in humans of different body mass indices [30]. In this randomized, controlled, cross-over study, eight normal-weight and eight obese age-matched men, ingested meals of varying fat content (10 *vs* 40 grams of fat) with blood samples, leukocytes, and chylomicron-rich fractions obtained during 8 hours. In addition, plasma LPS transporters (LBP and sCD14), and inflammatory mediators (interleukin-6 and nuclear factor-κB) were measured. They found that the obese cohort had higher postprandial endotoxemia after 40g ingestion of fat and their chylomicrons were more enriched with LPS compared to their normal weight counterpart. This led them to conclude that postprandial endotoxemia is modulated by the amount of ingested fat in obese men. In addition, LPS handling in plasma through chylomicrons and LBP appeared to drive the pro-inflammatory response. The mechanism for this may be explained by the fact that high-fat ingestion leads to adipocyte hypertrophy, which may be associated with local hypoxia and apoptosis [31]. Hypertrophic adipocytes secrete tumor necrosis factor-alpha in low quantities that stimulates a chemotactic response and attracts macrophages in response to the increase in adipocyte turnover.

Second, intestinal dysbiosis impacts obesity through the effect of impaired cellular immunity. Toll-like receptors (TLRs) are a type of pattern recognition receptor, which form a superfamily with interleukin-1 [1]. TLR-5 is a specific TLR that has been extensively studied as it has been demonstrated to have an essential role in the activation of innate immunity. By recognizing microbe-associated molecular patterns, as seen on bacteria, viruses, and fungi, TLR-5 interacts with the commensal microflora resulting in the induction of the pro-inflammatory cascade by activating pro-inflammatory mediators, most notable is nuclear factor-κB [1, 2, 32, 33]. Studies have also demonstrated that mice deficient in TLR-5 have a tendency to develop hallmark features of the obesity and the metabolic syndrome [34]. The role of TLRs-2 and -4 in the pathogenesis of obesity and the metabolic syndrome has also been described [35 - 38]. Loera-Rodriguez *et al*. recently evaluated the expression of TLR4 in a group of non-diabetic, obese Mexican patients [35]. A group of 210 patients were evaluated, 105 normal weight individuals and 105 non-diabetic obese patients. They found obesity to be strongly associated with the expression of TLR4 (77%, mean fluorescence index MFI) 7.70) compared to the normal weight cohort (70%, MFI 6.41). This led the authors to conclude that immune cells, *e.g.* TLR-4, stimulated by non-esterified fatty acids produce pro-inflammatory cytokines resulting in low-grade chronic inflammation, now described in the pathogenesis of obesity.

DATA AND OPTIONS FOR INTERVENTION

Clearly, the relationship between the gut microbiota and the development of obesity is multifactorial and we are only beginning to understand in intricacies of its pathogenesis. Current literature, while sometimes conflicting, does highlight some potential characteristic changes within the gut microbiota, which may represent potential therapeutic targets for the treatment of obesity. One such example is the increase in *Firmicutes* and decrease in *Bacteroidetes* that has been reported in obese individuals when compared to lean controls [3, 39 - 42]. Interestingly, the level of dysbiosis between these two phyla can be used to estimate a relative rate of energy harvest from diet; a study which examined the microflora of lean individuals demonstrated that a 20% relative change in the ratio of *Firmicutes:Bacteroidetes*, favoring an increased *Firmicutes* populous approximates a 150 kcal difference in energy harvest [43]. While there is some conflicting evidence that variations in the abundance of certain bacterial species may be more important than phylum level changes, these observed findings still highlight potential targets for intervention within the gut microbiotia. Other microbes have also been implicated in the pathogenesis of obesity. Several studies have demonstrated that an increase in *Proteobacteria* and *Bacteriodetes* coupled with decreased *Akkermansia muciniphilia*, is associated with increased obesity, insulin resistance, and inflammation [44, 45]. When combined, these alterations seen with obesity and the metabolic syndrome suggests that manipulation of the gut microbiome is a potential candidate for therapeutic intervention. This section seeks to explore the current evidence behind the use of antibiotics, probiotics, prebiotics, synbiotics, and fecal transplant as potential treatment options for obesity and the inherently linked metabolic syndrome.

Antibiotics

Antibiotics are commonly used to correct an underlying dysbiosis that occurs in certain disease states. As described earlier, there appears to be an underlying relationship between intestinal dysbiosis and the chronic low-grade inflammation that occurs in the pathogenesis of obesity and the metabolic syndrome. There are several overlapping pathways between the innate immune system and intestinal dysbiosis in the development of obesity, which may serve as potential targeted therapy.

The effects of antibiotics on the gut microbiome have been extensively studied, dating back to the early 1950s [46]. Recently, the attention has shifted onto the role of antibiotics to selectively modulate the gut microflora as a potential therapeutic option. Membrez *et al.* evaluated the role of antibiotics in combating diet-induced obesity (DIO) in mice [47]. Mice subjected to DIO were administered a combination of norfloxacin and ampicillin in their drinking water for 14 days, with results indicating that a dose of 1g/L resulted in maximal suppression of cecal aerobic and anaerobic bacteria. After two weeks of treatment, there were decreased blood glucose concentrations, increased liver glycogen stores, and decreased liver triglycerides. The authors concluded that while there appeared to be no reduction in body weight, antibiotics improved glucose tolerance in mice subjected to DIO. This study highlights the intricate nature of the metabolic pathways associated with obesity.

Rajpal *et al.* selectively manipulated the gut microflora in mice subjected to DIO [48]. Mice deficient of leptin were subjected to vancomycin (VAN) or ceftazidime (CEF) to modulate the gut microflora, with outcomes assessed using 16S rRNA sequencing techniques. These two antibiotics were allowed for distinct changes in gram-positive *versus* gram-negative bacteria as vancomycin inhibits the cell wall synthesis of gram-positive bacteria, whereas ceftazidime inhibits cell-wall synthesis in predominately gram-negative bacteria with minimal gram-positive coverage. Each antibiotic was given at three different doses (50 mg/kg, 150 mg/kg, or 500 mg/kg) daily over a two-week period and were then compared to mice fed normal chow (vehicle) and a prebiotic supplemented chow. At the end of two weeks, there were significant changes in weight in CEF150 mg/kg (p =0.004), CEF 500 mg/kg (p < 0.0001) and prebiotic (p < 0.0001) cohorts compared to baseline and the vehicle group. Mice in the prebiotics and CEF cohorts (irrespective of dose) exhibited decreased overall food intake, and decreased body fat percentage at 14 days in the prebiotic (p<0.0001) and CEF 500 mg/kg groups (p < 0.0001). In addition, the prebiotics and CEF 500mg/kg groups had decreased cytoplasmic lipid droplet content in the liver and brown adipose tissue. When comparing the biochemical changes, the CEF treated mice demonstrated a number of significant changes including improved hyperglycemic control and decreased plasma glucose and triglyceride levels.

These results suggest that specific antibiotics, in this case CEF, can alter the commensal microflora in a way that induces weight reduction and influences insulin signaling. VAN treated groups had a predominance in *Proteobacteria*, a gram-negative bacterial, whereas CEF treated groups demonstrated a skew towards increases in *Firmicutes*, a predominantly gram-positive bacteria. In addition, CEF treated groups had an overall increased abundance of *Lactobacillales* and decreased *Bacteroidetes* and *Clostridia*. One important observation from this study is that while mice treated with higher doses of CEF exhibited a greater change in body weight and fat compared to the lower dose group, pyrosequencing did not demonstrate there to be any significant differences in the gut microflora [48]. This suggests that microbial changes at a species and subspecies level need to be further investigated and may offer future research targets.

Despite promising results from rodent models, translational research does not support a beneficial effect for antibiotics in the treatment of obesity. While there are a number of studies that suggests early administration of antibiotics results in the development of childhood obesity [49 - 53], it is important to note that these studies are subjected to a significant number of potentially confounding factors that include maternal risk factors, socioeconomic status, delivery method, and breastfeeding status. A recent meta-analysis by Mikkelsen *et al*., which totaled 2 observational studies and 4 prospective trials, demonstrated there to be limited evidence to support a casual or mechanistic effect of antibiotics on body weight due to variation in study design, small sample sizes, and lack of significant changes in long-term outcomes data [49].

Recently, Reijnders et al. performed a double-blinded randomized placebo-control trial that compared the effects of antibiotics (administering amoxicillin, vancomycin, or placebo for 7 days) among 57 obese, pre-diabetic men on the gut microbiome [7]. The authors found that vancomycin ($p < 0.001$), but not amoxicillin ($p = 0.42$), resulted in decrease bacterial diversity compared to placebo. Vancomycin decreased the relative abundance of primarily gram-positive bacteria in the *Firmicutes* phylum; particularly affected groups were butyrate producing species such-as *Coprococcus eutactus, Faecalibacterium prausnitzii*, and *Anaerostipes caccae*. This was coupled with an increase in relative abundance of several gram-negative *Proteobacteria*. Furthermore, these changes were persistent for 8-weeks after the last dose of vancomycin. In contrast, there were no changes in the microbial composition in the amoxicillin cohort after 7-days of treatment and 8-weeks after their last dose of amoxicillin. To further assess the potential impact of microbial dysbiosis, the authors analyzed the effects of antibiotic therapy on insulin sensitivity, energy and substrate metabolism, gut permeability, systemic inflammatory markers, adipose gene tissue expression, and host metabolic parameters. There were no significant differences seen in sub-group analysis. This study highlights the fact not all intestinal dysbiosis produce a significant clinical effect. Clearly, the conflicting evidence between animal and human studies reinforces the need for further investigation on the role of antibiotics in the potential treatment of obesity before any firm conclusion can be drawn.

Another area of focus is deciphering the role of specific antibiotics that produce a clinically significant commensal change. The varying coverage of antibiotics used (gram-negative *vs.* gram-positive, aerobic *vs.* anaerobic) likely explains some of the variance in study outcomes. In addition, certain antibiotics appear to have a dose-dependent impact on the gut microbiota [7]. In the study by Reijnders *et al.*, oral vancomycin and amoxicillin were studied. Oral vancomycin primarily acts on the GI tract with limited systemic absorption, compared to amoxicillin, which has excellent bioavailability and would therefore exude a systemic effect. In addition, vancomycin covers gram-positive bacteria, compared to antibiotics used for gram-negative coverage (amoxicillin and ceftazidime), which also exerts an effect on gram-positive bacteria in addition to gram-negatives. Furthermore, several practical considerations must be addressed concerning the use of antibiotics for the treatment of obesity, namely antibiotic stewardship and antibiotic resistance. In addition, the use of antibiotics may potentially have deleterious outcomes (*e.g.* the development in antibiotic resistance that leads to the propagation of pathogenic strains such as vancomycin resistant enterococci (VRE) or extended-spectrum beta-lactamases (ESBL)). Certainly, the liberal use of antibiotics for the treatment of obesity would be against the varying premise of antibiotic stewardship, particularly if alternative measures were available. As such further research and insight is needed concerning the role of antibiotics in the treatment of obesity before they can be clinically recommended.

Overall, antibiotics clearly seem to have a profound effect on the gut microflora [1, 2]. These effects, be it long-term or short-term, can have marked inter-individual and intra-individual variations, and can significantly influence a variety of metabolic pathways [1, 2]. Certainly as the understanding of the gut microbiome continues to flourish, the role of antibiotic therapy in treating obesity and the metabolic syndrome will become more evident. Furthermore, antibiotics may be administered with other treatment modalities to offer a multifaceted treatment approach.

Probiotics

Probiotics are live microorganisms that, when administered in adequate quantities, can potentially reset the microbial imbalance in patients suffering from a host of disease [1, 54]. To date, there are a number of health benefits associated with probiotic use, which include symptomatic relief in those suffering from lactose intolerance [55], protection against or decreased duration of gastrointestinal infections [56 - 58], and a reduction of plasma cholesterol concentrations ultimately impacting coronary artery disease [59].

There are several mechanisms by which probiotics are thought to exert their beneficial effects, which include maintenance of the intestinal barrier integrity, competitive metabolic interactions against pathogens, production of anti-microbials, immune modulation, and the inhibition of adherence or translocation of pathogens [60]. As such, it is quite evident that probiotics play an influential role in gut microflora homeostasis and thus offer a potential target for therapeutic intervention.

Currently, there is limited data available on the use of prebiotics specifically for the treatment of obesity. Despite this, recent animal studies have shed light on the potential mechanisms through which probiotics exert influence on the pathways leading to obesity [61, 62].

One potential mechanism for probiotics in the treatment of obesity is improved metabolic and energy homeostasis. This has been suggested by studies in which mice subjected to DIO that were fed probiotics (*Lactobacillus rhamnosus PL60*) for a total of eight weeks demonstrated reduced body weight and white adipose tissue without decreased energy intake, an effect possibly mediated by alterations in the levels of conjugated fatty acids [61, 62]. These alterations in fatty acid metabolism and energy expenditure have also been seen with other probiotic strains. For example, a recent study investigated the role of three different probiotic strains (*Lactobacillus paracasei* CNCM I-4270, *Lactobacillus rhamnosis* I-3690, and *Bifidobacterium animalis* subsp. *Lacits* I-2494) in mice subjected to a high-fat diet (HFD) for a total of twelve weeks [63]. Each strain attenuated weight gain and macrophage infiltration into adipose tissue, while improving insulin sensitivity and hepatic steatosis. Interestingly, fecal rRNA analysis demonstrated that each probiotic strain resulted in a different alteration of the commensal microflora; such changes resulted in increased cecal acetate levels, altered lipopolysaccharide-binding protein, and decreased expression of TNF-α from adipose and hepatic tissue. Another recent study showed that a multi-strain probiotic (*Lactobacillys rhamnosus* LMG S-28148 and *Bifidobacterium animalis* ssp *lactis* LMG P-28149) led to decreased adipose tissue inflammation in mice on a HFD [64]. Additionally, there was modified fatty acid uptake and expression of SCFA receptor GPR43 (also known as FFAR-2). Next, there appeared to be relative compositional changes with restoration of the commensal gut microflora, which increased levels of *Akkermansia mucinophilia* and *Rikenellaceae* and decreased *Lactobacillaceae*. Finally, an *in vitro* model demonstrated that this probiotic mixture also altered the production of SCFAs leading to increased propionate and butyrate relative to acetate evidence by its influence on FFAR-2. Combined both these animal studies show that probiotics have the potential to regulate adipose tissue inflammation, alter or restore the composition of the gut microflora, and influence the production of SCFAs within the gut.

Probiotics have also been implicated in the complex regulation of fat storage. As previously discussed Fiaf is a circulating protein that inhibits LPL [1, 2]. Specific bacterial alterations, such as colonization of the gut microflora by *Bacteroides thetaiotaomicron* and *Methanobrevibacter smithii*, has been noted to cause suppression of Fiaf, which ultimately results in increased LPL and subsequent fat uptake and storage [4, 65]. Interestingly, Fiaf has been highlighted as a potential target for the treatment of obesity with use of probiotics containing the strain *Lactobacillus paracasei* ssp. *paracasei* F19 (F19) [66]. Mice subjected to a HFD supplemented with F19 demonstrated significantly reduced body fat and altered lipoprotein files, along with higher circulating levels of Fiaf compared to mice on a HFD without F19 supplementation. This was thought to be secondary to an increased activation of peroxisome proliferator-activated receptors (PPAR) alpha and gamma due to F19 secreted-factors.

Despite the many proposed pathways through which probiotics may exert a beneficial effect on weight loss and obesity, there is very little evidence supporting its use in humans. A recent systematic review and meta-analysis by Park *et al.* totaling four randomized control trials in humans, evaluated the efficacy of probiotics compared to placebo [67]. Overall, there were no significant differences in body weight, body mass index (BMI), or visceral fat. One should note the significant limitations in study design prior to dismissing any potential benefit of probiotics, which include treatment duration and the inability to account for any dietary modifications or exercise regimen in the trials. Table **1** lists a number of other studies on the role of probiotic in the development of treatment of obesity [61, 63, 64, 66, 68 - 72], however owing the widely varying study designs and outcomes, further investigation is required before probiotics can be recommended as a therapeutic option for the treatment of obesity.

Table 1. Summary of probiotic studies on the development and treatment of obesity [61 - 72].

Study	Probiotic Used	Study Group/Duration	Results	Comments
Lee et al. [61]	Lactobacillus rhamnosus PL60	DIO (diet-induced obesity) mice 8 weeks	Reduced energy intake and reduced white adipose tissue	Effect thought to be mediated by conjugated linoleic acid produced by the probiotic strain
Wang et al. [63]	Lactobacillus paracasei CNCM I-4270 Lactobacillus rhamnosis I-3690 Bifidobacterium animalis subsp. Lacits I-2494	HFD (high-fat diet) mice 12 weeks	Attenuated weight gain and macrophage infiltration into adipose tissue, while improving insulin sensitivity and hepatic steatosis	Each strain resulted in different microflora alterations which affected cecal acetate levels, altered LPS-binding protein, and decreased TNF-α
Alard et al. [64]	Lactobacillys rhamnosus LMG S-28148 Bifidobacterium animalis ssp lactis LMG P-28149	HFD mice 12-14 weeks	Decreased adipose tissue inflammation Modified FFAR-2 uptake and expression	Microflora showed increased levels of Akkermansia mucinophilia and Rikenellaceae and also decreased Lactobacillaceae
Aronsson et al. [66]	Lactobacillus paracasei ssp. paracasei F19	HFD mice 10 weeks	Reduced body fat Altered LPL profiles Increased Fiaf	Effects likely due to increased peroxisome proliferator-activated receptors (PPAR) alpha and gamma from probiotic secreted factors
Jung et al. [68]	Lactobacillus gasseri BNR17	62 obese volunteers Randomized double blind trial 12 weeks	A slight, but nonsignificant, weight loss in the probiotic group	Probiotic isolated from human breast milk
Kadooka et al. [69]	Lactobacillus gasseri SBT2055	210 healthy adults with large visceral fat areas 12 weeks	Decreased abdominal visceral fat areas as measured by CT scan	Beneficial effects attenuated 4 weeks after cessation of probiotic

(Table 1) contd.....

Study	Probiotic Used	Study Group/Duration	Results	Comments
Sharafedtinov et al. [70]	Lactobacillus plantarum TENSIA	40 obese and hypertensive patients Double-blind, placebo controlled randomized trial 3 weeks	Reduced body mass index	Probiotic administered in cheese Reduction in BMI closely associated with body water content
Sanchez et al. [71]	Lactobacillus rhamnosus CGMCC1.3274	125 obese adults Double-blind, placebo controlled randomized trial 24 weeks	No significant overall weight loss noted Subgroup analysis showed significant weight loss in women on probiotic	Weight loss in women was also associated with decreased circulating leptin levels
Zarrati et al. [72]	Lactobacillus acidophilus La5 Bifidobacterium BB12 Lactobacillys casei DN001	75 healthy overweight and obese adults assigned to probiotic, low-calorie diet, or both	Weight loss was greater when low-calorie diet was combined with probiotic then either alone	Probiotic administered in yogurt Noted effects on T-cell subset specific gene expression in peripheral blood mononuclear cells

Prebiotics

Prebiotics were originally defined as "non-digestible food ingredients that beneficially affect the host by selectively stimulating the growth and/or activity of one or a limited number of bacteria in the colon"; however, they are now more loosely defined as "selectively fermented ingredients that allow specific changes, both in the composition and/or activity in the gastrointestinal microflora, that confer benefits." [73 - 75] In order for a food to be classified as a prebiotic it must resist gastric acidity, hydrolysis by mammalian enzymes, and absorption in the upper gastrointestinal tract, in order to be fermented by the gut microbiota into SCFAs that can be used for energy [75, 76]. There are a number of prebiotic sources being studied for therapeutic use, however the predominant focus is on the use of the inulin-type fructans, oligofructose (OFS) and fructo-oligosaccharides [77 - 79].

While there is limited clinical evidence evaluating the role of prebiotics in the treatment of obesity, there are several metabolic pathways affected by prebiotics, which may become future therapeutic targets for obesity and metabolic syndrome including regulation of lipogenesis, inflammation, and satiety. Prebiotics are thought to alter gene expression of regulating enzymes involved in de novo lipogenesis as evidenced by animal studies that demonstrated decreased levels of lipogenic enzymes amongst animals fed a prebiotic supplemented diet [80].

As previously discussed, delivery of SCFAs into the liver is driven by inflammation and endotoxemia, both of which are significantly influenced by the commensal microflora. TLR-4, which is activated by LPS from gran-negative bacteria, appears to be significantly impacted by the gut microbiome [1, 2]. Activation of TLR-4 results in negative inhibition of insulin signaling, ultimately resulting in insulin resistance [81]. In addition, TLR-4 works in concert with other TLRs to maintain the integrity of the intestinal mucosa [82 - 85]. Mice treated with prebiotics have been shown to have decreased level of intestinal permeability and LPS absorption [86]. In particular, mice treated with OFS had decreased levels of pro-inflammatory cytokines and levels of endotoxemia, thought to be secondary to an increased concentration of *Bifidobacterium* [87].

Lastly, prebiotics are thought to regulate satiety. By definition, prebiotics must be fermentable into SCFAs by the gut microbiome. These SCFAs play a critical role in signaling pathways within the gut [1, 2]. Animal studies have shown that SCFAs regulate gut hormones by controlling satiety through the G-protein coupled receptors, FFAR 2 and 3 [13]. FFAR 2 and 3 work in concert with glucagon-like peptide 1 and peptide YY to modulate the release of digestive enzymes to help control intestinal motility and satiety [1, 2]. Mice deficient in either FFAR 2 or 3 have significantly less body fat, increased lean body mass, and lower triglyceride and cholesterol levels [1, 2]. In addition, prebiotic supplementation has been shown to increase levels of glucagon-like peptide 1 and peptide YY in both rodent and humans, while inhibiting the release of ghrelin (an appetite-stimulating hormone) [20, 88 - 94]. Prebiotic supplementation resulted in a slower and more sustained release of peptide YY, suggesting a potential role for appetite control [95, 96].

Cluny *et al*. evaluated the effects of OFS on DIO and diet-resistant (DR) mice [97]. The investigators supplements OFS daily for six weeks and noticed that OFS reduced the high-fat induced body weight by nearly 35% in both DIO and DR mice. In fact, DR mice in this study had lower body weight when compared to age-matched controls fed standard chow. Interestingly, a similar microbiota profile was seen in both DIO and DR mice that significantly differed from chow-fed rats, most notably *Clostridium* clusters I and XI (negated with prebiotic supplementation). Alterations in the gut microbiome were also noted in the study by Rajpal *et al*., which demonstrated that treatment with OFS resulted in significant weight loss and improved hyperglycemic control thought to be secondary to a relative increase in *Bacteroidetes* and decrease in *Clostridia* groups in the prebiotic treated group [48].

Parnell *et al.* randomized forty-eight healthy overweight adults (body mass index >25) to twelve weeks of daily prebiotics (OFS) or placebo [98]. Treatment with OFS was associated with a significant weight loss, 1.03 ± 0.43kg, compared to weight gain, 0.45 ± 0.31kg, in the placebo group (p = 0.01). The results also showed decreased caloric intake in the prebiotic group, along with decreased ghrelin and peptide YY levels, further supporting appetite regulation as a potential mechanism of prebiotics in the treatment of obesity.

Synbiotics

Synbiotics are a combination of prebiotics and probiotics, considered a new treatment strategy in obesity and the metabolic syndrome. There have been a few animal trials that have introduced this as a potential treatment option [63, 99, 100], however human data remains limited. Rabiei *et al.* performed a triple blind randomized controlled trial, which included 46 patients [101]. Patients were randomized to receive symbiotic therapy (2 capsules) or 2 placebo capsules daily for 3 months. They were both instructed on a proper weight loss diet per their adjusted ideal body weight. At weeks 0, 6, and week 12, anthropometric, body composition, blood pressure, and nutritional measurements were done. They found that these were reduced in all participants (p<0.05), however the trend of weight loss continued in the symbiotic group for at least 12 weeks, whereas they stopped at week 6 in the placebo cohort. This led the authors to conclude that symbiotic use can postpone the plateau phase of weight loss and ultimately prevent resistance to further weight loss.

Despite this supporting evidence, it is evident that further investigation into the role of synbiotics is required before advocating synbiotics as a treatment option for obesity.

The Role of Fecal Transplant

In 2004, Bäckhead *et al.* demonstrated that conventionalization of adult germ-free mice with microbiota from conventionally raised animals, despite decreased food intake, produced a 60% increase in body fat content within 14 days [3]. This landmark study proved the gut microflora to be an important environmental factor that plays a pivotal role in energy harvest, storage, and more importantly that these influences were transmissible. Subsequent studies have also demonstrated that germ-free mice colonized with 'obese microbiota' were more likely to have a significant increase in total body fat when compared to germ-free mice colonized with 'lean microbiota'. [5]

Recent studies have suggested that the effects of the gut microbiota may even be transmissible [6]. Ridaura *et al.* transplanted fecal microbiota from human twins discordant for obesity into germ-free mice, where they found that cohousing lean and obese mice prevented the development of increased adiposity and body mass in obese cage mates and transformed the microbiota metabolic profile to a lean like state; this transformation was related to a change in the prevalence of *Bacteriodales* species and in addition the bacterial invasion was diet-dependent. These results, therefore, suggest that the interactions between the gut microbiota and diet are both transmissible and modifiable and further support a role for the gut microbiota and fecal transplantation as a focal point for continuing research.

Clinical data thus far remains limited. Case reports of fecal microbiota transplant (FMT) performed for recurrent *Clostridium difficile* infection with donor samples procured from overweight donors with resultant new-onset obesity in the recipient have been described [102]. Vrieze *et al.* studied the effects of microbiota transplant from lean donors to male recipients with metabolic syndrome on the recipients' microbiota composition and energy homeostasis [103]. The study totaled 18 subjects, 9 of which received infusions from donors with a BMI <23 kg/m^2 while the other 9 underwent autologous transplant. 6-weeks post transfusion, lean donor recipients had a significant increase in insulin sensitivity and butyrate-producing microbiota. While early results are encouraging, large randomized-controlled trials and long term data are necessary to demonstrate the efficacy of FMT as a possible therapeutic intervention for obesity.

CONCLUSION

The obesity epidemic currently affects more than 1 in 3 American adults and 1 in 6 children and adolescents [104]. The economic burden from obesity and obesity-related diseases are currently in excess of $145 billion dollars [105]. The evidence presented strongly suggests there are several mechanisms in the pathogenesis of obesity, which are strongly influenced by intestinal dysbiosis. Thus, manipulation of the gut microflora appears to be a promising intervention in combating the obesity epidemic whether using antibiotics, probiotic, prebiotics, or fecal matter transplantation. Currently, there is much to be learned about the depth and breadth of the intestinal microbiome, specifically the role of specific bacterial strains in the pathogenesis of varying disease states. Further research is required before implementing gut microbial manipulation into standard clinical practice.

CONFLICT OF INTEREST

The authors confirm that they have no conflict of interest to declare for this publication.

ACKNOWLEDGEMENTS

Declared none.

REFERENCES

[1] Parekh PJ, Balart LA, Johnson DA. The Influence of the Gut Microbiome on Obesity, Metabolic Syndrome and Gastrointestinal Disease. Clin Transl Gastroenterol 2015; 6: e91.
[http://dx.doi.org/10.1038/ctg.2015.16] [PMID: 26087059]

[2] Parekh PJ, Arusi E, Vinik AI, Johnson DA. The role and influence of gut microbiota in pathogenesis and management of obesity and metabolic syndrome. Front Endocrinol (Lausanne) 2014; 5: 47.
[http://dx.doi.org/10.3389/fendo.2014.00047] [PMID: 24778627]

[3] Bäckhed F, Ding H, Wang T, et al. The gut microbiota as an environmental factor that regulates fat storage. Proc Natl Acad Sci USA 2004; 101(44): 15718-23.
[http://dx.doi.org/10.1073/pnas.0407076101] [PMID: 15505215]

[4] Bäckhed F, Manchester JK, Semenkovich CF, Gordon JI. Mechanisms underlying the resistance to diet-induced obesity in germ-free mice. Proc Natl Acad Sci USA 2007; 104(3): 979-84.
[http://dx.doi.org/10.1073/pnas.0605374104] [PMID: 17210919]

[5] Turnbaugh PJ, Ley RE, Mahowald MA, Magrini V, Mardis ER, Gordon JI. An obesity-associated gut microbiome with increased capacity for energy harvest. Nature 2006; 444(7122): 1027-31.
[http://dx.doi.org/10.1038/nature05414] [PMID: 17183312]

[6] Ridaura VK, Faith JJ, Rey FE, et al. Gut microbiota from twins discordant for obesity modulate metabolism in mice. Science 2013; 341(6150): 1241214.
[http://dx.doi.org/10.1126/science.1241214] [PMID: 24009397]

[7] Sayin SI, Wahlström A, Felin J, et al. Gut microbiota regulates bile acid metabolism by reducing the levels of tauro-beta-muricholic acid, a naturally occurring FXR antagonist. Cell Metab 2013; 17(2): 225-35.
[http://dx.doi.org/10.1016/j.cmet.2013.01.003] [PMID: 23395169]

[8] Prawitt J, Abdelkarim M, Stroeve JH, et al. Farnesoid X receptor deficiency improves glucose homeostasis in mouse models of obesity. Diabetes 2011; 60(7): 1861-71.
[http://dx.doi.org/10.2337/db11-0030] [PMID: 21593203]

[9] Li F, Jiang C, Krausz KW, et al. Microbiome remodelling leads to inhibition of intestinal farnesoid X receptor signalling and decreased obesity. Nat Commun 2013; 4: 2384.
[http://dx.doi.org/10.1038/ncomms3384] [PMID: 24064762]

[10] Gioiello A, Cerra B, Mostarda S, Guercini C, Pellicciari R, Macchiarulo A. Bile acid derivatives as ligands of the farnesoid x receptor: molecular determinants for bile acid binding and receptor modulation. Curr Top Med Chem 2014; 14(19): 2159-74.
[http://dx.doi.org/10.2174/1568026614666141112100208] [PMID: 25388535]

[11] Parséus A, Sommer N, Sommer F, et al. Microbiota-induced obesity requires farnesoid X receptor. Gut 2017; 66(3): 429-37.
[PMID: 26740296]

[12] Chakraborti CK. New-found link between microbiota and obesity. World J Gastrointest Pathophysiol 2015; 6(4): 110-9.
[http://dx.doi.org/10.4291/wjgp.v6.i4.110] [PMID: 26600968]

[13] Lin HV, Frassetto A, Kowalik EJ Jr, et al. Butyrate and propionate protect against diet-induced obesity and regulate gut hormones via free fatty acid receptor 3-independent mechanisms. PLoS One 2012; 7(4): e35240.
[http://dx.doi.org/10.1371/journal.pone.0035240] [PMID: 22506074]

[14] Harris K, Kassis A, Major G, Chou CJ. Is the gut microbiota a new factor contributing to obesity and its metabolic disorders? J Obes 2012; 2012: 879151.
[http://dx.doi.org/10.1155/2012/879151] [PMID: 22315672]

[15] Hartstra AV, Bouter KE, Bäckhed F, Nieuwdorp M. Insights into the role of the microbiome in obesity and type 2 diabetes. Diabetes Care 2015; 38(1): 159-65.
[http://dx.doi.org/10.2337/dc14-0769] [PMID: 25538312]

[16] Conterno L, Fava F, Viola R, Tuohy KM. Obesity and the gut microbiota: does up-regulating colonic fermentation protect against obesity and metabolic disease? Genes Nutr 2011; 6(3): 241-60.
[http://dx.doi.org/10.1007/s12263-011-0230-1] [PMID: 21559992]

[17] Schwiertz A, Taras D, Schäfer K, *et al.* Microbiota and SCFA in lean and overweight healthy subjects. Obesity (Silver Spring) 2010; 18(1): 190-5.
[http://dx.doi.org/10.1038/oby.2009.167] [PMID: 19498350]

[18] Darzi J, Frost GS, Robertson MD. Do SCFA have a role in appetite regulation? Proc Nutr Soc 2011; 70(1): 119-28.
[http://dx.doi.org/10.1017/S0029665110004039] [PMID: 21266094]

[19] Cuche G, Cuber JC, Malbert CH. Ileal short-chain fatty acids inhibit gastric motility by a humoral pathway. Am J Physiol Gastrointest Liver Physiol 2000; 279(5): G925-30.
[PMID: 11052989]

[20] Tolhurst G, Heffron H, Lam YS, *et al.* Short-chain fatty acids stimulate glucagon-like peptide-1 secretion *via* the G-protein-coupled receptor FFAR2. Diabetes 2012; 61(2): 364-71.
[http://dx.doi.org/10.2337/db11-1019] [PMID: 22190648]

[21] Samuel BS, Shaito A, Motoike T, *et al.* Effects of the gut microbiota on host adiposity are modulated by the short-chain fatty-acid binding G protein-coupled receptor, Gpr41. Proc Natl Acad Sci USA 2008; 105(43): 16767-72.
[http://dx.doi.org/10.1073/pnas.0808567105] [PMID: 18931303]

[22] Bjursell M, Admyre T, Göransson M, *et al.* Improved glucose control and reduced body fat mass in free fatty acid receptor 2-deficient mice fed a high-fat diet. Am J Physiol Endocrinol Metab 2011; 300(1): E211-20.
[http://dx.doi.org/10.1152/ajpendo.00229.2010] [PMID: 20959533]

[23] Shen J, Obin MS, Zhao L. The gut microbiota, obesity and insulin resistance. Mol Aspects Med 2013; 34(1): 39-58.
[http://dx.doi.org/10.1016/j.mam.2012.11.001] [PMID: 23159341]

[24] Vallès Y, Artacho A, Pascual-García A, *et al.* Microbial Succession in the Gut: Directional Trends of Taxonomic and Functional Change in a Birth Cohort of Spanish Infants. PLoS Genet 2014; 10(6): e1004406.
[http://dx.doi.org/10.1371/journal.pgen.1004406]

[25] Vallès Y, Gosalbes MJ, de Vries LE, Abellán JJ, Francino MP. Metagenomics and development of the gut microbiota in infants. Clin Microbiol Infect 2012; 18 (Suppl. 4): 21-6.
[http://dx.doi.org/10.1111/j.1469-0691.2012.03876.x] [PMID: 22647043]

[26] Yatsunenko T, Rey FE, Manary MJ, *et al.* Human gut microbiome viewed across age and geography. Nature 2012; 486(7402): 222-7.
[PMID: 22699611]

[27] Oldfield E IV, Johnson D. Nature *vs* Nurture: The Gut Microbiome and Genetics in the Development of Gastrointestinal Disease. J Hepatol Gastrointest Disord 2016; 2: 1-8.

[28] Lemas DJ, Yee S, Cacho N, *et al.* Exploring the contribution of maternal antibiotics and breastfeeding to development of the infant microbiome and pediatric obesity. Semin Fetal Neonatal Med 2016; 21(6): 406-9.
[http://dx.doi.org/10.1016/j.siny.2016.04.013] [PMID: 27424917]

[29] Cani PD, Bibiloni R, Knauf C, et al. Changes in gut microbiota control metabolic endotoxemia-induced inflammation in high-fat diet-induced obesity and diabetes in mice. Diabetes 2008; 57(6): 1470-81.
[http://dx.doi.org/10.2337/db07-1403] [PMID: 18305141]

[30] Vors C, Pineau G, Drai J, et al. Postprandial endotoxemia linked with chylomicrons and lipopolysaccharides handling in obese versus lean men: A lipid dose-effect trial. J Clin Endocrinol Metab 2015; 100(9): 3427-35.
[http://dx.doi.org/10.1210/jc.2015-2518] [PMID: 26151336]

[31] van Greevenbroek MM, Schalkwijk CG, Stehouwer CD. Obesity-associated low-grade inflammation in type 2 diabetes mellitus: causes and consequences. Neth J Med 2013; 71(4): 174-87.
[PMID: 23723111]

[32] Hayashi F, Smith KD, Ozinsky A, et al. The innate immune response to bacterial flagellin is mediated by Toll-like receptor 5. Nature 2001; 410(6832): 1099-103.
[http://dx.doi.org/10.1038/35074106] [PMID: 11323673]

[33] Rhee SH. Basic and translational understandings of microbial recognition by toll-like receptors in the intestine. J Neurogastroenterol Motil 2011; 17(1): 28-34.
[http://dx.doi.org/10.5056/jnm.2011.17.1.28] [PMID: 21369489]

[34] Vijay-Kumar M, Aitken JD, Carvalho FA, et al. Metabolic syndrome and altered gut microbiota in mice lacking Toll□like receptor 5. Science (80) 2010; 328: 228-31.

[35] De Loera-Rodriguez CO, Delgado-Rizo V, Alvarado-Navarro A, Agraz-Cibrian JM, Segura-Ortega JE, Fafutis-Morris M. Over-expression of TLR4-CD14, pro-inflammatory cytokines, metabolic markers and NEFAs in obese non-diabetic Mexicans. J Inflamm (Lond) 2014; 11(1): 39.
[http://dx.doi.org/10.1186/s12950-014-0039-y] [PMID: 25493077]

[36] Tsukumo DM, Carvalho-Filho MA, Carvalheira JB, et al. Loss-of-function mutation in Toll-like receptor 4 prevents diet-induced obesity and insulin resistance. Diabetes 2007; 56(8): 1986-98.
[http://dx.doi.org/10.2337/db06-1595] [PMID: 17519423]

[37] Tsukumo DM, Carvalho-Filho MA, Carvalheira JB, et al. Statement of Retraction. Loss-of-Function Mutation in Toll-Like Receptor 4 Prevents Diet-Induced Obesity and Insulin Resistance. Diabetes 2007;56:19861998. DOI: 10.2337/db061595. Diabetes 2016; 65(4): 1126-7.
[http://dx.doi.org/10.2337/db16-rt04a] [PMID: 27208024]

[38] Himes RW, Smith CW. Tlr2 is critical for diet-induced metabolic syndrome in a murine model. FASEB J 2010; 24(3): 731-9.
[http://dx.doi.org/10.1096/fj.09-141929] [PMID: 19841034]

[39] Gangarapu V, Yıldız K, Ince AT, Baysal B. Role of gut microbiota: obesity and NAFLD. Turk J Gastroenterol 2014; 25(2): 133-40.
[http://dx.doi.org/10.5152/tjg.2014.7886] [PMID: 25003671]

[40] Goel A, Gupta M, Aggarwal R. Gut microbiota and liver disease. J Gastroenterol Hepatol 2014; 29(6): 1139-48.
[http://dx.doi.org/10.1111/jgh.12556] [PMID: 24547986]

[41] Ley RE, Bäckhed F, Turnbaugh P, Lozupone CA, Knight RD, Gordon JI. Obesity alters gut microbial ecology. Proc Natl Acad Sci USA 2005; 102(31): 11070-5.
[http://dx.doi.org/10.1073/pnas.0504978102] [PMID: 16033867]

[42] Duncan SH, Lobley GE, Holtrop G, et al. Human colonic microbiota associated with diet, obesity and weight loss. Int J Obes 2008; 32(11): 1720-4.
[http://dx.doi.org/10.1038/ijo.2008.155] [PMID: 18779823]

[43] Jumpertz R, Le DS, Turnbaugh PJ, et al. Energy-balance studies reveal associations between gut microbes, caloric load, and nutrient absorption in humans. Am J Clin Nutr 2011; 94(1): 58-65.
[http://dx.doi.org/10.3945/ajcn.110.010132] [PMID: 21543530]

[44] Festi D, Schiumerini R, Eusebi LH, Marasco G, Taddia M, Colecchia A. Gut microbiota and metabolic syndrome. World J Gastroenterol 2014; 20(43): 16079-94.
[http://dx.doi.org/10.3748/wjg.v20.i43.16079] [PMID: 25473159]

[45] Le Chatelier E, Nielsen T, Qin J, et al. Richness of human gut microbiome correlates with metabolic markers. Nature 2013; 500(7464): 541-6.
[http://dx.doi.org/10.1038/nature12506] [PMID: 23985870]

[46] Gillings MR, Paulsen IT, Tetu SG. Ecology and evolution of the human microbiota: Fire, farming and antibiotics. Genes (Basel) 2015; 6(3): 841-57.
[http://dx.doi.org/10.3390/genes6030841] [PMID: 26371047]

[47] Membrez M, Blancher F, Jaquet M, et al. Gut microbiota modulation with norfloxacin and ampicillin enhances glucose tolerance in mice. FASEB J 2008; 22(7): 2416-26.
[http://dx.doi.org/10.1096/fj.07-102723] [PMID: 18326786]

[48] Rajpal DK, Klein J-L, Mayhew D, et al. Selective Spectrum Antibiotic Modulation of the Gut Microbiome in Obesity and Diabetes Rodent Models. PLoS One 2015; 10(12): e0145499.
[http://dx.doi.org/10.1371/journal.pone.0145499] [PMID: 26709835]

[49] Mikkelsen KH, Allin KH, Knop FK. Effect of antibiotics on gut microbiota, glucose metabolism and body weight regulation: a review of the literature. Diabetes Obes Metab 2016; 18(5): 444-53.

[50] Trasande L, Blustein J, Liu M, Corwin E, Cox LM, Blaser MJ. Infant antibiotic exposures and early-life body mass. Int J Obes 2013; 37(1): 16-23.
[http://dx.doi.org/10.1038/ijo.2012.132] [PMID: 22907693]

[51] Ajslev TA, Andersen CS, Gamborg M, Sørensen TI, Jess T. Childhood overweight after establishment of the gut microbiota: the role of delivery mode, pre-pregnancy weight and early administration of antibiotics. Int J Obes 2011; 35(4): 522-9.
[http://dx.doi.org/10.1038/ijo.2011.27] [PMID: 21386800]

[52] Azad MB, Bridgman SL, Becker AB, Kozyrskyj AL. Infant antibiotic exposure and the development of childhood overweight and central adiposity. Int J Obes 2014; 38(10): 1290-8.
[http://dx.doi.org/10.1038/ijo.2014.119] [PMID: 25012772]

[53] Saari A, Virta LJ, Sankilampi U, Dunkel L, Saxen H. Antibiotic exposure in infancy and risk of being overweight in the first 24 months of life. Pediatrics 2015; 135(4): 617-26.
[http://dx.doi.org/10.1542/peds.2014-3407] [PMID: 25825533]

[54] Sanders ME. Probiotics: definition, sources, selection, and uses. Clin Infect Dis 2008; 462: S58-61. discussion S144–51.
[http://dx.doi.org/10.1086/523341]

[55] de Vrese M, Stegelmann A, Richter B, Fenselau S, Laue C, Schrezenmeir J. Probiotics compensation for lactase insufficiency. Am J Clin Nutr 2001; 73(2) (Suppl.): 421S-9S.
[PMID: 11157352]

[56] Marteau PR, de Vrese M, Cellier CJ, Schrezenmeir J. Protection from gastrointestinal diseases with the use of probiotics. Am J Clin Nutr 2001; 73(2) (Suppl.): 430S-6S.
[PMID: 11157353]

[57] Verna EC, Lucak S. Use of probiotics in gastrointestinal disorders: what to recommend? Therap Adv Gastroenterol 2010; 3(5): 307-19.
[http://dx.doi.org/10.1177/1756283X10373814] [PMID: 21180611]

[58] Ritchie ML, Romanuk TN. A meta-analysis of probiotic efficacy for gastrointestinal diseases. PLoS One 2012; 7(4): e34938.
[http://dx.doi.org/10.1371/journal.pone.0034938] [PMID: 22529959]

[59] Ooi LG, Liong MT. Cholesterol-lowering effects of probiotics and prebiotics: a review of *in vivo* and *in vitro* findings. Int J Mol Sci 2010; 11(6): 2499-522.

[http://dx.doi.org/10.3390/ijms11062499] [PMID: 20640165]

[60] Yan F, Polk DB. Probiotics: progress toward novel therapies for intestinal diseases. Curr Opin Gastroenterol 2010; 26(2): 95-101.
[http://dx.doi.org/10.1097/MOG.0b013e328335239a] [PMID: 19952741]

[61] Lee HY, Park JH, Seok SH, et al. Human originated bacteria, Lactobacillus rhamnosus PL60, produce conjugated linoleic acid and show anti-obesity effects in diet-induced obese mice. Biochim Biophys Acta Mol Cell Biol Lipids 2006; 1761: 736-44.

[62] Rosenbaum M, Knight R, Leibel RL. The gut microbiota in human energy homeostasis and obesity. Trends Endocrinol Metab 2015; 26(9): 493-501.
[http://dx.doi.org/10.1016/j.tem.2015.07.002] [PMID: 26257300]

[63] Wang J, Tang H, Zhang C, et al. Modulation of gut microbiota during probiotic-mediated attenuation of metabolic syndrome in high fat diet-fed mice. ISME J 2015; 9(1): 1-15.
[http://dx.doi.org/10.1038/ismej.2014.99] [PMID: 24936764]

[64] Alard J, Lehrter V, Rhimi M, et al. Beneficial metabolic effects of selected probiotics on diet-induced obesity and insulin resistance in mice are associated with improvement of dysbiotic gut microbiota. Environ Microbiol 2016; 18(5): 1484-97.
[http://dx.doi.org/10.1111/1462-2920.13181] [PMID: 26689997]

[65] Arslan N. Obesity, fatty liver disease and intestinal microbiota. World J Gastroenterol 2014; 20(44): 16452-63.
[http://dx.doi.org/10.3748/wjg.v20.i44.16452] [PMID: 25469013]

[66] Aronsson L, Huang Y, Parini P, et al. Decreased fat storage by Lactobacillus paracasei is associated with increased levels of angiopoietin-like 4 protein (ANGPTL4). PLoS One 2010; 5(9): 1-7.
[http://dx.doi.org/10.1371/journal.pone.0013087] [PMID: 20927337]

[67] Park S, Bae J-H. Probiotics for weight loss: a systematic review and meta-analysis. Nutr Res 2015; 35(7): 566-75.
[http://dx.doi.org/10.1016/j.nutres.2015.05.008] [PMID: 26032481]

[68] Jung S-P, Lee K-M, Kang J-H, et al. Effect of Lactobacillus gasseri BNR17 on Overweight and Obese Adults: A Randomized, Double-Blind Clinical Trial. Korean J Fam Med 2013; 34(2): 80-9.
[http://dx.doi.org/10.4082/kjfm.2013.34.2.80] [PMID: 23560206]

[69] Kadooka Y, Sato M, Ogawa A, et al. Effect of Lactobacillus gasseri SBT2055 in fermented milk on abdominal adiposity in adults in a randomised controlled trial. Br J Nutr 2013; 110(9): 1696-703.
[http://dx.doi.org/10.1017/S0007114513001037] [PMID: 23614897]

[70] Sharafedtinov KK, Plotnikova OA, Alexeeva RI, et al. Hypocaloric diet supplemented with probiotic cheese improves body mass index and blood pressure indices of obese hypertensive patients a randomized double-blind placebo-controlled pilot study. Nutr J 2013; 12: 138.
[http://dx.doi.org/10.1186/1475-2891-12-138] [PMID: 24120179]

[71] Sanchez M, Darimont C, Drapeau V, et al. Effect of Lactobacillus rhamnosus CGMCC1.3724 supplementation on weight loss and maintenance in obese men and women. Br J Nutr 2014; 111(8): 1507-19.
[http://dx.doi.org/10.1017/S0007114513003875] [PMID: 24299712]

[72] Zarrati M, Salehi E, Nourijelyani K, et al. Effects of probiotic yogurt on fat distribution and gene expression of proinflammatory factors in peripheral blood mononuclear cells in overweight and obese people with or without weight-loss diet. J Am Coll Nutr 2014; 33(6): 417-25.
[http://dx.doi.org/10.1080/07315724.2013.874937] [PMID: 25079040]

[73] Gibson GR, Roberfroid MB. Dietary modulation of the human colonic microbiota: introducing the concept of prebiotics. J Nutr 1995; 125(6): 1401-12.
[PMID: 7782892]

[74] Gibson GR, Probert HM, Loo JV, Rastall RA, Roberfroid MB. Dietary modulation of the human colonic microbiota: updating the concept of prebiotics. Nutr Res Rev 2004; 17(2): 259-75.
[http://dx.doi.org/10.1079/NRR200479] [PMID: 19079930]

[75] Slavin J. Fiber and prebiotics: mechanisms and health benefits. Nutrients 2013; 5(4): 1417-35.
[http://dx.doi.org/10.3390/nu5041417] [PMID: 23609775]

[76] Miura K, Ohnishi H. Role of gut microbiota and Toll-like receptors in nonalcoholic fatty liver disease. World J Gastroenterol 2014; 20(23): 7381-91.
[http://dx.doi.org/10.3748/wjg.v20.i23.7381] [PMID: 24966608]

[77] Sabater-Molina M, Larqué E, Torrella F, Zamora S. Dietary fructooligosaccharides and potential benefits on health. J Physiol Biochem 2009; 65(3): 315-28.
[http://dx.doi.org/10.1007/BF03180584] [PMID: 20119826]

[78] Macfarlane S, Macfarlane GT, Cummings JH. Review article: prebiotics in the gastrointestinal tract. Aliment Pharmacol Ther 2006; 24(5): 701-14.
[http://dx.doi.org/10.1111/j.1365-2036.2006.03042.x] [PMID: 16918875]

[79] de Jesus Raposo MF, de Morais AM, de Morais RM. Emergent Sources of Prebiotics: Seaweeds and Microalgae. Mar Drugs 2016; 14(2): 27.
[http://dx.doi.org/10.3390/md14020027] [PMID: 26828501]

[80] Parnell JA, Raman M, Rioux KP, Reimer RA. The potential role of prebiotic fibre for treatment and management of non-alcoholic fatty liver disease and associated obesity and insulin resistance. Liver Int 2012; 32(5): 701-11.
[http://dx.doi.org/10.1111/j.1478-3231.2011.02730.x] [PMID: 22221818]

[81] Oldfield E IV, Dong R, Johnson D. Non-alcoholic Fatty Liver Disease and the Gut Microbiota: Exploring the Connection. Gastro Open J 2015; 1: 30-43.
[http://dx.doi.org/10.17140/GOJ-1-107]

[82] Ehses JA, Meier DT, Wueest S, et al. Toll-like receptor 2-deficient mice are protected from insulin resistance and beta cell dysfunction induced by a high-fat diet. Diabetologia 2010; 53(8): 1795-806.
[http://dx.doi.org/10.1007/s00125-010-1747-3] [PMID: 20407745]

[83] Rivera CA, Gaskin L, Allman M, et al. Toll-like receptor-2 deficiency enhances non-alcoholic steatohepatitis. BMC Gastroenterol 2010; 10: 52.
[http://dx.doi.org/10.1186/1471-230X-10-52] [PMID: 20509914]

[84] Szabo G, Velayudham A, Romics L Jr, Mandrekar P. Modulation of non-alcoholic steatohepatitis by pattern recognition receptors in mice: the role of toll-like receptors 2 and 4. Alcohol Clin Exp Res 2005; 29(11) (Suppl.): 140S-5S.
[http://dx.doi.org/10.1097/01.alc.0000189287.83544.33] [PMID: 16344599]

[85] Cario E, Gerken G, Podolsky DK. Toll-like receptor 2 controls mucosal inflammation by regulating epithelial barrier function. Gastroenterology 2007; 132(4): 1359-74.
[http://dx.doi.org/10.1053/j.gastro.2007.02.056] [PMID: 17408640]

[86] Cani PD, Possemiers S, Van de Wiele T, et al. Changes in gut microbiota control inflammation in obese mice through a mechanism involving GLP-2-driven improvement of gut permeability. Gut 2009; 58(8): 1091-103.
[http://dx.doi.org/10.1136/gut.2008.165886] [PMID: 19240062]

[87] Cani PD, Neyrinck AM, Fava F, et al. Selective increases of bifidobacteria in gut microflora improve high-fat-diet-induced diabetes in mice through a mechanism associated with endotoxaemia. Diabetologia 2007; 50(11): 2374-83.
[http://dx.doi.org/10.1007/s00125-007-0791-0] [PMID: 17823788]

[88] Delzenne NM, Cani PD, Daubioul C, Neyrinck AM. Impact of inulin and oligofructose on gastrointestinal peptides. Br J Nutr 2005; 93 (Suppl. 1): S157-61.
[http://dx.doi.org/10.1079/BJN20041342] [PMID: 15877889]

[89] Reimer RA, Maurer AD, Eller LK, *et al.* Satiety hormone and metabolomic response to an intermittent high energy diet differs in rats consuming long-term diets high in protein or prebiotic fiber. J Proteome Res 2012; 11(8): 4065-74.
[http://dx.doi.org/10.1021/pr300487s] [PMID: 22788871]

[90] Cani PD, Lecourt E, Dewulf EM, *et al.* Gut microbiota fermentation of prebiotics increases satietogenic and incretin gut peptide production with consequences for appetite sensation and glucose response after a meal. Am J Clin Nutr 2009; 90(5): 1236-43.
[http://dx.doi.org/10.3945/ajcn.2009.28095] [PMID: 19776140]

[91] Nilsson A, Johansson E, Ekstrom L, *et al.* Effects of a Brown Beans Evening Meal on Metabolic Risk Markers and Appetite Regulating Hormones at a Subsequent Standardized Breakfast: A Randomized Cross-Over Study. PLoS One 2013. Epub ahead of print.
[http://dx.doi.org/10.1371/journal.pone.0059985]

[92] Parnell JA, Reimer RA. Prebiotic fibres dose-dependently increase satiety hormones and alter Bacteroidetes and Firmicutes in lean and obese JCR:LA-cp rats. Br J Nutr 2012; 107(4): 601-13.
[http://dx.doi.org/10.1017/S0007114511003163] [PMID: 21767445]

[93] Kellow NJ, Coughlan MT, Reid CM. Metabolic benefits of dietary prebiotics in human subjects: a systematic review of randomised controlled trials. Br J Nutr 2014; 111(7): 1147-61.
[http://dx.doi.org/10.1017/S0007114513003607] [PMID: 24230488]

[94] Gee JM, Johnson IT. Dietary lactitol fermentation increases circulating peptide YY and glucagon-like peptide-1 in rats and humans. Nutrition 2005; 21(10): 1036-43.
[http://dx.doi.org/10.1016/j.nut.2005.03.002] [PMID: 16157241]

[95] Karhunen LJ, Juvonen KR, Flander SM, *et al.* A psyllium fiber-enriched meal strongly attenuates postprandial gastrointestinal peptide release in healthy young adults. J Nutr 2010; 140(4): 737-44.
[http://dx.doi.org/10.3945/jn.109.115436] [PMID: 20147463]

[96] Jakobsdottir G, Nyman M, Fåk F. Designing future prebiotic fiber to target metabolic syndrome. Nutrition 2014; 30(5): 497-502.
[http://dx.doi.org/10.1016/j.nut.2013.08.013] [PMID: 24262515]

[97] Cluny NL, Eller LK, Keenan CM, Reimer RA, Sharkey KA. Interactive effects of oligofructose and obesity predisposition on gut hormones and microbiota in diet-induced obese rats. Obesity (Silver Spring) 2015; 23(4): 769-78.
[http://dx.doi.org/10.1002/oby.21017] [PMID: 25820256]

[98] Parnell JA, Reimer RA. Weight loss during oligofructose supplementation is associated with decreased ghrelin and increased peptide YY in overweight and obese adults. Am J Clin Nutr 2009; 89(6): 1751-9.
[http://dx.doi.org/10.3945/ajcn.2009.27465] [PMID: 19386741]

[99] De Preter V, Hamer HM, Windey K, Verbeke K. The impact of pre- and/or probiotics on human colonic metabolism: does it affect human health? Mol Nutr Food Res 2011; 55(1): 46-57.
[http://dx.doi.org/10.1002/mnfr.201000451] [PMID: 21207512]

[100] Lesniewska V, Rowland I, Cani PD, Neyrinck AM, Delzenne NM, Naughton PJ. Effect on components of the intestinal microflora and plasma neuropeptide levels of feeding Lactobacillus delbrueckii, Bifidobacterium lactis, and inulin to adult and elderly rats. Appl Environ Microbiol 2006; 72(10): 6533-8.
[http://dx.doi.org/10.1128/AEM.00915-06] [PMID: 17021202]

[101] Rabiei S, Shakerhosseini R, Saadat N. The effects of symbiotic therapy on anthropometric measures, body composition and blood pressure in patient with metabolic syndrome: a triple blind RCT. Med J Islam Repub Iran 2015; 29: 213.
[PMID: 26478871]

[102] Alang N, Kelly CR. Weight gain after fecal microbiota transplantation. Open Forum Infect Dis 2015; 2(1): ofv004-4.
[http://dx.doi.org/10.1093/ofid/ofv004] [PMID: 26034755]

[103] Vrieze A, Van Nood E, Holleman F, *et al.* Transfer of intestinal microbiota from lean donors increases insulin sensitivity in individuals with metabolic syndrome. Gastroenterology 2012.Epub ahead of print.
[http://dx.doi.org/10.1053/j.gastro.2012.06.031]

[104] Flegal KM, Carroll MD, Kit BK, Ogden CL. Prevalence of obesity and trends in the distribution of body mass index among US adults, 19992010. JAMA 2012; 307(5): 491-7.
[http://dx.doi.org/10.1001/jama.2012.39] [PMID: 22253363]

[105] Tsai A, Williamson D, Glick H. Direct medical cost of overweight and obesity in the United. Int Assoc Study Obes 2011; 12: 50-61.
[http://dx.doi.org/10.1111/j.1467-789X.2009.00708.x]

SUBJECT INDEX

A

Abnormal adipose tissue enlargement 41
Abnormalities, valvular 9
Adeno-associated virus (AAV) 74
Adipocyte differentiation 80, 96, 108, 110, 120
Adipogenesis 99, 104, 108, 109, 110, 111, 113, 114
Adipokines 69, 73, 82, 108, 111, 112, 114, 118, 120, 153, 157, 161, 169
  novel 112
Adiponectin 102, 105, 106, 108, 109, 110, 111, 117, 149, 154, 155, 156, 157, 159, 173
  secretion of 105, 109, 155
Adipose tissue 3, 11, 14, 17, 21, 31, 32, 33, 39, 40, 41, 69, 71, 80, 81, 87, 88, 96, 97, 101, 118, 120, 149, 150, 153, 154, 155, 156, 157, 158, 159, 160, 161, 162, 164, 168, 173, 179, 207, 213, 214, 215
  dysfunctional 153
  tissue nesfatin-1/NUCB-2 expression 69
  visceral 39, 87, 164
  white 40, 41, 155, 159, 160, 213
Adiposity, truncal 164
Adrenalectomy 170
Adrenal glands 6, 14, 154, 159, 168, 170, 172
Aldosterone concentrations 169
Amoxicillin 212
AMP-activated protein kinase 107, 207
Amphetamine 6, 7, 9, 13
Androgens 168, 174, 178, 179
  free 179
Annexin 118
Anorexia nervosa 65, 72, 74
Anorexigenic effects 65, 67, 70, 73, 74, 207
Antibiotics 120, 204, 210, 211, 212, 213, 219
  effects of 210, 212
  role of 210, 212, 213
  use of 210, 212
Antibiotic stewardship 212
Anti-obesity agent 10
Anti-obesity drugs 3, 4, 5, 20, 28, 33, 40, 69
  candidate 69
  novel 4, 40
Anti-obesity effects 8, 11, 15, 19, 21, 22, 23, 28, 31, 32, 36, 38, 39

Anti-obesity treatment 65, 69, 74
Antioxidants 150, 161, 166, 169, 170, 175, 176, 177, 178, 179, 180, 181, 182, 184
  natural 150, 181, 183, 184
Antioxidant systems 150, 157, 162, 163, 165, 170, 181
Apolipoprotein A-IV 118
Apoptosis 99, 112, 114, 116, 117, 162, 209
Appetite suppression 8, 12, 13, 14, 156
Atherosclerosis 11, 31, 44, 113, 157, 158, 166, 175, 176

B

Bacteroidetes 206, 209, 217
BAT 100, 105
  mitochondria 105
Beloranib 27, 28
  effects of 27
Blood-brain barrier 156
Blood glucose levels 43
Body mass index (BMI) 4, 7, 17, 25, 27, 71, 72, 83, 85, 98, 101, 108, 119, 150, 152, 154, 161, 167, 182, 214, 216, 218, 219
Body weight loss 9, 17, 28
  induced sustained 9
  significant 17
Body weight 26, 86, 101, 117, 181
  reductions 26, 181
  regulation 86, 101, 117
Brain-derived neurotrophic factor (BDNF) 24
Brain ventricle 66
Brown adipose tissues 40, 211
Buffers, rehydration 96, 97
Bupropion 19, 20, 22, 23
Butyrate 204, 206, 207, 212, 214

C

Caloric restriction 5, 7, 118, 162

Canagliflozin 38, 39
Carbonic anhydrases 23, 106
Cardiovascular 12, 14, 81, 87, 106, 107, 113, 116, 149, 150, 157, 160, 169, 171, 174, 180, 183
  disease (CVD) 12, 81, 87, 106, 107, 113, 116, 149, 150, 157, 169, 171, 180, 183
  risk 12, 160, 174, 180
Catalase 165, 166, 176, 177, 180, 181
Catecholamines 6, 13, 155, 169
Catecholestrogens 176
CB1 receptor 14, 15
  antagonists, selective 14
Ceftazidime 210, 212
Cerebro-spinal fluid (CSF) 69, 156
Cetilistat 3, 21, 22
  administration group 21
  treatment 21, 22
  treatment groups 22
Characteristics, phenotypic 84, 85, 173
Chemical derivatization 93, 94
Childhood obesity 81, 83, 84, 86, 87, 109, 116, 119, 150, 152, 160, 162, 167, 172, 173, 174, 182, 183, 208, 211
  examining 116
  oxidative stress in 160, 183
Children and adolescents 96, 101, 103, 104, 118, 219
Chip array technologies 91
Cholesterol, total 12, 45, 166
Chronic sibutramine treatment 13
Chylomicrons 34, 208
Circulation, hepatic portal 207
Combination therapies 17, 19, 39, 121
Co-morbidities 44, 87, 89, 97, 100, 101, 104, 106, 108, 111, 115
  associated 44, 104, 106, 108, 111, 115
  obesity-associated 87, 89, 97, 100, 101
Composition, bile acid 206
Computed tomography (CT) 44, 45, 103
Copy number variation (CNV) 85
Coronary artery disease (CAD) 151, 174, 175
Cortex, adrenal 169
Corticotropin-releasing factor (CRF) 66, 67, 68
Cortisol 156, 169, 170, 171, 172, 173
  associations of 173
C-reactive protein (CRP) 101, 149, 172

CRF2 67, 68
  antagonist 68
  receptors 67, 68
CRF neurons 68, 69
Cushing's syndrome (CS) 170, 171, 172, 173
Cysteines 114
Cytokines 111, 116, 149, 153, 154, 157, 158, 160, 165, 169, 172, 173, 209, 217
  pro-inflammatory 111, 153, 154, 157, 209, 217

D

Damage, endothelial 158, 160, 161
Dapagliflozin 39
Dexfenfluramine 5, 6, 9, 10
D-fenfluramine 9
DGAT1 21, 31, 32, 33
  inhibitors 21, 31, 32, 33
DGAT inhibitor 3, 33
Diabetes mellitus 3, 42, 72, 81, 157, 171
Diet 10, 17, 23, 25, 34, 44, 45, 46, 82, 119, 150, 154, 167, 178, 180, 181, 182, 183, 184, 209, 219
  enriched 180, 181
  high-fat/sucrose 44, 45, 46
Dietary 32, 33, 34, 182, 205, 206
  fat content 32, 33, 34
  fibers 182
  polysaccharides 205, 206
Diet-induced obesity (DIO) 8, 34, 36, 40, 44, 181, 206, 207, 210, 213, 215, 217
  high-fat 34
  high-fat western 207
Discoveries, biomarker 95, 115, 116
Diseases 3, 44, 119, 151, 219
  obesity-associated renal 119
  obesity-related 3, 44, 151, 219
DNA microarrays 94
Drugs 3, 4, 5, 6, 7, 8, 9, 10, 12, 14, 16, 17, 19, 20, 21, 22, 23, 24, 27, 28, 29, 36, 38, 39, 40, 94, 104, 119
  anti-diabetic 36
  anti-epileptic 16
  combination 19, 22
Dysbiosis 204, 205, 206, 208, 209, 210, 212, 219

Dyslipidemia 3, 12, 15, 16, 17, 43, 44, 149, 151, 152, 157
Dysregulation 114, 116, 120, 153, 172

E

Electron 91, 93, 94
   capture dissociation (ECD) 94
   spray ionization (ESI) 91, 93
Elevation, catecholamine 6
Endocannabinoids 14
Endothelial dysfunction 149, 150, 161, 169, 170
Endotoxemia 204, 208, 217
   metabolic 204, 208
Energy 3, 4, 6, 8, 11, 12, 13, 14, 21, 27, 30, 31, 36, 39, 69, 70, 73, 81, 82, 85, 86, 102, 103, 104, 113, 156, 160, 179, 206, 207, 208, 209, 213, 218, 219
   consumption 31, 39
   expenditure 3, 4, 6, 8, 13, 27, 30, 36, 39, 69, 70, 85, 86, 103, 104, 156, 213
   harvest 206, 208, 209, 218
   homeostasis 3, 14, 73, 81, 82, 85, 86, 102, 113, 160, 179, 206, 207, 208, 213, 219
   intake 3, 11, 12, 21, 39, 85
Energy balance 34, 67, 69, 70, 81, 85, 86, 120, 154, 155, 159, 162, 167
   long-term 154
Enterocytes 28
Enzymatic digestion 93
Enzyme-linked immuno sorbent assay (ELISA) 93
Epidermal growth factor receptor (EGFR) 169
Estrogens 168, 174, 175, 176, 177, 178
Extended-spectrum beta-lactamases (ESBL) 212

F

FABP4 for pediatric obesity 100
Fat 32, 33, 108
   cell numbers 108
   energy content diet 32, 33
Fat absorption 10, 21, 22, 31, 32, 33
Fatty acid binding protein 98
Fecal microbiota transplant (FMT) 204, 219

Fenfluramine 5, 6, 9, 10, 13
   effects of 9, 10
Fenfluramine treatment 10
Fetal programming 114, 115, 116
Fiaf expression 207
Follicle-stimulating hormone (FSH) 179
Food intake 7, 8, 9, 10, 15, 17, 18, 25, 26, 29, 36, 37, 38, 65, 66, 67, 68, 69, 70, 71, 72, 73, 74, 108, 159, 179, 211
   normal 9, 10
   reduced 15, 17, 18, 66
   regulating 3, 65, 67, 71
Fourier-transform ion-cyclotron resonance (FTICR) 93
Free-fatty acid (FFAs) 80, 87, 204, 207, 217
   receptors (FFAR) 204, 207, 217

G

Gamma-amino butyric acids (GABAs) 16
Geldanamycin derivatives 99
Genes 40, 42, 85
   obesity-associated 85
   yellow obese 40, 42
Genome-wide association studies (GWAS) 85
Gestation 115, 155
GH, maximal secretory capacity of 164
GH concentrations, lower 164
GH secretion 164, 165
Glomerular hyper filtration 101
Glucocorticoids 86, 108, 110, 155, 156, 168, 171
Gluconeogenesis 157, 158, 181, 207
Glucose 12, 22, 26, 30, 38, 42, 44, 46, 67, 120, 155, 156, 158, 159, 206
   impaired 30, 206
   urinary 42
Glucose homeostasis 72, 87, 88, 59, 100, 160
   normal 87, 88, 100
Glucose tolerance, impaired 43, 44
Glutathione peroxidase (GPx) 163, 181
Glutathione-reductase (GR) 171
Glutathione S-transferase (GST) 171
Glyceroneogenesis 105
Growth hormone (GH) 28, 32, 154, 156, 162, 163, 164, 165, 217
Gut microbiome 210, 212, 213, 217

Gut microbiota 120, 121, 204, 205, 208, 209, 212, 216, 218, 219

H

Haptoglobin 117
Heat shock proteins (HSPs) 98, 99, 111
Hepatocytes 28, 158, 160
Hepatotoxicity 28, 176
High density lipoprotein (HDL) 87, 97, 178
High fat diet (HFD) 99, 102, 214, 215
Hirsutism 178, 179
Hormonal derangement 150
Hormones, adrenal 170, 171, 172
Hormone sensitive lipase (HSL) 105
Hydroperoxides 165
Hyperglycemia 38, 41, 42, 43, 72, 98, 152
Hyperinsulinemia 32, 38, 41, 42, 43, 44
Hyperlipidemia 7, 15, 32, 38, 42, 44, 46, 151
Hyperphagia 41, 42
Hyperplasia 89, 107, 108
Hyperthyroidism 165, 166, 172
　secondary 172
Hypocaloric diet 12, 22, 181, 182
Hypogonadism 84, 174, 175
Hypothalamic-hypophyseal-adrenal (HHA) 171
Hypothalamus 7, 9, 14, 17, 18, 26, 36, 66, 69, 70, 71, 72, 73, 86, 154, 155, 156, 159
Hypothyroidism 165, 166, 167, 172
　overt 166
　subclinical 166, 167

I

Immobilized metal affinity chromatography (IMAC) 113
Immobilized pH gradient (IPG) 91
Impaired glucose tolerance (IGT) 43, 44, 87, 88, 100
Inflammation, obesity-induced adipose 101
Inhibition of lipid absorption 20, 21
Injection, intracerebroventricular 68, 70
Insomnia 6, 7, 17, 23, 25
Insulin 12, 16, 32, 41, 43, 44, 80, 81, 83, 88, 97, 98, 99, 101, 102, 107, 109, 112, 113, 114, 115, 117, 120, 149, 150, 151, 153, 154, 155, 157, 158, 159, 160, 162, 167, 173, 174, 178, 180, 181, 206, 210, 212, 214, 215, 217, 219
　levels 12, 44, 154, 206
　receptor 157, 158, 160
　-related substrate (IRS) 181
　resistance 16, 32, 41, 43, 44, 80, 81, 83, 88, 97, 98, 99, 101, 102, 107, 109, 112, 113, 114, 115, 117, 120, 149, 151, 153, 155, 158, 159, 160, 162, 167, 173, 174, 178, 206, 210, 217
　sensitivity 83, 112, 150, 154, 158, 159, 160, 180, 212, 214, 215, 219
　sensitivity improving 214, 215
　sensitivity systemic 159, 160
　stimulation 113, 114
　tolerance 206
　treatments 102, 113, 162
Intestinal dysbiosis 204, 205, 206, 208, 210, 212, 219
Isotope-coded affinity tags (ICAT) 94

J

Janus Kinase (JAK) 104

K

Key anti-obesity strategy 108, 110
Kidney disease 101, 119
　obesity-induced chronic 101

L

Lactation 86, 87, 115
Lateral hypothalamic area (LHA) 70
Lepob mutations 41
Leptin 3, 4, 6, 17, 20, 21, 22, 36, 40, 41, 43, 67, 70, 73, 74, 86, 101, 106, 111, 154, 155, 156, 157, 160, 161, 168, 178, 179, 182, 210
　levels 6, 22
　receptor dysfunction 40, 41
　receptors 17, 43, 156, 168
　secretion 155, 156, 168
　treatment 36
　absorption 3, 4, 20, 21

Lipid peroxidation 163, 165, 170, 174, 176
  reduced 163
Lipogenesis 80, 96, 106, 120, 154, 216, 217
Lipoperoxides 163
Lipoxins 101
Liraglutide treatment 26
Long-evans tokushima otuska (LETO) 27
Lorcaserin treatment 18
Lorcaserin treatment groups 18
LPL activity in adipose tissue 207
Luteinizing hormone (LII) 178, 179
Lymphocytes 106, 153, 157, 158, 162

M

Macrophages 106, 153, 157, 158, 160, 177, 209
Magnetic resonance imaging (MRI) 103
Markers, fetal-programming-related obesity 116
Mass spectrometry (MS) 90, 92, 93, 94, 96, 97, 105, 120, 161, 180
Maternal food restriction 115, 116
Matrix-assisted laser desorption ionization (MALDI) 93
Mazindol treatment 8
Mechanisms 4, 5, 10, 21, 23, 24, 39, 66, 67, 69, 71, 74, 86, 112, 156, 161, 163, 165, 168, 169, 171, 178, 181, 205, 207, 208, 209, 213, 218, 219
  leptin-independent 67, 69
  potential 213, 218
  regulatory 66, 207
  underlying 205
Melanin-concentrating hormone (MCH) 66
Metabolic 34, 65, 155, 156, 179, 180, 207
  disorders 34, 65
  functions 155, 156, 207
  Kisspeptin actions 179, 180
Metabolism, bile acid 205, 206
Metformin 22, 104, 181
MGAT2 inhibitors 21, 34, 35
MGAT inhibitor 3
Microbiota 120, 204, 205, 208, 218, 219
  commensal 204, 205, 208
Microbiota transplant, fecal 204, 219

Microflora 204, 205, 206, 208, 209, 211, 214, 215, 217
  commensal 204, 205, 209, 211, 214, 217
Mitochondrial respiratory chain 161, 166, 168
Mitogen-activated protein kinase (MAPK) 169
Monoacylglycerol 11, 33
Monoamine-reuptake inhibitor 4, 5
Monogenic obesity 84, 85
  non-syndromic 84
Motility, gastroduodenal 70, 71
mRNA levels 17
MTP inhibitors 3, 20, 28, 29, 31, 39

N

Naltrexone 19, 20
Nesfatin 69, 71, 73
Nesfatin-1 68
Nesfatin-1 66, 67, 68, 69, 71, 72, 73
  and anti-obesity treatment 69
  anorexigenic effect of 68
  antiserum 66
  intracerebroventricular 68
  levels 72
  neurons 67, 71, 72, 73
Neurons 6, 66, 68, 69, 70, 156
  central 69
Neuropeptide 6, 66, 67, 70, 73
Neurotransmitters 6, 12, 14, 16, 67
Neutrophil granulocytes, human 177
Next generation sequencing (NGS) 85, 122
Noradrenaline 12, 24
Nuclear factor-κB 208, 209
Nucleobindin 65, 66
Nucleus 26, 66, 67, 68, 71, 73, 154, 156, 157
  arcuate 26, 66, 67, 157
  paraventricular 66, 71, 73
Nutrition, maternal 114, 115

O

Obese 154, 156, 207, 208
  adolescents 154, 156
  cohorts 207, 208
Obesity 8, 13, 26, 82, 83, 85, 86, 87, 98, 102, 104, 107, 114, 115, 149, 152, 153, 156, 161, 205, 206

abdominal 98, 152, 156, 161
adolescent 152
ameliorated impaired 13, 26
android 87
central nervous system-induced 8
developing 83, 102
epidemic 149
global 85
hyperplastic 153
hypertrophic 107
maternal 86, 115
modulating 206
morbid 104
parental 82, 83, 114
phenotypes 85
polygenic 85
potential mechanism linking 149
prevention 83
/proteomics 96
-related disorders 112
-related problems 81, 83
resistance 89
severe 152
suggesting 205
therapy 106
treatment 25
trends 81, 85
Omentin 107
Orlistat 3, 4, 5, 6, 10, 11, 12, 20, 21, 119
  effect of 11, 12
Orlistat treatment 12
Orphan G-protein-coupled-receptor 159
OSBP-related proteins (ORPs) 111
Ovariectomy 169, 176, 177
Overweight adolescents 112, 164, 173
Oxidative stress 97, 113, 116, 149, 150, 152, 165, 170, 172, 180, 183
Oxytocin 67, 68, 73

P

Pancreatic lipases 11, 21
Pediatric obesity 80, 81, 83, 84, 96, 99, 100, 102, 103, 106, 107, 108, 113, 114, 115, 116, 117, 119, 120, 121, 208
  parallels adults 96
  prevalence rates 119
  proteomic characterization of 80, 120
Pediatric population 80, 81, 83, 97, 112, 116
Peritoneum 87
Peroxisome proliferator-activated receptor (PPAR) 40, 99, 165, 180, 214, 215
Phentermine 3, 5, 6, 7, 9, 13, 16, 17
  /topiramate 5, 16, 17
Phentermine treatment 7
Phosphorylation 17, 89, 113, 158, 160
  inhibiting secondary protein 17
Pigment epithelium-derived factor (PEDF) 112
Pioglitazone treatment group 38
Plasma proteome 116, 117
Post translational modifications (PTMs) 89, 90, 92, 94, 95, 113, 114, 120
Preadipocytes 88, 96, 106, 108, 111, 112, 153, 154, 173
Prebiotics 120, 204, 210, 211, 213, 216, 217, 218, 219
Prebiotic supplementation 217
Prepubertal children 161, 173
Proapolipoprotein A-1 97
Probiotics 120, 204, 210, 213, 214, 215, 216, 218, 219
Production 16, 18, 42, 69, 150, 153, 157, 158, 159, 160, 161, 162, 177, 207, 213
  hepatic glucose 157, 158
  superoxide anion 177
Pro-inflammatory cascade 208, 209
Proprionate 204
Protective effects 162, 174, 178, 179, 180, 206
Protein 4, 14, 36, 90, 91, 92, 93, 94, 95, 98, 99, 105, 113, 114, 122
  carbonylation 114
  -coupled receptor family 14
  detection 91, 92
  expression 93, 94
  expression profile 90
  kinase 99, 105, 113, 122
  kinase A (PKA) 105, 122
  synthesis 95, 98
  tyrosine phosphatase 4, 36
Protein modifications 90, 113, 162
  oxidative liver 162
Protein-protein interactions 95, 100

Proteins 4, 17, 28, 71, 80, 83, 97, 99, 100, 101, 102, 103, 105, 108, 111, 114, 115, 116, 118, 149, 165, 172, 173
   adipocyte 97, 114
   candidate 118
   cytoskeletal 111, 114
   diet-associated 118
   domain-containing 108
   identified 71, 80, 83, 105
   identifying 97, 115
   microsomal triglyceride transfer 4, 28
   mitochondrial 105, 165
   reactive 149, 172
   serum 102, 116
   target 97, 100, 101
   uncoupling 17, 103, 165, 173
   zinc finger 99
Proteome 83, 89, 90, 95, 97, 104, 105, 106
   mitochondrial 104
Proteome profiling 97
Proteomic(s) 80, 82, 83, 89, 90, 93, 96, 100, 101, 102, 104, 107, 109, 114, 115, 116, 120, 121
   investigations 115, 116
   profiling 114, 115
   shotgun 93
Pyruvate carboxylase 110

R

Radical nitrogen species (RNS) 150, 153
Radical oxygen species (ROS) 122, 150, 153, 168, 169, 171, 176
Reactive oxygen intermediate (ROI) 162
Receptors, amine-associated 5, 6
Reduced white adipose tissue 215
Regenerating system 169
Regulating nascent protein folding 99
Relationship, symbiotic 205
Resistance 99, 120, 212
   antibiotic 212
   obesity-related insulin 120
   particular obesity-associated insulin 99
Retinol binding protein (RBP) 102, 159, 160
Rimonabant 4, 5, 6, 14, 15, 16, 24
   effects of 15
   in obesity (RIO) 15
   treatment 15, 16
RIO-diabetes 15, 16
Rosiglitazone 104

S

SCFAs, production of 214
Search tool for the retrieval of interacting genes/proteins (STRING) 102
Secretomes 80, 101, 102, 103
Serotonin receptor 5, 9
Sex hormone binding globulin (SHBG) 179
SGLT2 Inhibitors 21, 38, 39
Short chain fatty acids (SCFAs) 204, 206, 207, 216, 217
Sibutramine cardiovascular outcomes (SCOUT) 14
Sibutramine treatment 12, 13, 14
Signal transducer and activator of transcription (STAT) 104
Slow wave sleep (SWS) 66
Sodium-dodecyl sulphate (SDS) 90, 91
Stem cells 107, 111
Steroids, gonadal 174, 175

Stress 67, 98, 171, 172
   hormones 171, 172
   response 67, 98, 172
Syntaxins 111
Systemic inflammation 117, 150, 152, 183
   obesity-associated 117

T

Tesofensine 24, 25
   treatment 25
Testosterone 174, 175, 177, 179
TG-rich lipoproteins 28
TG synthesis 31, 33, 34
THA neurons 66
Therapy 10, 16, 22, 40, 65, 74, 80, 109, 151, 204, 205, 210, 212, 213
   antibiotic 204, 212, 213
   anti-obesity 16

obesity-associated 109
Thiazolidinediones 103, 104
Thyroid hormones 155, 161, 165, 166, 167, 168, 172, 182, 183
Tomography, computed 44, 45, 103
Total 12, 45, 166, 172, 175, 180, 181
    antioxidant capacity (TAC) 166, 172, 175, 180, 181
    antioxidant status (TAS) 166
    cholesterol (TC) 12, 45, 166
Transthyretin 117
Triglycerides 11, 15, 21, 23, 28, 31, 45, 89, 155, 160, 163, 166, 174, 207
Tsumura suzuki obese diabetes (TSOD) 40, 42
Tuberal hypothalamic area (THA) 66
Tumor necrosis factor (TNF) 101, 153, 209

U

Uncoupling protein (UCP) 17, 103, 165, 173
Unsaturated fatty acids (UFAs) 115

V

Vancomycin 210, 212
    oral 212
Vancomycin resistant enterococci (VRE) 212
VAT 97, 98, 100
    depots 97, 98, 100
    overexpression of heat shock proteins 98
Very low-density lipoprotein (VLDL) 28
Visceral 39, 40, 44, 87, 97, 98, 99, 100, 101, 102, 103, 106, 111, 164, 178
    adipose tissue (VAT) 39, 87, 97, 98, 99, 100, 101, 102, 103, 106, 111, 164
    obesity 40, 44, 178
Vitamin D binding protein (VDBP) 103, 117
VMH obesity 8

W

Weight loss effects 7, 8, 10, 38, 107

Z

Zonisamide 22, 23, 107
Zucker diabetic fatty (ZDF) 40, 41

www.ingramcontent.com/pod-product-compliance
Lightning Source LLC
Chambersburg PA
CBHW051909210526
45473CB00006B/1959